Promoting Men's Mental Health

Promoting Men's Mental Health

Edited by

DAVID CONRAD

Specialty Registrar in Public Health, Liverpool PCT
Associate Member, Centre for Men's Health
Leeds Metropolitan University

and

ALAN WHITE

Professor of Men's Health, Centre for Men's Health
Leeds Metropolitan University

Forewords by

ALASTAIR CAMPBELL

Mind Champion 2009, author of All In The Mind
Spokesman and Chief Strategist to the Prime Minister, 1994–2003

and

LOUIS APPLEBY

National Clinical Director for Mental Health

Radcliffe Publishing
Oxford • New York

Radcliffe Publishing Ltd
18 Marcham Road
Abingdon
Oxon OX14 1AA
United Kingdom

www.radcliffe-oxford.com
Electronic catalogue and worldwide online ordering facility.

British Library Cataloguing in Publication Data
A catalogue record for this book is available from the British Library.

ISBN-13: 978 184619 331 6

The paper used for the text pages of this book is FSC
certified. FSC (The Forest Stewardship Council)
is an international network to promote responsible
management of the world's forests.

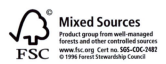

Mixed Sources
Product group from well-managed
forests and other controlled sources
www.fsc.org Cert no. SGS-COC-2482
© 1996 Forest Stewardship Council

Typeset by Pindar NZ, Auckland, New Zealand
Printed and bound by TJI Digital, Padstow, Cornwall, UK

Contents

Foreword

Alastair Campbell

This book is a welcome and important contribution to a thankfully growing debate. Mental illness remains in some ways the last great taboo in our society, a taboo which leads directly to stigma and discrimination which for some can be even worse than the symptoms of their illness. If it is true that one in four of us will at some point have direct experience of mental illness – and sometimes I believe this widely quoted figure is an underestimation – then as a society we have to be far more open and honest about the issues that flow from that. It is also the case, in very general terms, that men are more likely than women not to be open, and not to reach out for help when they may need it. Good mental health isn't simply an absence of mental health problems, but a positive state of well-being that enables us to realise our own abilities, contribute productively to society and cope with the normal stresses of life. The term 'mental health' for many people though is simply another way of talking about mental illness; something which, for men especially, largely remains off limits. Men's reluctance to acknowledge emotional pressures to others, or frequently even to themselves, can create a build-up of pressure which often only finds release at the point of crisis. When the crisis hits, the stigma of mental illness and its incompatibility with dominant notions of masculinity mean that men are more reluctant than women to seek the help that they may need.

This book in part is about encouraging men who have reached crisis point to seek help. Equally it's about prevention, and sets out some of the excellent work being done on that.

As well as practical work which is happening in communities around the country, there is also much work to be done to change representations of mental health issues in the media – to help de-stigmatise mental illness. Too often, mental illness in the media is linked to violence, whereas in truth the mentally ill are more likely to be the victim than perpetrator of violence.

While a lot of good work is already being done, the targeted promotion of mental health to men and boys is still in its infancy. In highlighting some of the work already being done, I hope it can inspire practitioners and policy-makers to initiate similar interventions, develop new ones and lift the promotion of men's mental health much higher up the agenda, both in the UK and abroad.

Alastair Campbell
Mind Champion 2009, author of *All In The Mind*
Spokesman and Chief Strategist to the Prime Minister, 1994–2003
March 2010

Foreword

Louis Appleby

Men's health in general is poor in comparison to women's. Male life expectancy at birth in England is five years less than women. Men are worse at using the health service than women, and more likely to use anonymous sources of health advice like websites. Our challenge is persuading men to take their health more seriously, and to make better use of the services available.

We also know that men are three times more likely than women to take their own lives. From the 1970s to the 1990s, whilst the suicide rate fell in older men and in women it was rising in men under the age of 35. That is why, in developing our national suicide prevention strategy, we made sure it included measures aimed at young men. We set out to tackle risk factors such as depression; alcohol problems; drug misuse; unemployment; family and relationship breakdown. The suicide rate in men under 35 is now falling.

However, we still need to know more about why men find it difficult to talk about their problems; why they are more resistant to health promotion messages; and why they were reluctant to seek help when in distress. We need to be more innovative in the way we try to reach men. We can do this by moving out from more traditional health settings – I have seen mental health teams working in sports halls and high streets. Most importantly, we need to listen to what men, and young men in particular, are saying to us so that we can provide services that they will access when they need them.

This book will help stimulate further discussion and hopefully encourage men to seek help or support. It also highlights some positive work going on in the United Kingdom and elsewhere which could be replicated further.

Professor Louis Appleby
National Clinical Director for Mental Health
March 2010

Preface

Good mental health is much more than simply the absence of mental illness. It's easy, of course, to think of men who have a diagnosable mental disorder as being in poor mental health. There are countless others though whose state of mental well-being is severely hampering their ability to live a happy, well-balanced and fulfilled life who will never be offered (or seek) professional help, or whose problems will unnecessarily be left to escalate to a point where they qualify for medical intervention. Health promotion of all types is about enabling people to get the most from their lives, for as much of their lives as possible – to participate in society, to build positive relationships with others, to experience satisfying and meaningful work, and to make the most of one's potential unhampered by the restraints of avoidable physical or psychological impairment. Although very important, a reduction in the prevalence of illness is just one outcome of this work and thus mental health promotion is about more than simply preventing mental disorders. Its aim is to promote positive mental health in a broad sense by increasing psychological well-being, competency and coping skills, and by creating supportive living and working environments (WHO 2004).

Our aim with this book has been to highlight the breadth of the challenges to achieving mental well-being that men are facing and, through examples of good practice, provide a guide for those working in primary care on how best to target and help those men who need support. It should be noted that this book does not address working with men with a diagnosis of mental illness who are already under the care of mental health services. Rather, it responds to the increasing recognition, as the costs associated with mental distress become realised, that restricting activity to just managing those who have developed a mental illness is too limited an approach. The influential Sainsbury Centre for Mental Health produced a policy report (2006) that had as its vision for 2015 a world in which the promotion of the mental health and well-being of the population was a key component of all public service delivery. The World Health Organization summary report (WHO 2004) on promoting mental health has a similar quest. The need for a cross-cutting approach has also been emphasised by the Men's Health Forum's report on the mental health of men and boys, *Untold Problems* (Wilkins 2010). This vision is starting to materialise at the policy level, with the launch in 2009 of a series of EU Presidential conferences to support the development of the 'European pact on mental health and well-being' (EC 2008).

In our first book, *Men's Health – How to Do It* (Conrad and White 2007), the focus was on trying to capture the work of the Bradford Health of Men team, who had been developing outreach services specifically aimed at men across a broad range of health issues. In this book we have returned to some of the team for their expert knowledge on working with men with mental and emotional problems, but we have also moved further afield to capture best practice in the rest of the United Kingdom as well as examples from Europe and America.

Within the book there are chapters that explore the state of our understanding of men's mental health and discuss specific mental health issues faced by different groups of men, along with some of the contemporary cultural and other societal factors that have an influence on men's mental well-being. There are also chapters that demonstrate how some of these many challenges to men's mental well-being can be addressed through practically focused initiatives and male-friendly ways of working.

The main message that we hope comes from this book is that many men are finding the world a stressful and emotionally draining place and that this is causing problems for them and for those who live and work with them. If there is a serious wish to improve the health and well-being of men then we have to accept that relying on the current orthodoxy on mental ill-health will not be enough. For real progress to be made we have to become more aware of and responsive to men's emotional and mental health needs.

David Conrad
Alan White
March 2010

REFERENCES

Conrad D, White A (2007) *Men's Health – How to Do It*. Oxford: Radcliffe Publishing.

European Commission (EC) (2008) European Pact for Mental Health and Well-being 'Together for Mental Health and Well-being', Brussels, 13 June 2008, Slovenia Presidency of the EU. Available at: http://ec.europa.eu/health/ph_determinants/life_style/mental/docs/pact_en.pdf (Accessed 1 May 2009).

Sainsbury Centre for Mental Health (2006) *The Future of Mental Health: a Vision for 2015*. Policy paper. London: Sainsbury Centre for Mental Health.

Wilkins D (2010) *Untold Problems: a review of the essential issues in the mental health of men and boys*. London: Men's Health Forum.

World Health Organization (WHO) (2004) *Prevention of Metal Disorders*. Geneva: WHO.

About the editors

David Conrad

David is a Specialty Registrar in Public Health and an Associate Member of the Centre for Men's Health, Leeds Metropolitan University. He is a co-editor of the book *Men's Health – How to Do It*, a hands-on guide to setting up and delivering community-based health services for men and boys, which was published by Radcliffe Publishing in 2007. He has an MA in Visual Culture, an MSc in Health Promotion and a Masters in Public Health.

Alan White

Alan is Professor of Men's Health at Leeds Metropolitan University. He has been a pioneering academic working in the field of men's health for 14 years. He has delivered over 80 invited and peer-reviewed papers and has had over 60 books, journal articles and reports published nationally and internationally on the state of men's health.

Professor White is the Director of the Centre for Men's Health, Leeds Metropolitan University and Chair of the Board of Trustees for the Men's Health Forum and a member of the Executive of the European Men's Health Forum. His research includes the 'Scoping Study on Men's Health' for the Department of Health in the UK; the 'Report on the State of Men's Health across 17 European Countries'; and an epidemiological study on men and cancer. Alan is working this year on the First European State of Men's Health Report for the European Commission. His research also includes work on men's experiences of illness including coronary heart disease, diabetes and prostate cancer; the evaluation of the national pilots for Self Care as part of the NHS WiPP and a study on the Bradford Health of Men initiative, the latter being the subject of the first book by Conrad and White, *Men's Health – How to Do It* (Radcliffe Publishing, 2007). He is also a co-editor of the book *Hazardous Waist: tackling male weight problems* (Radcliffe Publishing, 2007) and the medical text *Men's Health*. Recently Alan has been working with Headingley Stadium in Leeds to establish health checks for the supporters of the Leeds Rhinos, Leeds Carnegie and Yorkshire Cricket and is undertaking an evaluation study with the football Premier League in England on men's health.

About the authors

Stephen Anderson

Stephen is the Service Manager for the Breathing Space out-of-hours helpline service in Scotland. Breathing Space is a free and confidential service for any individual who is experiencing low mood or depression, or is in need of someone to talk to. Stephen has worked for Breathing Space for over 8 years, seeing the service develop from a small pilot service to a full national service as part of the NHS and Scottish Government strategies.

Prior to working for Breathing Space, Stephen worked for the Essentia Group, where he gained wide experience on different helpline services, including the Campaign Against Living Miserably (CALM) service, which provided an early template for Breathing Space.

Steve Boorman

Steve is a specialist occupational physician, with long experience of working in Royal Mail Group – the UK's largest single employer of men. Since 2003 he has been Royal Mail's Corporate Responsibility Director, developing approaches to individual and organisational well-being in a complex and fast-changing business environment. Royal Mail has developed innovative approaches to occupational health, demonstrating the commercial advantage that improved workforce health can deliver.

Steve is Chief Examiner to the Diploma in Occupational Medicine examination, an Honorary Senior Clinical Lecturer to Birmingham University, and an ex-President of the Royal Society of Medicine's Occupational Medicine section. In 2009 he was appointed to lead the review, commissioned by the Health Secretary, of Health and Well-being for the NHS workforce.

Peter Branney

Peter is a Research Fellow in the Centre for Men's Health, Leeds Metropolitan University. His research is concerned with critically exploring contemporary issues around gender and health while developing and evaluating methods for doing so. He is editor of the *QMiP Bulletin* and has published (with David Wilkins, Sarah

Payne and Gillian Granville) the Department of Health *Gender and Health Services Study* (2009). Current research includes constructions of decisions to use (or not use) health services, experiences of illness, and participative qualitative methodologies.

Before taking on his first post-doctoral position at the Centre for Men's Health, Peter had held an ESRC studentship at the University of Leeds and was a visiting doctoral student at Massey University, Aotearoa/New Zealand. He holds a BSc in psychology and philosophy, an MSc in psychological approaches to health and a PhD in psychology from the University of Leeds.

Adrienne Burgess

Adrienne is Research Manager at the UK think tank, the Fatherhood Institute. Her research summaries on fatherhood topics are widely used by policy-makers and practitioners alike. Her book *Fatherhood Reclaimed: the making of the modern father*, published by Vermilion in 1997, helped set a new agenda on fatherhood in the UK and has been published in translation throughout the world, as has *Will You Still Love Me Tomorrow?* (Vermilion, 2002), in which she presented, in an accessible form, the huge body of research on couple relationships. Adrienne is also co-author, with other Fatherhood Institute trainers, of its highly regarded *Toolkit for Father-Inclusive Practice* and *Invisible Fathers: working with young dads*, a resources pack for practitioners. Adrienne speaks and trains on fatherhood in the UK, the US and Australia.

Mike Bush

Mike has worked in the social healthcare area for over 38 years, mainly in Community Mental Health Teams as a mental health social worker. He is a member of the Samaritans National Advisory Group and attends the All Party Parliamentary Group on Suicide Prevention. He has been an advisor to the Yorkshire and Humberside Regional Mental Health Promotion and Suicide Prevention Forum. Mike is also a member of the Department of Health National Suicide Prevention Strategy Working Party, responsible for developing the 'Help is at Hand' National Suicide Bereavement Information Pack. He is a member of the Leeds National Service Framework Standard 7 Group, responsible for the local suicide prevention strategy.

Mike has been a speaker at national and regional conferences concerning suicide issues and men's mental health. He has appeared as a panellist on the Radio 4 'You and Yours' programme concerning mental health issues regarding suicide and stigma. He has also been involved with local radio and television regarding mental health issues.

Walter Busuttil

Walter served for 16 years in the Royal Air Force, where he was instrumental in the setting up of mental health rehabilitation services for servicemen returning from the first Gulf War. He was also part of the clinical team that rehabilitated the released British Beirut Hostages. He is a Consultant Psychiatrist and is the Medical Director of the national charity Combat Stress, which looks after ex-servicemen and combat veterans with mental health difficulties. He has published and lectured internationally about treatment and rehabilitation of chronic and complex presentations of post-traumatic stress disorder and has helped to set up services for its treatment nationally.

Ruth Coombs

Ruth joined Mind Cymru in July 2004. She heads up the Influence and Change Team, which includes the Social Justice and Rural Affairs Officer. Ruth has a health and social care focus, working on all aspects of adult mental health in Wales, supporting, challenging and lobbying national movers and shakers on mental health policy and implementation. She is a member of the Mental Health Research Network Cymru steering group, with the brief to enable and support the inclusion of service users and carers in mental health clinical research in Wales.

Nick Davy

Nick qualified as a Registered Nurse in 1987 and has worked in general medicine, oncology and terminal care in England and abroad. He moved to Yorkshire in 1997 and worked in genito-urinary medicine before starting work in men's health in 2001. Nick's main area of focus is around sexual health.

Pete Dominey

Pete is a BACP Accredited Counsellor and group facilitator who has been working with men individually and in groups for 10 years. He has an MA in Cultural Studies, in which he focused his studies on men, masculinities and violence. Pete is also a core team member of Mandorla, a group of men committed to working with men (www.mandorla-menswork.org).

Sue Dominey

Sue is a BACP Accredited counsellor and group facilitator, with 8 years' experience of managing The Brave Project, a violence prevention/anger management group for men in Bradford (www.brave-project.org). She is also a Churchill Fellow, having researched violence prevention work with boys and young men in Australia and New Zealand. Sue and Pete Dominey can be contacted at thebraveproject@hotmail.com.

Tricia Dressel

Tricia is the Director of Prevention and Education at the Mazzoni Center, one of the oldest HIV/AIDS service organisations in the US. In her current role, Tricia oversees local and federally funded programmes promoting the health and well-being of young men. She has over 10 years' experience in the public health field as a researcher, educator, advocate, counsellor and administrator. Tricia studied international development at Middlesex University in London, earned her BA in sociology from the State University of New York, and a MS in Organizational Dynamics from the University of Pennsylvania.

Keith Elder

Keith's interest in mental health issues began in Wolverhampton in the 1970s when he observed the damaging impact of a mental health system that relied at that time almost entirely on institutional care. In 1982, he was appointed the first West Midlands Director of Mind, a post he held until 2001 when Mind's regional structure was dismantled. During the early 1990s he became aware of mental distress in the countryside and has championed rural issues within Mind ever since. During the last few years he has coordinated the quality review of Mind's affiliated local Mind association network, as well as leading Mind's rural team. He is currently undertaking an MSc by research in Health Services Management at the University of Birmingham.

Paul Hopkins

Paul is a Health Improvement Specialist working for NHS Gloucestershire. He is coordinator of the Gloucestershire Boys and Young Men Network, and co-founder of The Red Knob, a social marketing initiative committed to authentic and culturally relevant approaches to young men's health. Paul is currently undertaking an MSc in Men's Health at Leeds Metropolitan University.

Dennis Jones

After finishing a degree in Humanities in 1977, Dennis worked as an electricity meter reader in Derby, farmer and fisherman in the Orkney Islands, barman in Barcelona, window cleaner in Rotterdam and comic artist in Yorkshire. While unemployed in the early 1980s he became a volunteer and later a volunteer coordinator at Mind, where he ran groups for men who had been in the mental health system to help them regain lost skills through voluntary activity in the community. He subsequently developed advocacy programmes and programmes to resettle long-stay patients from the old Victorian psychiatric institutions back into the communities of Dewsbury in West Yorkshire.

Dennis joined the Health Promotion Service in Bradford nine years later as a specialist in sexual health and began the Bradford Health of Men project in 1998 with a group of male health visitors, developing male friendly services and interventions (www.healthofmen.com). He currently works part-time for the Health of Men project, concentrating on men and mental well-being.

Andrew Kinder

Andrew is a Chartered Counselling and Chartered Occupational Psychologist, the Chair Emeritus of the Association for Counselling at Work (a Division of the British Association for Counselling and Psychotherapy, www.counsellingatwork.org.uk), and an Associate Fellow of the British Psychological Society. He has an MSc in Occupational Psychology, holds three diplomas in counselling and a certificate in Cognitive Behavioural Therapies.

He has worked in the area of stress, trauma and employee assistance within organisations for over 12 years and has run numerous courses for all levels on managing stress, maximising performance under pressure, advanced telephone skills, coping with change and trauma support as well as having his own case-load of clients, many of whom have stress-related issues. He has contributed to various government consultations on stress and was a member of the steering group which produced the 'Mind Out for Mental Health' line managers' resource, *A Practical Guide to Managing and Supporting Mental Health in the Workplace*.

Andrew has published widely and is particularly interested in the management of stress and trauma within an occupational health context. He is currently responsible operationally and professionally for a large employee assistance programme which delivers training, counselling and coaching products to increase the psychological health of individuals and organisations. He has been instrumental in the introduction of early intervention programmes in a number of large organisations relating to employee engagement and employee well-being. His latest book, *Employee Wellbeing Support: a workplace resource*, co-edited with Professor Cary Cooper and Rick Hughes, was published by John Wiley & Sons in March 2008. He has also co-written, with Rick Hughes, *Guidelines for Counselling in the Workplace*, which is published by BACP and available free via www.counsellingatwork.org.uk

Barry Langham

Barry is a Harm Reduction Worker at the Bridge Project, a Bradford-based drug treatment charity. Bridge was established more than 20 years ago and offers a range of services for drug users residing in Bradford (as well as their parents, partners and carers), including a men's clinic and a needle exchange.

Svend Aage Madsen

Svend Aage is currently Head of the Department of Psychology, Play Therapy and Social Counselling, research leader at the Centre for Knowledge on Support for Patients and leader of the Psychological and Psychosocial Research Unit at Copenhagen University Hospital, Rigshospitalet, Denmark. He has recently led several research projects, including 'Men as patients', 'Men and fatherhood', 'The meaning of gender in professional work with victims of rape' and 'Men's mental health and psychotherapy'.

Dr Madsen has been a member of several governmental committees and think tanks, developing guidelines for health services around pregnancy and birth, the obesity epidemic, child obesity and men and gender. Current research activity includes the Nordic and European research and development projects 'Men's psychological transition to fatherhood under the community framework strategy on gender equality (2001–2005)' and 'Violence intervention in specialist healthcare' under the 'Daphne III Programme 2007–2013 to Prevent and Combat Violence Against Children, Young People and Women and to Protect Victims and Groups at Risk'.

Jo McCullagh

Jo is a Tobacco Control Programme Manager for Cheshire and Merseyside. Formerly, Jo was a Health Promotion Specialist working in Health Improvement at NHS Sefton in Merseyside. Her specialist areas were men's health, cancer prevention and tobacco control. She developed a number of health improvement initiatives to facilitate men's access to information, empower them to be health aware and access health and leisure services, in order to improve key lifestyle behaviours. Activities have been undertaken at a diverse range of workplace sites, leisure centres and barber shops, targeting population groups, including taxi, bus and lorry drivers, seafarers, police and firemen, construction workers and dockers. For further information, please email jo.mccullagh@heartofmersey.org.uk

Martin Neal

Having initially worked as a painter and decorator, Martin began his career in health and social care 30 years ago, working with the National Autistic Society. Following this he trained to be a mental health nurse; upon completing his training in 1985 he held a number of posts, culminating in becoming a Clinical Nurse Advisor. From there he went on to manage the research portfolio within an NHS trust. He moved into nurse education at Leeds Metropolitan University through a secondment and took up a permanent post of Senior Lecturer in 2004. He held the post of Course Leader for the BSc (Hons) Nursing Mental Health branch for three and a half years, before moving on to a new role within the faculty. He is currently undertaking a PhD looking at how younger people with chronic lymphocytic leukaemia deal with the impact of having chronic cancer.

Merv Pemberton

Merv is a men's health advisor for Bradford and Airedale Community Health Services. Working as part of the Bradford Health of Men services (www.healthofmen. com), he devised an innovative and successful programme of anti-bullying intervention which has been delivered in schools, places of worship and other community venues. Along with his anti-bullying work, Merv has been involved in projects targeted towards the Afro-Caribbean community, as well as helping in the delivery of a range of other Health of Men services.

Jane Powell

Jane has spent over 20 years organising campaigns within the voluntary and statutory sectors. She was responsible for initially launching CALM, a cutting edge campaign for young men aged 15–35, as a Department of Health pilot in 1997, working with it until its expansion into Liverpool in 2000. In 2004–05 she was approached to close the campaign down, but, with the encouragement of Tony Wilson (music mogul and founding Trustee of CALM), instead launched it as a charity. The campaign offers help, information and advice to young men via a helpline and website. 'CALMzones' have also been set up in East Lancashire and Merseyside, working with local authorities to promote CALM regionally in consultation with Primary Care Trusts. For further information please visit www.thecalmzone.net

Steve Robertson

Steve is a Reader in Men's Health at the Centre for Men's Health, Leeds Metropolitan University. He worked in the UK National Health Service for over 20 years as a nurse and health visitor before commencing a career in research in 1999. He completed his PhD at Lancaster University in 2003 and has since been involved in a variety of research and evaluation projects.

His main interests and publications are around social theories of masculinity and their application to aspects of health and illness but he has also worked on masculinity and disability; the sociology of (male) bodies; fathers and fatherhood; men, masculinity and mental well-being; evaluating men's health programmes, and men's engagement (or not) with health services. His first book, *Understanding Men and*

Health: Masculinities, Identity and Well-Being, was published by OU Press in Autumn 2007 and his second, edited text, *Men, Masculinities and Health: Critical Perspectives*, was published by Palgrave in 2009. Steve has an increasing international reputation, having worked and produced publications with fellow academics, policy-makers and practitioners from Australia, the United States and Canada. He was a founding member of the European Men's Health Development Foundation, where he continues to sit as a co-director, and he has also acted as a consultant on gender and men's health to the UK Department of Health and the World Health Organisation (Europe).

Pete Sayers
Pete has spent his career within the NHS, working for almost 15 years with emotionally disturbed adolescents. He then went on to manage an alcohol treatment unit and practised as a Community Psychiatric Nurse before managing It's a Goal! (www.itsagoal.org.uk), a mental health intervention delivered at football grounds aimed at tackling depression and suicide among young men aged 16–35.

Christian Scambor
Christian is a clinical and health psychologist and a founder member of the NPO Men's Counselling Centre in Graz, Austria. There he has worked as a psychologist, project manager and researcher within various European and national projects, specialising in gender and men's studies, gender mainstreaming, health, and evaluation methodology. He is a member of the interdisciplinary expert network GenderWerkstätte, Austria, and a trainer in gender analysis and gender mainstreaming. His former roles include psychosocial work in a home for youngsters in crisis and HIV prevention for Styrian AIDS Support.

Justin Varney
Justin is a Consultant in Public Health Medicine working in outer East London. Prior to this he had experience in a range of acute and primary care specialties. He has worked for many years as a visible community activist on lesbian, gay, bisexual and transgender (LGBT) health issues as well as stints as an advisor to the Department of Health and Metropolitan Police on sexual orientation and gender identity. He is the author of the NHS LGBT health site www.healthwithpride.nhs.uk and led the development of the first NHS-funded resources for LGBT people on domestic violence.

Jeremy Voaden
Jeremy has worked in the field of mental health, community development and recovery for over 20 years, as a mental health nurse and public health specialist. In the early 1990s, he worked as a nurse and health promotion specialist for people living with HIV. This led to an interest in public mental health and he subsequently worked as Mental Health Promotion Lead in Gloucestershire and Public Mental Health Specialist with NIMHE. Currently he is Senior Services Manager: Community Development and Response with the British Red Cross in Herefordshire, Shropshire and Worcestershire. He is a founding member of Gloucestershire Boys and Young Men Network.

Louise Warwick-Booth

Louise is a Senior Lecturer at Leeds Metropolitan University with specific interests in health policy and social policy. She is currently the course leader for the BSc Public Health – Health Studies programme. Her book *Researching with Communities: Community Based Research for Regeneration* was published by VDM Verlag in 2009.

Toby Williamson

Toby is Head of Development at the Mental Health Foundation, where he also takes a lead on older people's mental health projects. The Foundation is a UK-wide charity that works in the field of mental health for people of all ages and on issues affecting people with learning disabilities. Toby has extensive experience of working in adult mental health services in both the voluntary and statutory sectors and has been involved in setting up and managing a variety of services for people with severe and enduring mental health problems living in the community.

James Woodall

James is a Lecturer in Health Promotion at Leeds Metropolitan University. He has conducted a number of research projects in prisons and is also currently completing a PhD on health promotion and public health in prison settings at Leeds Met's Centre for Health Promotion Research. James has published research on the barriers to promoting positive mental health in young offenders' institutions and the role that prison visitors' centres can play in addressing the government's health inequalities agenda.

April MW Young

April is Vice President for Justice Initiatives at the Collins Center for Public Policy, an action-oriented think tank based in Florida, USA. She designed the Overtown Men's Health Study, gathering extensive data on residents of this distressed Miami neighbourhood. In addition to research on the social determinants of poor men's health, April works on related issues of juvenile justice, adult incarceration and community re-entry. She has a PhD in Social Anthropology from Harvard University and an AB from Princeton University's Woodrow Wilson School of Public and International Affairs.

About the Men's Health Forum

THE CENTRE OF EXCELLENCE FOR MEN'S HEALTH POLICY AND PRACTICE

MHF is a charity that provides an independent and authoritative voice for male health in England and Wales and tackles the issues and inequalities affecting the health and well-being of men and boys.

MHF's vision is a future in which all boys and men in England and Wales have an equal opportunity to attain the highest possible level of health and well-being.

We work to achieve this through:

➤ policy development, research and lobbying
➤ supporting other organisations and services to engage more effectively with boys and men on health issues
➤ leading the annual National Men's Health Week
➤ publishing the award-winning range of 'mini manual' health booklets for men
➤ running the unique 'consumer' website for men – www.malehealth.co.uk
➤ working with MPs and government
➤ developing innovative and imaginative best practice projects
➤ training service providers and others
➤ collaborating with the widest possible range of interested organisations and individuals.

MHF was founded by the Royal College of Nursing in 1994 and became an independent charity in 2001. The Forum works across a number of health and related issues.

These include:

➤ physical activity
➤ cancer
➤ workplace health
➤ mental health
➤ access to primary care.

Our work focuses particularly on those groups of men with the worst health and we are striving to ensure that we take account of the diversity of men and their needs.

Men's mental well-being

We have a sustained programme of work on men's mental well-being, including a series of projects on young men and suicide. In 2006 men's mental well-being was the theme of National Men's Health Week.

In 2010 we published *Untold Problems*, a review of the key issues in male mental health, for the National Mental Health Development Unit, and we completed a project on black and minority ethnic men's mental health.

For more about our work on men's mental well-being and other issues visit www. menshealthforum.org.uk

Men's Health Forum, 32 Loman Street, London SE1 0EH

office@menshealthforum.org.uk

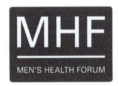

CHAPTER 1

Introduction

Alan White

Go along to any sporting event and you'll find no shortage of men giving vivid displays of their current mental state! But in other settings we see a very different picture – we see boys having difficulty sharing their grief over bereavement, we see sadness erupting as anger, or unexpected suicide in men who were found to have hidden depths of despair. This book seeks to unravel the complexities of men's mental health and offer practical guidance on how services can be developed that can reach out to men at the most vulnerable times of their lives.

Though the book is aimed specifically at practitioners, its message also needs to be heard by those setting health policy and strategy, as we have to see a shift in the way that health services are provided for men with emotional and mental health problems – something that cannot happen without their support. We also hope that this book is not just of interest to those working in the health and social care sector. Men themselves have to become more aware of their mental and emotional health needs and so do their families and friends. It's necessary for us to get the messages out to teachers and others who work with boys and men as well, such that they can, perhaps, interpret behaviour in a different light and offer support and guidance to those boys and men who are experiencing difficulties.

The World Health Organization (WHO) has a broad definition of mental health, describing it as a state of well-being in which the individual realises his or her own abilities, can cope with the normal stresses of life, can work productively and fruitfully and is able to make a contribution to his or her community (WHO 2002). This definition neatly reflects the range of issues that make up mental health, but can also be broken down further into more specific elements. In 1997, the 'Key Concepts' project (EC 2004) was set up by the European Commission to look at how mental health is conceptualised and concluded that mental health is best considered as including positive (mental well-being) and negative (mental ill-health) elements. Positive mental health, or mental well-being, is not merely the absence of mental ill-health but the ability to cope with adversity. Negative mental health, or mental ill-health, can be further divided into psychological distress and psychiatric disorders. Psychological distress is a continuum of mental health difficulties often associated with common negative and stressful life events that would not meet the diagnostic criteria for discrete psychiatric disorders. As such, psychiatric disorders are not necessarily worse than psychological distress but they may be chronic, whereas distress may be transient.

Whichever way you look at it, it's apparent that the mental health of the population is increasingly being recognised as one of the most important areas of public health.

WHO have estimated that unipolar depression will be the second most significant contributor to the global burden of disease by 2030 (Mathers and Loncar 2006). The case for the new European Pact on Mental Health and Well-being is in part based on the recognition that mental disorders are on the rise in the EU, with almost 50 million citizens (about 11% of the population) estimated to experience mental disorders and depression – the most prevalent health problem in many EU-Member States (EC 2008). In the UK, one in four people suffer some form of mental illness at some point in their lives and at any one time one sixth of the population are suffering from a common mental health problem (DH 2009).

The high cost of mental health problems can be seen not only in the misery of the disrupted lives of those affected on a day-by-day basis, but also starkly through the mortality data. The inability to deal with problematic emotions is seen as a major contributing factor in the continued high numbers of suicides, with 2481 men (and 684 women) dying from intentional self-harm in England and Wales in 2007, the majority of these deaths occurring in middle-aged men (ONS 2008). If the deaths that are categorised as 'event of undetermined cause', which are often seen as unproven suicides, are included (men with 827 deaths and women with 333 deaths recorded) then some 3304 male deaths have as a core an emotional cause. This is not just a problem in the UK; across the world men's suicide levels are extremely high, such as in Lithuania where the suicide rate is over 10 times higher than that for women in the 35–44 age range (White and Holmes 2006).

The problems of mental health go well beyond the mortality data. The Sainsbury Centre for Mental Health (2007) has estimated that in the UK alone mental health problems account for:

➤ £8.4 billion a year in sickness absence. The average employee takes seven days off sick each year, of which 40% are for mental health problems. This adds up to 70 million lost working days a year, including one in seven directly caused by a person's work or working conditions.
➤ £15.1 billion a year in reduced productivity at work. 'Presenteeism' accounts for 1.5 times as much working time lost as absenteeism and costs more to employers because it is more common among higher-paid staff.
➤ £2.4 billon a year in replacing staff who leave their jobs because of mental ill-health.

A recent Kings Fund report on the cost of mental health care in England to 2026 (McCrone *et al.* 2008) forecasts that the combined cost of lost productivity due to mental health problems and the direct cost of health and social care will double in real terms.

MEN AND MENTAL HEALTH

It has been suggested that the way that men present with mental or emotional difficulties is different from women and that this also causes problems in the effective diagnosis of the problem and referral on for effective treatment (Brownhill *et al.* 2005, White 2006). This was recognised within the European Mental Health report, where it is noted that whilst women have higher levels of depression and anxiety (or internalising disorders) men have higher levels of substance abuse and antisocial disorders (or externalising disorders) (EC 2004) which can be detrimental for men, their friends and family, and their community (Stewart and Harmon 2004, Kupers 2005, Winkler *et al.* 2006).

In England and Wales, for the category of deaths 'Mental and Behavioural causes' (ONS 2008) there were 5390 male and 11 192 female deaths recorded in 2007, but if you break these down by age you find that in the 15–64 (working) age range there are 1034 male deaths, compared to 331 female deaths (a ratio of 3:1). These deaths do not include suicide and in this younger age group are predominately made up of accidental deaths due to psychoactive substance use (alcohol, opioids and dependence). It is also salutary to note that a recent large-scale study from Denmark (Nielsen *et al.* 2008) has shown that chronic long-term stress can affect life expectancy, the effects being most pronounced amongst younger and healthier men.

In 2001, White (2001) undertook Scoping Study on Men's Health for the then Minister for Public Health. Four key areas emerged as the most relevant in understanding men's health problems: men's access to health services; men's lack of awareness of their health needs; men's seeming inability to express emotions; and men's lack of social networks. All of these were interlinked in terms of how men have been socialised to manage their health and well-being, but they also reflect a society that has not given sufficient attention to targeting men, either through services that reflect their needs or through the enablement of men to manage their health more effectively. As Micale (2008) notes, it is often the case that men's emotional problems are explained away rather than being seen as the cry for help they often are. As we come to recognise the complex pathways men take to get help for their emotional and mental health difficulties, we need to be able to identify ways in which public health interventions can be made more accessible (Möller-Leimkühler 2002; Brownhill *et al.* 2002; Brownhill *et al.* 2005; Emslie *et al.* 2006; White 2006; Payne 2008).

In 2006, the Men's Health Forum focused their National Men's Health Week on men's mental health. In their accompanying policy document 'Mind Your Head' (Wilkins 2006) and through the collaboration of over 41 organisations for the development of the 'Brain Manual' (Banks 2006) there was the first national recognition of the state of men's problems with their emotional and mental health. More recently a principal mental health charity, Mind, focused their 2009 mental health week onto 'Men and Mental Health', accompanied by their report 'Get It Off Your Chest' (Mind 2009). Both these campaigns have called for a more proactive approach to reaching out to men.

POLICY DEVELOPMENTS

The wish to see a broader approach to men's mental health has come at a good time with regard to health policy developments, both in the UK and across the globe. In the UK there have been significant changes to the way healthcare is being viewed, one of the main catalysts being the publication of Lord Darzi's 'High Quality Care For All' report (DH 2008), which advocates that comprehensive well-being and prevention services should be commissioned to meet the specific needs of local populations, with family doctors being encouraged to help individuals and their families stay healthy. The report also notes the benefits to general well-being from stronger mental health promotion.

In the UK, the National Service Framework for Mental Health (DH 1999) has been the main guide for how services should be configured. It is now being replaced by the 'New Horizons' strategy,* which aims to promote good mental health and well-being whilst also improving the services for people who have mental health problems. Its ten-year goal is to reduce the stigma associated with mental health and to promote a whole-population approach to the challenges posed by an increasingly stressed community. It is important that this new strategy coincides with the European Pact on Mental Health and Well-being, the focus of which is also on trying to reduce the burden of mental distress on the state, the individual and their families.

There is an added impetus for this text and that is to help guide those tasked with meeting the needs of the Equality Act of 2006, which has placed a gender equality duty on all those providing services that have to meet the needs of men and women. The basis of this duty is that the legal responsibility has moved to the provider to ensure that they have considered whether their population group has had their specific needs incorporated within the design and delivery of their provision. For men, with regard to their mental health, this must include an understanding of their differing presentation of mental health problems, their specific needs with regard to their help-seeking behaviour and the type of approach that would be most effective in reaching out to them.

Taking on a whole-population approach to mental health, as advocated within the UK Government's 'New Horizons', requires us to look beyond mental illness into those aspects of our lives that affect our emotional stability. As these are many and varied, we need to be looking for a complex solution to what is obviously a complex problem. It requires us to understand how men manage their mental and emotional health if we wish to fully comprehend the genesis of the difficulties that they face. We then need to adopt a much broader strategy in tackling men's mental health needs.

---

* www.newhorizons-mentalhealth.co.uk

REFERENCES

Banks I (2006) Brain Manual: *The Step-By-Step Guide for Men to Achieving and Maintaining Mental Well-Being*. Sparkford: JH Haynes & Co Ltd.

Brownhill S and Wilhelm K (2002) Detecting depression in men: a matter of guesswork. *Int J Men's Health*. 1(3): 259–280.

Brownhill S, Wilhelm K, Barclay L and Schmied V (2005) 'Big build': hidden depression in men. *Aus and NZ J Psychiatry*. 39: 921–931.

Department of Health (DH) (1999) *National Service Framework for Mental Health*. London: DH.

Department of Health (DH) (2008) *High Quality Care for All*. London: DH.

Department of Health (DH) (2009) *A New Vision for Mental Health and Well-being*. London: DH.

European Commission (EC) (2004) Action for Mental Health: activities co-funded from European Community Public Health Programmes 1997–2004. Available at: http://ec.europa.eu/health/ph_determinants/life_style/mental/docs/action_1997_2004_en.pdf (Accessed 1 May 2009).

European Commission (EC) (2008) European Pact for Mental Health and Well-being 'Together for Mental Health and Well-being', Brussels, 13 June 2008, Slovenia Presidency of the EU. Available at: http://ec.europa.eu/health/ph_determinants/life_style/mental/docs/pact_en.pdf (Accessed 1 May 2009).

Emslie C, Ridge D, Ziebland S and Hunt K (2006) Men's accounts of depression: reconstructing or resisting hegemonic masculinity? *Social Science & Medicine*. 62: 2246–57.

Kupers TA (2005) Toxic masculinity as a barrier to mental health treatment in prison. *J Clin Psych*. 61(6): 713–724.

Mathers CD and Loncar D (2006) Projections of Global Mortality and Burden of Disease from 2002 to 2030. *PLoS Med* 3(11): e442.doi:10.1371/journal.pmed.0030442.

McCrone P, Dhanasiri S, Patel A, Knapp M and Lawton-Smith S (2008) *Paying the Price: the cost of mental health care in England to 2026*. London: Kings Fund.

Micale MS (2008) *Hysterical Men: the hidden history of male nervous illness*. Harvard: Harvard University Press.

Mind (2009) *Get It Off Your Chest: men and mental health*. London: Mind.

Möller-Leimkühler AM (2002) Barriers to help seeking by men: a review of sociocultural and clinical literature with particular reference to depression. *J Affective Disorders*. 71: 1–9.

Nielsen NR, Kristensen TS, Schnohr P and Grønbæk M (2008) Perceived Stress and Cause-specific Mortality Among Men and Women: results from a prospective cohort study. *Am J Epidemiol*. 168(5): 481–491.

Office for National Statistics (ONS) (2008) *Mortality Statistics: deaths registered in 2007*. DR07. London: ONS.

Payne S (2008) Mental Health. In: Wilkins, D, Payne, S., Granville, G., and Branney, P (eds), *The Gender and Access to Health Services Study*. London: Men's Health Forum/Department of Health.

Sainsbury Centre for Mental Health (2006) *The Future of Mental Health: a Vision for 2015*. London: Sainsbury Centre for Mental Health.

Sainsbury Centre for Mental Health (2007) *Mental Health at Work: developing the business case*. [Policy papers]. London: Sainsbury Centre for Mental Health.

Stewart D and Harmon K (2004) Mental health services responding to men and their anger. *Int J Mental Health Nursing.* **13**: 249–254.

White AK (2001) *Report on the Scoping Study on Men's Health.* London: Department of Health.

White AK and Holmes M (2006) Patterns of mortality across 44 Countries among men and women aged 15–44. *J Men's Health & Gender.* **3**(2): 139–151.

White AK (2006) Personal Perspective: Men and mental well-being: encouraging gender sensitivity. *Mental Health Review J.* **11**(4): 3–6.

Wilkins D (2006) *Mind Your Head: men, boys and mental well-being.* London: Men's Health Forum.

Winkler D, Pjrek E and Kasper S (2006) Gender-specific symptoms of depression and anger attacks. *J Men's Health & Gender.* **3**(1): 19–24.

World Health Organization (2002) *The World Health Report 2001: mental health: new understanding, new hope.* WHO: Geneva.

CHAPTER 2

On the edge? An introduction to men's mental health

Peter Branney and Alan White

INTRODUCTION

This chapter aims to outline three main issues in men's mental health:

1 conceptions of mental health marginalise the difficulties that men have with emotional and mental well-being.
2 referral and diagnostic procedures exclude many of men's mental health difficulties.
3 mental health services fail to reach many of the groups where there may be men with mental health difficulties.

ARE MEN ON THE EDGE?

'Mental disorders', 'mental illness', 'mad', 'insane', 'troubled' and even 'neuropsychiatric disorders'; the terms for mental health are manifold and this is in a large part because it can cover such a wide range of issues. There is depression, anxiety, and psychosis. Along with these three, there are many others that can be included; alcoholism, epilepsy, dementia, learning disorders and violence to name but a few. Combine the breadth of issues of mental health with those associated with gender and there is a great deal to consider. An overview such as this cannot give adequate attention to all of the issues related to and on the margins of mental health and, if it intends to remain true to the practical focus of this book, nor should it. Practitioners have a difficult job; they have numerous demands on their time and when it comes to working with either a specific issue or a particular person it is likely that the problem will be complex, involving many difficult decisions. As such, a practitioner will have to take stock of what they know and decide on the main issues and it seems sensible that this chapter should have the same scope.

Our aim is to delineate the main issues for promoting men's mental health and in doing so we have to make a number of choices. In making our choices we are ignoring other issues but we want to clarify three points about our decision-making process. First, we have selected three issues because we think they are particularly important but this does not mean that they will always be important. Indeed, the hope behind a practical-based book such as this is that it will result in changes to how mental health in men is managed, which should therefore alter the main issues that need tackling. Second, issues related to mental health will differ across the globe and within countries. Our hope is that exploring the large-, or macro-scale issues will help when it comes to defining and dealing with issues at a local, or micro, level. It is important to remember that context does affect gendered differences in mental health (Emslie *et al.* 2002). Finally, the main issues of men's mental health that we are presenting are specific to the context of this book, which is the promotion of mental health.

The title of this chapter provides a hint at what we think are the main issues, which we present as three partial answers to the question, 'are men on the edge?'. Asking such a question will annoy many because it is representative of a somewhat dated and negative view of mental ill-health as contained within individuals who have lost control. Unfortunately, such a view predominates and if we are to promote men's mental health then we need to be aware of how it is manifest. In the Introduction, Alan White defined mental health as both positive (emotional well-being) and negative (what is usually meant by the term 'mental health'). Structures that deal with mental health explicitly are largely, if not always, focused on the negative aspects. These 'structures' are mental health services that are along a continuum from those that are run in the community to those that are in the hospital, with a variety of services in between. The question 'are men on the edge?' also provides a metaphor of teetering on the edge of a precipice that encapsulates the three answers to the questions that we are going to present. We hope to show that this precipice is not one of individual rational control but it is the services that are designed to tackle mental ill-health.

Answer 1: men are on the edge of conceptions of mental health

Mental ill-health is a substantial problem and can be expressed in terms of what's referred to as 'Disability Adjusted Life Years' (DALYs), which are a combination of the years of life lost due to premature mortality and the years of life spent living in disability due to a specific condition. Across the world, mental ill-health accounts for almost a third of the DALYs from non-communicable disease (Prince *et al.* 2008) and just over a tenth of the DALYs from all diseases (WHO 2001). There are a wide variety of mental illnesses and it will be easier if we focus on those that cause the most disability, which will be expressed as the greatest proportion of DALYs. The World Health Organization (WHO) annually publishes statistics on health from across the world. In 2001 WHO focused on mental health, providing statistics for the top 20 causes of disability for those aged 15 to 44 years old. These statistics are particularly useful here because they help us compare mental ill-health to other causes of disability, such as traffic accidents, asthma and HIV/AIDS, and they exclude children, where mental ill-health may be categorised in very different ways.

Unipolar depressive disorders emerge as a major cause of disability and in both sexes it is second only to HIV/AIDS in terms of DALYs. In women depression accounts for a little over one in ten of all DALYs but in men it is a little less at one in fifteen. Schizophrenia and bipolar affective disorder are the eight and ninth causes of disability but there is little difference between men and women. Depression, bipolar disorder and schizophrenia are some of the more traditional mental ill-health diagnoses because they attempt to define an internal problem of the individual, particularly, but not exclusively, with how they feel. Combined, they account for 15.9% of DALYs in women and 11.6% in men, which means that women have greater disability from these internal mental ill-health conditions.

There are two other mental ill-health problems that are within the top 20 causes of disability, which do not fit easily with the focus on the internal functioning of an individual. Alcohol-use disorders are the fifth leading cause of disability in those aged 15 to 44 years. When considering men and women separately however, alcohol misuse shows big differences. For men, alcohol misuse is the fourth leading cause of disability but does not even enter into the top 20 causes of disability for women. Self-inflicted injuries are, after alcohol, the sixth main cause of disability although there is little difference between men (3.0%) and women (2.4%). As a condition of mental ill-health these two stand out because they are concerned not with the inner working of the individual but with what they do. That is, not with how they feel but with how much alcohol they drink, not with how they perceive the world but with how they (mis)treat their body. Combined, these behavioural mental health conditions account for well over three times more DALYS in men (8.1%) than in women (2.4%).

The differences between internal and behavioural mental ill-health – confirmed by a review of mental health in the European Union (EC 2004) – are important because the condition with which someone is classified can determine the options available to them, and to health professionals, when faced with services for mental health. However, there is a need to stop to think about these for a while. At their most basic, aren't the differences between internal and behavioural merely conceptual? Someone can feel deeply sad or anxious and there may be many ways, including drinking too much or inflicting damage on the body, in which they may mistreat themselves. It is therefore possible that it is not just a fact that women have more internal problems and men have more behavioural difficulties but rather that we have different ways for conceptualising the mental ill-health of men and women. Yes, these problems can occur together – they can be co-morbid – as someone can be diagnosed as both depressed and as an alcoholic but this does not explain the conceptual differences.

You may notice something a little confusing about the distinction between internal and behavioural and this explains why it seems that men are on the edge of conceptions of mental health. 'Internal' and 'mental' both refer to the inner workings of the individual, particularly the individual's mind, and so it seems that internal mental ill-health is simply mental ill-health. This means that conceptually the behavioural mental ill-health, focusing on the actions of the individual, seems to suggest that the workings of the inner mind are less relevant. As the greatest proportion of those with DALYs due to internal mental ill-health are women and those with DALYS due to behavioural mental ill-health are men it seems that men's mental ill-health somehow fails to fit with understandings of mental health. A more applied way to consider conceptions of mental health is to explore practices for deciding what, if any, mental health difficulties an individual has.

Answer 2: men are on the edge of processes of referral and diagnosis

While the conceptions of mental health considered above sound like something that only interests academics they are particularly important in practice. The relevance of such conceptions for practitioners emerges when we start to consider whether someone should be seen by a mental health service. In this context, another term for 'conception' would be 'diagnosis'. In the academic and clinical domains, diagnosis can mean a specific procedure which identifies a discrete mental illness. In practice, however, it can be difficult to decide which diagnosis is most appropriate and often someone does not necessarily need a formal diagnosis to be referred to or be seen by a mental health service. As such, our focus is on the broader processes of referral and diagnosis. Unfortunately, focusing on something so broad means that it is difficult to identify such processes with any certainty and then to make any comment on it. Looking at depression may help us along our way because there is a body of research that is linked to referral and diagnostic procedures but also because depression is one of those internal mental health difficulties that affects women more than men.

In terms of depression there is a well-documented disparity between clinical (Office of National Statistics 2000; ISD Scotland 2004) and community (Bland *et al.* 1988; Wells *et al.* 1989; Blazer *et al.* 1994; Meltzer *et al.* 1995; Singleton *et al.* 2000; Wilhelm *et al.* 2002) samples in the rate of depression in men. That is, when we look at clinical samples – those containing people who are under the care of a (mental) health service and have a diagnosis of depression – we find many more women with depression than men. When we look at community samples the differences in rates of diagnosis between men and women are smaller. In the UK, for example, nationally collected figures show that for every four men diagnosed with depression in general practice there are ten women with the same diagnosis (Office of National Statistics 2000). This contrasts with a national household survey in the UK, which found that there were eight men for every ten women with depression (Singleton *et al.* 2000). Putting aside complexities of this research, there are at least three possible explanations for this disparity; first, that there is an under-diagnosis of men; second, that there is an over-diagnosis of women; and last, that there are systematic biases in the diagnoses of both men and women. The last answer is potentially more accurate as it would allow for over-diagnoses of groups of men, such as has been found in relation to black and minority ethnic groups (Keating *et al.* 2002; Bhui *et al.* 2003; Healthcare Commission 2007).

Looking at classification systems offers the potential for further insight into bias in the diagnosis of depression. These systems – specifically the tenth edition of the *International Statistical Classification of Diseases and Related Health Problems* (ICD-10) and the fourth edition of the *Diagnostic and Statistical Manual of Mental Disorders*

(DSM-IV) – define clusters of symptoms as specific disorders (depressive episode, recurrent depressive disorder, dysthymia, etc). In practice, health professionals can draw upon the list of symptoms for each disorder to help them diagnose the difficulty a specific individual has and then subsequently to make the most appropriate referral or devise a treatment plan. As such, the classification systems are like a top-down protocol guiding practitioners in how to understand the difficulties their patients present with. Research has taken a bottom-up approach and looked at people who have been diagnosed as depressed and asked them to list their symptoms (including symptoms that are not listed as diagnostic of depression). Box 2.1 is taken from a review of approaches to depression and men (Branney and White 2008) and shows the diagnostic and non-diagnostic criteria and highlights those symptoms that occur most often in men or women. Symptoms that have been shown to occur more frequently in depressed men are slow movements, scarcity of gestures and slow speech (Kivelä and Pahkala 1988), non-verbal hostility (Katz *et al.* 1993), trait hostility (Fava *et al.* 1995) and alcohol dependence during difficult times (Angst *et al.* 2002), which are not common to diagnostic criteria for (adult) depression. Increased hostility might be indicative of a conduct disorder mixed with depression but is limited to onset in early childhood. It appears that the symptoms that are indicative of depression in men are absent from classification criteria for depression.

BOX 2.1 Diagnostic criteria for depression

ICD-10 F32 Depressive Episode

➤ Depressed mood

➤ Loss of interest or enjoyment

➤ Reduced energy leading to increased fatigability and diminished activity

➤ Marked tiredness after slight effort

➤ Reduced concentration and attention

➤ Reduced self-esteem and self-confidence*

➤ Ideas of guilt and unworthiness

➤ Bleak and pessimistic views of the future

➤ Ideas or acts of self-harm or suicide*

➤ Disturbed sleep

➤ Diminished appetite.*

DSM-IV Major Depressive Episode

➤ Depressed mood

➤ Loss of interest or enjoyment

➤ Weight loss

➤ Insomnia or hypersomnia

➤ Psychomotor agitation

➤ Fatigue

➤ Feelings of unworthiness*

➤ Reduced concentration.

Non-diagnostic

➤ Alcohol dependence during difficult times[†]

➤ Bodily pains*

➤ Hostility (non-verbal)[†]

➤ Hostility (trait)[†]

➤ Scarcity of gestures[†]

➤ Slow movements[†]

➤ Slow speech[†]

➤ Stooping posture.*

---

* Shown to discriminate between sex, occurring more frequently in women.
[†] Shown to discriminate between sex, occurring more frequently in men.
Source: Branney and White (2008)

We are not trying to say that classification systems are the only reason for the disparity between depression in men in the clinic and in the community. Nor are we suggesting that they explain the difference in the effect of internal and behavioural mental illnesses on men and women. In practice there is often more fluidity in diagnosis and referral than these systems suggest. For example, aggression may be recognised as part of depression by many practitioners. It is very difficult to explore referral and diagnostic processes as they occur to explain the clinic-community disparity, which means that studying classifications systems is one, if imperfect, approach. At the very least, the approach we have taken allows us to move on from conceptions of mental health to the more practical concern with referral and diagnosis, where it seems that men are on the edge.

It is also noteworthy that there seems to be an overlap with the conceptions of mental illness that affect men more than women – that is, behavioural mental ill-health such as substance misuse and suicide – and symptoms that differentiate men and women with depression. It appears that the symptoms men have are predominantly concerned with their behaviour; that is, how men move and talk, how they (violently) interact, and how they use alcohol. There is also an overlap between the internal conceptions of mental health that affect women more than men and the symptoms that women with depression have more often than men. In particular, the symptoms for women are concerned with their internal mental states – with self-esteem, self-confidence and feelings of unworthiness. This is where we can move to a distinction that sits a bit better (than the internal behavioural distinction) alongside mental health. This distinction is between problem-focused and emotion-focused difficulties, which is often used when referring to the way men and women experience and express mental ill-health (e.g. Busfield 1996). What we are suggesting, therefore, is that processes of referral and diagnosis seem to focus on emotion, which means that those whose difficulties are problem-focused are under-served by mental health services. This leads us onto questions of whether services are managing to reach men who have mental health difficulties.

Answer 3: men are on the edge of the reach of mental health services

In the Introduction, we pointed out that structures that explicitly target mental health largely limit themselves to the negative aspects. That is, mental health services focus on ill-health and one way to consider if men are on the edge is to explore whether services reach men with such difficulties. Even the best evidence-based service is little use if it cannot persuade relevant people to use it. There are three different bodies of information that we can draw upon to consider the reach of mental health services in relation to men.

First, the starting point is to ask if there are people with difficulties that would be classified as having a mental disorder who are not under the care of a specific service. Another way of putting this is to ask if there are people who fit a service's inclusion or referral criteria but who are not using the service. That there are fewer men with depression in clinical samples than there are in the community suggests a specific area where services are failing to reach men. The difficulty with this approach is that it is usually limited to the notions of mental ill-health that are given in formal classification systems. We have already suggested that conceptions of mental health and processes of referral and diagnosis do not adequately fit many men so they could easily be missed by such an approach. It is also possible to argue that mental health services do not have to reach everybody who would get a diagnosis but only those that want help. Unfortunately, if those that want to promote mental health only concern themselves with people who want good emotional well-being they may find that they end up working only with the converted.

Second, it is possible to look at aspects that are related to a service's work that are not specific referral criteria. Many mental health services are directly or indirectly concerned with helping to prevent harm but it can be difficult to pick up individuals before they have, for example, actually harmed themselves. Suicide is a key here because nothing can be done once it has been completed. Globally the rate of suicide mortality for men is four times higher than that for women (White and Holmes 2006) – China is the only country where women's suicide mortality is greater than men's (Hawton 2000). Many people who complete suicide have never been in contact with a mental health service and it is possible that they have never shown any signs that would have resulted in a referral to such a service and in these cases it may be that there is little that could have been done to prevent it occurring. Alternatively, because conceptions of mental health somewhat marginalise behavioural or problem-focused difficulties it could be that mental health services do not currently deal with problems that could lead up to suicide.

The last approach is to look at information that is indicative, rather than diagnostic, of mental ill-health. Given the importance that problem-focused difficulties seem to have with men and their mental ill-health, there is a great deal to which we can turn. For every 100 000 people in the world about 140 are imprisoned (this includes those at pre-trial stages; Tkachuk and Walmsley 2001) and these people are usually men. In prison populations, the proportion of men ranges from 95% (England) to 90% (US).[*] This is such a well-recognised gender gap that it is extraordinarily difficult to find statistics on global crime levels that separate figures for male and female perpetrators (the assumption being that there are too few female criminals to justify the extra work). Some, such as the Men's Health Forum (Wilkins 2006) want to suggest that these crime figures are, at the very least, indicative of low-level mental distress but they have to tread carefully for two reasons. First, it is unlikely that any evidence will unequivocally prove that crime is underlined by mental ill-health. Second, suggesting that all criminals (whether male or female) are mentally ill risks pathologising a large proportion of the population as both bad and mad. Looking at crime rates in more detail demonstrates that men tend to commit offences that endanger people, or what would be called violent crimes (CrimeInfo 2008),[†] which includes common assault (i.e. no injury), harassment, homicide, serious or less serious wounding, and sexual offences. Posing a risk to others is one of those signs that would concern many mental health professionals and, indeed, is often one of the key referral criteria for mental health services.

Each of these three different approaches points towards groups of men that mental health services are failing to serve. In relation to mental health, these groups seem to be defined by their focus on problems rather than emotions. It is little surprise that mental health services fail to serve groups that are defined by their outward behaviour, such as violent criminals. Unfortunately, it is extremely difficult to imagine how services could be transformed to provide for these groups while ensuring that they do not criminalise people with mental health difficulties or pathologise criminals. A focus group study by Brownhill and colleagues (2005) on depression in men and women is instructive because it provides a framework, called the 'Big Build', (*see* Figure 2.1) to understand problem-focused difficulties in terms that relate well to mental health. The difference with depression in men and women that seemed most important was not how depression was experienced but how it was expressed. Their study seems to suggest that depression is part of an inner emotional world that is contained, constrained or set free by gendered practices. The model explains how masculine practices in relation to depression result in a debilitating trajectory of destructive behaviour and emotional distress. These practices start as avoidance, numbing and escaping behaviours that may escalate to violence and suicide. The point seems to be that emotional difficulties are aligned with the enactment of what may be termed antisocial behaviours.

---

[*] World Prison Brief, International Centre for Prison Studies, Kings College, London. Downloaded 1 August 2008 from www.kcl.ac.uk/depsta/law/research/icps/worldbrief/.

[†] www.crimeinfo.org.uk/servlet/factsheetservlet?command=viewfactsheet&factsheetid=110&category=factsheets

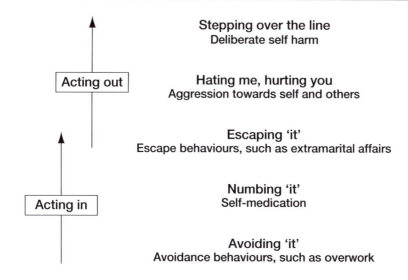

Stepping over the line
Deliberate self harm

Acting out   **Hating me, hurting you**
Aggression towards self and others

Escaping 'it'
Escape behaviours, such as extramarital affairs

Numbing 'it'
Self-medication

Acting in

Avoiding 'it'
Avoidance behaviours, such as overwork

FIGURE 2.1 'Big Build'
Source: Brownhill *et al.* (2005)

CONCLUSION: A NOTE OF CAUTION

The aim of this chapter is to delineate the main issues for promoting men's mental health and we have tried to achieve this by providing three different answers to the question, 'are men on the edge?'. As men are worst affected by behavioural mental health difficulties where the inner mental world is seen as less relevant, the first answer was to say that men are on the edge of conceptions of mental health. It is in referral and diagnostic procedures that conceptions of mental health become relevant for practice and these seem to focus on emotions rather than the problems that many men would evidence. As such, the second answer was that men are on the edge of processes of referral and diagnosis. This led onto further questions about whether mental health services are reaching people, particularly men, with problem-focused difficulties. There are many groups that are defined by their problems where men predominate, such as violent criminals. As such, the final answer was that men are on the edge of the reach of mental health services. The last answer also brought us full circle because it provides a potential way of conceptualising mental health difficulties where the inner emotional world is aligned with outward signs of antisocial behaviour in what is termed a 'Big Build' (Brownhill *et al.* 2005).

In taking a renewed focus on outward problems, such as in the Big Build, forward into the promotion of men's mental health, there are two cautionary notes that must be added. First, focusing on antisocial behaviour or, more broadly, outward signs of mental health difficulties should not be at the expense of dealing with emotional difficulties. Second, neither should a focus on outward behaviour be seen as merely a way of reaching men so as to tackle their inner mental health. Both risks highlight that it is important that any attention on the individual should not be at the expense of considering the social structures that make problem-focused mental health difficulties a possibility in contemporary society. If, for example, a particular man's abusive behaviour is underlined by emotional difficulties then we need to find ways to support him while also challenging the social edifice for making abuse a way of being (mentally ill) for him.

ACKNOWLEDGEMENTS

The authors would like to thank Karl Witty and Steve Robertson for feedback on an earlier draft of this chapter.

REFERENCES

American Psychiatric Association (2000) *Diagnostic and Statistical Manual of Mental Disorders* (4th ed, text revision). Washington, DC: APA.

Angst J, Gamma A, Gastpar M, Lepine J-P, Mendlewicz J and Tylee A (2002) Gender differences in depression: epidemiological findings from the European DEPRES I and II studies. *European Archives of Psychiatry & Clinical Neuroscience*. **252**: 201–209.

Bhui K, Standeld SA, Holt S, Priebe S, Mole F and Feder G (2003) Ethnic variations in the pathways to and use of specialist mental health services. *Br J Psychiatry*. **182**: 105–116.

Bland R, Newman SC and Orn H (1988) Period prevalence of psychiatric disorders in Edmonton. *Acta Psychiatrica Scandinavica*. **77**: 33–42.

Blazer D, Kessler R, McGonagle K and Swartz M (1994) The prevalence and distribution of major depression in a national community sample: the National Comorbidity Survey. *Am J Psychiatry*. **151**: 979–986.

Branney PE and White AK (2008) Big boys don't cry: men and depression. *Advances in Psychiatric Treatment*. **14**: 256–262.

Brownhill S, Wilhelm K, Barclay L and Schmied V (2005) 'Big build': hidden depression in men. *Australian & NZ J Psychiatry*. **39**: 921–931.

Busfield J (1996) *Men, Women and Madness: understanding gender and mental disorder*. London: Palgrave Macmillan.

CrimeInfo (2008) *Women, Gender and Crime*: England and Wales. http:/crimeinfo.org.uk

Emslie C, Fuhrer R, Hunt K, Macintyre S, Shipley M and Stansfeld S (2002) Gender differences in mental health: evidence from three organisations. *Social Science & Medicine*. **54**: 621–624.

European Commission (EC) (2004) *The State of Mental Health in the European Union*. Geneva: Health & Consumer Protection Directorate General, European Commission.

Fava M, Nolan S, Kradin R and Rosenbaum J (1995) Gender differences in hostility among depressed and medical outpatients. *J Nervous & Mental Disease*. **183**: 10–14.

Hawton K (2000) Sex and suicide: gender differences in suicidal behaviour. *Br J Psychiatry* 177: 484–485.

Healthcare Commission (2007) *Count Me In: results of the 2006 national census of inpatients in mental health and learning disability services in England and Wales.* London: Commission for Healthcare Audit and Inspection.

ISD Scotland (2004) *Practice Team Information.* Edinburgh: Scottish Health Statistics.

Katz M, Wetzler S, Cloitre M, Swann A, Secunda S, Mendels J and Robins E (1993) Expressive characteristics of anxiety in depressed men and women. *J Affective Disorders.* 28: 267–277.

Keating F, Robertson D, McCulloch A and Francis E (2002) *Breaking the Circles of Fear: A Review of the Relationship between Mental Health Services and African and Caribbean Communities.* London: Sainsbury Centre for Mental Health.

Kivelä S-L and Pahkala K (1988) Clinician-rated symptoms and signs of depression in aged Finns. *International J Social Psychiatry.* 34: 2229–2235.

Meltzer H, Gill B, Petticrew M and Hinds K (1995) *The Prevalence of Psychiatric Morbidity among Adults in Private Households, 1995.* London: The Stationary Office.

Office of National Statistics (2000) *Key Health Statistics from General Practice 1998.* London: The Stationary Office.

Prince M, Patel V, Saxena S, Maj M, Maselko J, Phillips MR and Rahman A (2008) Global mental health 1: no health without mental health. *Lancet.* 370: 859–877.

Singleton N, Bumpstead R, O'Brien M, Lee A and Meltzer H (2000) *Psychiatric Morbidity among Adults Living in Private Households.* London: The Stationary Office.

Tkachuk B and Walmsley R (2001) World Prison Population: Facts, Trends and Solutions. HEUNI Paper No. 15. Helsinki: The European Institute for Crime Prevention and Control (affiliated with the United Nations). Available at: www.heuni.fi/uploads/6mq2zlwaaw3ut. pdf (Accessed 4 October 2008).

Wells J, Bushnell J, Hornblow A, Joyce P and Oakley-Browne M (1989) Christchurch psychiatric epidemiology study, Part I: methodology and lifetime prevalence for specific psychiatric disorders. *Aus & NZ J Psychiatry.* 23: 315–326.

White AK and Holmes M (2006) Patterns of mortality across 44 countries among men and women aged 15–44 years. *J Men's Health & Gender.* 3: 139–151.

Wilhelm L, Mitchell P, Slade T, Brownhill S and Andrews G (2002) Prevalence and correlates of DSM-IV major depression in an Australian national survey. *J Affective Disorders.* 75: 155–162.

Wilkins D (2006) *Mind Your Head: men, boys and mental well-being.* London: Men's Health Forum.

World Health Organization (WHO) (1992) The International classification of disease (ICD-10): classification of mental and behavioural disorders. *Clinical Descriptions and Diagnostic Guidelines.* Geneva: WHO

World Health Organization (WHO) (2001) *The World Health Report 2001 – Mental Health: New Understanding, New Hope.* Geneva: WHO.

CHAPTER 3

Cultural representations of masculinity and mental health

David Conrad and Louise Warwick-Booth

INTRODUCTION

In the field of men's health we talk a lot about how a large proportion of men are trapped in a traditional masculine identity which is detrimental to their health and discourages them from addressing health problems. Men in Western post-industrial society have been described as being in a state of crisis – struggling to find meaning and identity in a world where women are breadwinners too and stable jobs based purely on male muscle are harder to come by than ever before (e.g. Clare 2000). There's the idea that while new and alternative masculinities are on offer to men, the majority cling pointlessly but relentlessly to their 'old man' gender roles, spiralling into torment as they become increasingly anachronistic. There may not be much evidence that men themselves are experiencing this sense of crisis (Gauntlett 2008) but there is evidence that traditional notions of masculinity still play a major role in how men behave and wish to be perceived by their peers. O'Brien and colleagues (2005) conducted focus groups with men to discuss a range of aspects of health, including the issue of consulting the GP about depression. Even in this context, with the discussion of mental health legitimised by the research setting, most of the groups responded to the topic with an impenetrable wall of machismo. When there were hints from the discussion that one or more of the group participants had experienced problems with depression there was often a strong resistance to exploring the issues on any kind of personal level, particularly among the group comprised of younger men.

But where do our notions of masculinity come from? Who sets the rules about how men should behave, how they should feel about mental health issues and how they should deal with their own? Of course, gender roles are largely self-replicating, as each generation is socialised into them by the one before. But we also know that gender roles can change – women are no longer just seen as housewives and that's something that has to varying degrees changed across the social spectrum in the UK. Representations of women in the media have also changed, partly in response to the changes in society but also partly as a cause of those changes.

Popular culture can play a big role in steering the attitudes of each generation in a particular direction, whether that be in reinforcing existing values and beliefs or promoting new ones. Whole books have been written on debates around the construction of gender identities and representations of gender and health in the media, but we aim in this chapter to touch on just a few of the key themes that partly help us understand how men's attitudes to masculinity and mental health might be formed.

WHERE DO CULTURAL NORMS OF MASCULINITY COME FROM?

Let's first focus on cultural representation as a concept. Culture is about shared meanings embodied in collective practices, specifically relating to identity and formed through the social interactions in which we participate. We demonstrate cultural representation when we express ourselves and carry out our everyday practices. Indeed, cultural representation is also a form of regulation in terms of social conduct. These cultural representations appear normal but they actually position subjects in certain societal roles (Hall 1997).

All men are socialised with regards to gender roles and this influences how they see themselves in terms of masculinity and expectations of how they should behave, what they should wear, work roles and activities such as drinking and sexual conduct. Boys and girls are treated differently from birth and messages about gendered actions are reiterated via the media (White 2007). The dominant (hegemonic) cultural representation of being male and masculine is of being independent, powerful, physically strong and almost invincible (see Newman 1997). Furthermore, the dominant construct of masculinity is not associated with feeling or indeed expressing emotions, which doesn't make it conducive to encouraging men to seek help with mental health problems. For the majority of men in Western culture being masculine is about being healthy in a physical sense but also being emotionally strong and it's this model of masculinity which they measure themselves against.

Social constructionist theories of masculinity recognise that gender is not individual but rather something 'done' and achieved in the context of social interactions. The construction of gender identity is a joint effort and the role of the peer group is key. People's ideas about health and illness are an example of what Berger and Luckman (1971) term objectifications of the social world. Through language and their everyday practices, men order their social world in terms of gender roles and expectations; this becoming internalised as an objective fact.

Queer theorists see gender as a performance (though not necessarily a conscious one) which is continuously reinforced through repetition. They consider the masculine/feminine divide to be a social construction, resulting from the man/woman divide which is itself a social construction. They see the notion of fixed identity as an illusion, thus laying open the possibility of change. The lifelong playing out of hegemonic masculinity by the majority of men is therefore not regarded as something inevitable that we can't do anything about (Gauntlett 2008).

MASCULINITY IN THE MEDIA

There's been much criticism of media representations of mental health issues, which frequently focus on violent and criminal acts conducted by the mentally ill (Wahl 2003). The resulting stigmatisation of the mentally ill has compounded the effects of hegemonic masculinity on men's willingness to even discuss mental well-being issues, let alone acknowledge a diagnosable mental illness.

Crawshaw (2007) looked at representations of health in the mainstream UK magazine *Men's Health*. He found that a neo-liberal model of health was promoted in which men were constructed as active and entrepreneurial citizens able to take charge of maintaining their own health through self-management in ways that fitted with a hegemonic masculine identity.

As such, there was no acknowledgement of other masculinities and non-heterosexual desires or relationships were excluded from the picture.

One could argue, of course, that the magazine is not setting out to foist hegemonic masculine values onto the nation's men, merely to address the issues which are relevant for that portion of the male population who already subscribe to these values and are the target audience of the publication. A magazine like *Men's Health* will, to a large extent, be preaching to the converted in terms of its messages around masculinity and what it is to be a healthy man. However, in failing to acknowledge alternative masculinities or to frame hegemonic masculinity as just that, the exclusion of anything (or anyone) that fails to conform to the heterosexual, visibly physically fit, independent, groomed and well-self-managed macho stereotype sends the message that anything else is, if not unacceptable, at the very least not healthy.

Crawshaw points out that *Men's Health* presents self-help strategies as the means by which health is achieved. While there's nothing wrong with encouraging men to access information which they can work through by themselves, this should really be presented as one of a range of ways of accessing help and advice. Otherwise, rather than being encouraged to make use of appropriate services when necessary, the message that men should always be able to manage their own health without having to involve other people could hinder rather than improve their health. The reality is that a state of mental well-being is not something that we can achieve and maintain in isolation. The hegemonic construct of masculinity has been built on concepts of self-reliance and the notion that strength is a refusal to show weakness; informing men in a publication dedicated to their pursuit of health that this is indeed the road to perfect well-being has dangerous implications.

It wouldn't be accurate, however, to suggest that the mainstream press have only presented a single stereotype of masculine identity with any consistency. The shift from the post-industrial 'new man' of the 1980s to the 'new laddism' of the 1990s shows how the media have the capacity to foist onto their audiences alternative masculinities of their choosing when they see fit. In terms of mental well-being the 'new man' seemed to have a lot more going for him than the emotionally stifled paranoid macho 'old man' that he superseded (Beynon 2004). 'New man' rejected sexism, embraced his nurturing side, was in touch with his emotions and wasn't afraid to express them. But just how many new men were out in the real world as opposed to posing on the pages of glossy magazines is open to question (Nixon 1996).

Whilst media representations of men may have blurred the boundaries between masculine and feminine, gay and straight, these changes were and still are mostly irrelevant for the bulk of the UK population, whose lives bear little relation to the metropolitan lifestyles of which certain sections of the press present an almost pornographic depiction. The post-industrial 'new man' was a middle class, educated and very much Western-centric figure who had little connection to the traditional blue-collar man whose job may have disappeared but whose lifestyle and culture largely remained the same (Beynon 2004). Working-class men were suddenly unfashionable, but they were still there. The portrayal of 'new man' may have pointed a way for 'old men' to be reborn as emotionally sensitive champions of equality, liberated from the shackles of their traditional values and all set to do the washing-up, but how many of them were equipped with the means to get to the starting post, or even accepted the notion of a need to get there?

Like the 'new man', that other prominent 1980s characterisation of masculine identity, the 'Yuppie', sent a clear message to the traditional working-class male that he was no longer relevant. But he also had another message for 'old man' – that he was a failure. Accumulating financial wealth, not producing commodities, was the new mark of a man's success. It didn't matter how you achieved it or whether you'd gone to a good school. It was OK to be a barrow boy who'd made good as long as you flashed the cash and a suitably bulging Filofax to prove it. Just as the 'new man' had been comically portrayed by some as a tree-hugging wimp who'd lost all dignity, the Yuppie was also lampooned in popular culture, but the difference was that this became seen as a celebration of this form of masculinity rather than undermining it. The TV portrayal of the obnoxious wad-waving 'Loadsamoney' character by comedian Harry Enfield, which satirised the values and aspirations of the unsophisticated and uneducated male whose sense of self-worth seemed to rest entirely on his ability not only to accumulate wealth but to belittle every man around him by thrusting it about in a primeval show of one-upmanship, became more of a mascot than an embarrassment for those it set out to ridicule.

This was also true of Michael Douglas' famous portrayal of the ruthless red-braces-clad bond-trader character of Gordon Gekko in the 1987 film 'Wall Street'. The film perfectly portrayed the clash between old industrial man, whose life had become an anachronism and who was set to be thrown on the scrap heap with his masculinity and sense of self-worth in tatters, and the emotionally sterile, unashamed selfishness of the Yuppie for whom even his own well-being, let alone that of others, was insignificant in comparison with the quest to achieve ever greater status through the accumulation of money for its own sake. 'Greed is good' and 'lunch is for wimps' became proud slogans for those who sought to emulate the character of Gekko (Jennings 2005), whose creation probably did more to encourage young men into a career in the financial markets than it did to put them off from it.

When 'new laddism' took hold in the 1990s with the arrival of 'Loaded' magazine, it seemed like a resurgence, a reinvigoration and proud return to glory, for the kind of juvenile, un-politically correct, unashamedly sexist, loud, drunken yobbish masculinity that had fallen out of favour in popular culture but which, in reality, had never gone anywhere. It was essentially a working-class masculine identity, but one which also fitted easily with the student lifestyle of binge drinking and skirt chasing, valuing play over work and baring your arse to authority without ever threatening to put down that traffic cone and get serious for long enough to overturn it. Young middle-class men were now quite happy to be mistaken for working class. Bettering yourself meant lowering yourself, not donning a sharp suit and an aluminium briefcase to show that you'd risen above the masses. With the likes of the band Oasis, radio host Chris Moyles and the famously wealthy TV and radio presenter Chris Evans seemingly never off the air, there was no shortage of reminders that now you didn't have to behave yourself in order to get ahead and become sexually successful, admired, socially accepted and rich.

Eventually even new laddism began to grow stale and fell out of favour, but new types of men are constantly being invented and offered up by the media (Beynon 2004). Some have the memetic qualities to take off and remain in the collective consciousness for years (especially if they can be used to sell products); others never get beyond wrapping the next day's chips.

So hegemonic masculinity isn't the be all and end all – alternative masculinities have been popularised by the media. But at every turn men are burdened by them. The 'old (industrial) man', who bears the closest resemblance to what still stands as the hegemonic construct of masculinity, has his behaviour and attitudes mocked in certain circles as some kind of outdated circus performance of hyper-masculinity. At the same time he has to maintain that identity in order to avoid being mocked by his peers. He's no longer valued by wider society and in many cases also has to deal with the stresses of having his livelihood taken away. The heterosexual 'new man' may be in touch with his emotions and keen to express them in a healthy way but ultimately hegemonic masculinity holds sufficient sway for him to be labelled a tree-hugger and his sexuality to be called into question. Although the broadsheet press are more likely to reflect on hegemonic masculinity and acknowledge it as problematic to mental health, it will still be promoted as a more desirable alternative when compared to 'feminised' masculinities (Coyle and Sykes 1998). The unfeeling 'Yuppie', who disregards his own emotional needs and those of everyone else in the pursuit of wealth, is now especially vilified in the credit-crunch era and anyway is probably heading for an ulcer, a heart attack, a breakdown, or is setting up a catalogue of future mental health problems for his children.

MEN UNDER PRESSURE

There is a danger that in attempting to explain men's attitudes and behaviours, and in promoting men's health, we portray men as passive and naïve (Gough 2006). In truth, gender identities arise from a combination of structural- and individual-level influences (Giddens 1986) and the balance and relationship between the two is what determines men's gender practices. Men therefore shouldn't be seen as mere unthinking recipients of whatever popular culture throws their way, but at the same time we have to acknowledge that men's identity and their attitudes to mental health are formed and performed within an arena of cultural influences (Beynon 2004).

Even those who reject hegemonic notions that men shouldn't show emotion or ask for psychological support may still feel restricted in how they can behave for fear of the reactions of men who don't. Whether or not men conform to the dominant construct of masculinity, they are still measured against it (White 2007). Examples of this in action were found in O'Brien and colleagues' (2005) focus groups. The authors reported how men describing episodes of severe depression seemed to fear being exposed as weak by the group. Conscious of the power of other men to define and police their masculinity, they framed their depressive symptoms as 'workplace stress' – a more 'manly' term which suggests the battle-weariness of the dedicated macho breadwinner, rather than a 'feminine' emotional collapse. This fits with the finding of Emslie and colleagues (2006) that some men will discuss depression in the context of a 'heroic' struggle with the more feminine aspects of their identity.

We can't really blame men for feeling the need to protect themselves from negative judgements in this way. The tendency in Western society to see outpourings of emotion as undesirable on the basis that they represent a failure in reasoning (Crossley 1998), coupled with perceptions of 'inappropriate' emotions related to gender roles, both in terms of 'masculine' displays of emotion by women and 'feminine' displays of emotion by men, create a very real pressure to internalise our feelings. There are certain circumstances in which a show of emotion by a man which breaks from the hegemonic construct of masculinity is considered acceptable, as long as it remains within certain parameters of intensity and duration. Men are allowed to step quietly outside the rules for a brief period of time in what society deems exceptional circumstances, but not to skip away from them naked with their arms waving and blowing a kazoo just whenever they feel like it. We don't think less of a man crying in a TV interview over the death of hundreds of colleagues in the World Trade Center attacks of 9/11, for example, but we almost see it as our collective duty to ridicule Tom Cruise for whooping, jumping on a couch and repeatedly punching the floor on a TV talk show to express joy about finding romance. Ironically, had Tom been exhibiting the same behaviour at a bar to express joy about his favourite sports team winning a tournament we'd probably see this as acceptable masculine behaviour – even if he'd burst into tears. It may seem far more rational to be jumping around and crying tears of joy over finding romance than over watching a bunch of total strangers winning a football match, but if you're a man only the latter is culturally acceptable. Of course, this would depend on the sport. In the UK it's OK to be a man crying over a soccer match because the sport has such a strong and longstanding association with hegemonic masculinity. Publicly getting emotional over it just goes to show your fellow men how committed you are to this manly interest and how important you see it as being to your life. But if you're a man crying over a lacrosse tournament, you might want to do it in private. Lacrosse, like romance, is labelled as a feminine pursuit in our culture. The same goes for emotional problems and mental ill-health.

We can't tear down hegemonic masculinity overnight, but we can work to encourage men to see mental well-being as something that's a normal aspect of everyday living, not something embarrassing, wimpish or just a politically correct way of referring to serious mental illness. We also know that we need to do more to get men who are experiencing mental health problems to seek medical help early on. Traditional 'masculine' ideas about being able to cope in the face of problems, dealing with pain and not being weak are often cited by men as reasons why they don't seek medical help when feeling ill (O'Brien *et al.* 2005). When they are in a healthcare setting, men will typically do their best to control their emotions (Moynihan 1998), emphasising physical symptoms over psychological ones even if the underlying issue is a mental health problem. Common perceptions of GPs in terms of leadership, medical arrogance and omnipotence create consultations in which male sexuality, embarrassment and personal relationships are all evaded (Banks 2001), and that's if men actually attend a consultation to begin with. We certainly shouldn't dump the whole problem onto doctors, but they do have a crucial role to play in allowing their male patients to partly release themselves from the constraints of hegemonic masculinity (at least for the duration of the consultation).

CONCLUSION

Despite representations of various alternative masculinities in popular culture over time, the dominant perception of masculine identity still demands a lifelong performance of self-control, independence, emotional strength and self-management of physical and mental health problems. In a culture in which the popular press associate mental illness with criminal acts of violence or public displays of extremely unusual behaviour, and in which it's more acceptable for men to cry over a football match than it is for them to cry over a relationship, it's little wonder that they're reluctant to access health services to own up to symptoms of depression.

Gender identities are changeable and it's certainly tempting to dream of a future where men are freed from the shackles of constructed masculinities which set them up to ruthlessly police their own (and each other's) behaviours for signs of 'feminine' deviance. Such a world may be achievable, but we're not there yet. However much some may be understandably alarmed by health promotion tactics which makes use of hegemonic masculine stereotypes to engage men, and thus arguably reinforce them (Scott-Samuel 2006), we owe it to men to find ways to make mental health accessible to them, whatever construct of masculinity they subscribe to and however much we might wish that they didn't.

REFERENCES

Banks I (2001) No Man's Land: men, illness and the NHS. *BMJ.* **323**: 1058–1060.

Berger P and Luckman T (1971) *The Social Construction of Reality.* Harmondsworth: Penguin.

Beynon J (2004) The commercialisation of masculinities: from the 'New Man' to the 'New Lad'. In C. Carter and L. Steiner (eds), *Media and Gender*. Maidenhead: Open University Press, pp. 198–291.

Clare A (2000) *On Men: masculinity in crisis*. London: Chatto and Windus.

Coyle A and Sykes C (1998) Troubled men and threatening women: The construction of crisis in male mental health. *Feminism & Psychology*. **8**: 263–284.

Crawshaw P (2007) Governing the healthy male citizen: Men, masculinity and popular health in Men's Health magazine. *Social Science & Medicine*. **65**: 1606–1618.

Crossley N (1998) Emotions and communicative action. In G Bendelow and SJ Williams (eds). *Emotions in Social Life: critical themes and contemporary issues*. London: Routledge, pp. 16–38.

Emslie C, Ridge D, Zeeland S and Hunt K (2006) Men's account of depression: reconstructing or resisting hegemonic masculinity? *Social Science and Medicine*. **62**: 2246–57.

Gauntlett D (2008) *Media, Gender and Identity: an introduction*. Abingdon: Routledge.

Giddens A (1986) *The Constitution of Society: outline of the theory of structuration*. Berkeley, CA: University of California Press.

Gough B (2006) 'Try to be healthy, but don't forgo your masculinity': deconstructing men's health discourse in the media. *Social Science & Medicine*. **63**: 2476–2488.

Hall S (1997) *Representation: cultural representation and signifying practices*. Newbury Park, CA: Sage.

Jennings MJ (2005) *A Business Tale: a story of ethics, choices, success and a very large rabbit*. New York: AMACOM.

Moynihan C (1998) Theories in health care and research: theories of masculinity. *BMJ*. **317**: 1072–1075.

Newman S (1997) Masculinities, men's bodies and nursing. In J Lawler (ed), *The Body in Nursing*. Melbourne: Churchill Livingstone, pp. 135–153.

Nixon S (1996) *Hard Looks: masculinity, spectatorship and contemporary consumption*. London: UCL Press.

O'Brien R, Hunt K and Hart G (2005) 'It's caveman stuff, but that is to a certain extent how guys still operate': men's accounts of masculinity and help seeking. *Social Science & Medicine*. **61**: 503–516.

Scott-Samuel A (2006) Mixed messages: Should health promotion messages use content which might reinforce gender stereotypes? *MHF*. Issue 9.

Wahl OF (2003) *Media Madness: public images of mental illness*. New Brunswick, New Jersey: Rutgers University Press.

White A (2007) Men's health – what's it all about? In D Conrad and A White (eds). *Men's Health – How to Do It*. Oxford: Radcliffe Publishing, pp. 9–26.

CHAPTER 4

Social capital and men's mental health

David Conrad

INTRODUCTION

Positive, mutually beneficial and sustainable relationships are an important aspect of good mental health which can be easily taken for granted. At both an individual and a community level, good social relations are good for health and negative relations are bad for health. As well as helping to protect us from the onset or recurrence of mental ill-health, strong social networks can also help us to recover from mental disorders (Whiteford *et al.* 2005).

The concept of 'social capital' captures the value of good social networks and the trust and norms of reciprocity which are required for developing and sustaining mutually beneficial relationships. Although it's been around in different forms for some time, it was Robert Putnam's book *Bowling Alone*, charting the decline of community in the US over the latter half of the 20th century, that first popularised the concept in 2000. Since then, there has been a rapid growth in social capital research, with academics from a range of fields attempting to further clarify it, measure it, quantify its effects and understand how it works. As the evidence base has grown, the importance of social capital for public health and community building has become increasingly reflected in government health policies. In the UK, the Government has highlighted the development of social capital as an important feature of mental health promotion and local authorities have been encouraged to implement measures which improve people's social networks and increase community participation as part of their efforts to improve mental health (see De Silva 2005).

This chapter provides a brief introduction to social capital, its importance for mental well-being and the implications for promoting men's mental health.

WHAT IS SOCIAL CAPITAL?

The term 'social capital' was first coined by LJ Hanifan, state supervisor of rural schools in West Virginia, US in 1916, who used it to refer to the benefits for people in being part of a group. Since then, a wide range of definitions have been put forward (see Halpern 2005), often less straightforward than Hanifan's original explanation. Putnam's definition is the most widely accepted in the field of public health (Muntaner *et al.* 2001), but incorporates a broad range of factors, defining it as 'features of social organisation such as networks, norms and social trust that facilitate coordination and cooperation for mutual benefit' (Putnam 1995).

A key issue in the different approaches to social capital is the question of whether it operates at an individual or community level. In other words, is it about how the nature of our connections to others affects us as individuals, or how the way that a community is connected as a whole affects those living in it, regardless of their own individual connectedness? Thinking about the benefits of social support steers us more toward the individual approach, but thinking about norms of cooperation, such as strangers helping each other out or people doing things that benefit their whole neighbourhood, steers us toward the community approach. The reality, though, is that social capital incorporates both these aspects (Kawachi *et al.* 2004).

Distinctions have also been drawn between 'structural' and 'cognitive' social capital. Structural social capital is that which exists in formal social structures with established roles, rules and procedures and is enabling of beneficial cooperative behaviour (Hitt *et al.* 2002). Cognitive social capital includes the shared norms and attitudes that predispose people towards beneficial cooperative behaviour (Krishna and Uphoff 1999).

The number of competing definitions can make the concept of social capital seem rather confusing, but each is really just focussing on different pieces of the same puzzle. Whether we think of social capital as being comprised of networks, trust and norms of reciprocity, social support, the things that we can access through our networks, or simply as a resource comprised of the benefits of social connections and relationships (Conrad 2008), all definitions are based on the principle that social capital provides advantages to those who have access to it (Burt 2000). These advantages can range from better prospects in finding a job (Granovetter 1973) to more mundane things which enable the functioning of our everyday lives. For this reason, social capital is a concept that's used in a range of fields, including public health, business, economics, political studies and sociology. There are books about how to use it to build stronger communities (e.g. Leonard and Onyx 2004) and books about how to use it to get ahead in your work and career (e.g. Baker 2000).

WHERE DOES SOCIAL CAPITAL COME FROM?

Social capital-rich relationships are built on a principle of generalised reciprocity. Rather than a tit-for-tat exchange in which favours are counted and tracked, help is accessible from each party without expectation of some specific and equal return. In order to be willing to help others we need to be able to trust that norms of reciprocity will be adhered to. Trust can be divided into two types: thick trust and thin trust. Thick trust is the kind that we have in our close relationships and thin trust applies to our weaker relationships – the people that we don't know very well – and to the wider community. Feeling safe without locking your front door is an example of thin trust. Trusting that your wife or business partner won't run away with your life's savings or tell your most embarrassing secrets to the neighbours are examples of thick trust.

There are two main types of social capital: bonding and bridging. Bonding social capital is generated by our relationships with people who'd be considered our natural social acquaintances because of shared or common circumstances. Typical sources would be relationships with family members or friendships with colleagues that are based on working in the same office, sharing similar backgrounds or doing similar kinds of jobs. Harvard sociologist Xavier de Souza Briggs (1998) said that bonding social capital is good for 'getting by'. In other words, bonding with our natural neighbours and acquaintances is useful for the smooth running of our everyday lives. It gives us a feeling of belonging and provides a reliable stock of resources that we can draw on to fulfil our established roles. Bridging social capital is generated by relationships with people who are outside of our normal social circle. Whereas bonding social capital is good for getting by, bridging social capital is good for getting ahead. Instead of enabling us to function in our current circumstances, it enables us to change those circumstances. Woolcock (1998) also introduced the idea of 'linking social capital' to distinguish connections formed across formal or institutionalised strata of power or authority from bridging connections with people outside of our personal social arena but of roughly equal status.

SOCIAL CAPITAL AND MENTAL WELL-BEING

First, it's important to acknowledge that there is a need to exercise caution when interpreting the research evidence around social capital due to the variety of definitions and research methods being used. You can find two papers on social capital and discover that they're actually measuring quite different phenomena. The different methods and approaches used by researchers have also made the published studies difficult to synthesise in a truly meaningful way. Another limitation is that studies looking at social capital often focus on networks within a geographical space, but with the rapidly increasing usage and normalising of web-based social networking we may need to look beyond just those relationships which are based primarily on face to face interactions.

In *Bowling Alone* Putnam (2000) detailed an array of research evidence that suggests that our social connectedness impacts on our mental and physical health. A significant body of research now exists linking access to social support and illness. Mortality rates for people with fewer social relationships have been shown to be many times higher than for those with larger social networks (McKenzie and Harpham 2006) and a study of social capital indicators across 50 countries found a significant association with lower suicide rates and higher life satisfaction (Helliwell 2004). Although the mechanisms by which social capital affects our health are not fully understood, better social networks are believed to help the spread of health education messages and improve access to informal caring. Social capital has also been shown to facilitate better access to health services (Hendryx *et al.* 2002). A case control study in the Netherlands, for example, found that strong trust and social cohesion within a neighbourhood mitigate the effect of socioeconomic deprivation on children's mental health service use (van der Linden *et al.* 2003). Strong social networks may also help changing societal norms which have an impact on health to take hold, such as stigmatising of drink-driving (Whiteford *et al.* 2005).

The strongest evidence linking *social capital and mental health* is around aspects of social support, the health impact of which was being researched long before the concept was entwined with social capital. We know that people who suffer from poor mental health tend to report smaller social networks, with fewer intimate relationships and a lower quality of support (see Halpern 2005). The findings of studies looking at multiple indicators of *social capital and mental health* have been less consistent, however.

A study by Pevalin and Rose (2003) published by the Health Development Agency (HDA) investigated the links between social capital and health using the British Household Panel Survey (BHPS). Social capital was measured in four ways: social participation, level of contact with friends, extent of crime in neighbourhood and level of attachment to neighbourhood. Social participation was found to reduce the likelihood of an onset of common mental illness and low social support reduced the likelihood of a recovery. However, they concluded that social capital played only a minor role in the processes leading to the onset of and recovery from common mental illness and poor self-rated health.

De Silva and colleagues (2005) conducted a systematic review of research on social capital and mental illness, looking at data from 21 quantitative studies. Fourteen measured social capital at the individual level and seven at an ecological level. The former offered evidence for an inverse relation between cognitive social capital and common mental disorders. There was also moderate evidence for an inverse relation between cognitive social capital and child mental illness, and combined measures of social capital and common mental disorders. The authors' overall conclusion though was that current evidence is inadequate to inform the development of specific social capital interventions to combat mental illness.

Rather than focussing solely on how social capital links with definable mental illnesses, however, we need to think much more in terms of its impact on mental well-being. Good mental health is not simply the absence of mental illness. People who live their lives in a state of unhappiness, stress, frustration or anxiety who wouldn't meet the criteria to be diagnosed with a mental illness could not be described as mentally healthy either. Some might argue that in our world of limited resources for health interventions it's not the role of the health promoter or clinician to help to make people happy when there is still so much work to be done in treating and preventing defined illnesses. Let's consider, though, some of the things that can result from being in these negative states – repressed anger; insecurity that prevents people from having the confidence to make the most of their lives (or to access health services); alcohol and drug abuse; violence and threatening behaviour; bullying; domestic violence; lack of emotional intelligence that makes people into bad workmates and bad parents; risk-taking behaviour; and the sense of demotivation and lack of self-worth that makes people resistant to health promotion messages. Should we really say that these issues aren't public health concerns because they can't be found in the pages of the DSM-IV?*

Social capital, with its entanglement of confused definitions, may not instinctively seem like a concept that has much to offer those seeking to understand and address problems of mental well-being on the ground, especially when the evidence is unclear. But when we think of what it means to be without access to social capital – to be isolated; to have no one to trust in a moment of crisis or to turn to for sympathy at the end of a tough working day; to feel disconnected and distrustful of those around you; to face life's challenges without reliable sources of help and advice; to doubt your place in your community and in wider society – then its relevance to promoting mental well-being becomes clear.

The importance of these things is felt by us all. Surveys conducted in Scotland which asked members of the public aged 16 and over about mental health issues found that good relationships with family and friends and a social life were considered to have positive effects on mental health. Also, younger and middle-aged people were more likely to say that relationship problems affected mental health negatively (Braunholtz *et al.* 2004). In an analysis of US data from 1952–1993 Twenge (2000) identified low social connectedness and high environmental threat as the factors which most contributed to a sense of anxiety in young people. The (2008) NICE guidance on 'Occupational therapy interventions and physical activity interventions to promote the mental well-being of older people in primary care and residential care' states that social activities, social networks and family contact are among the factors most frequently mentioned by older people as important to their mental well-being.

The impact of adverse life events is modulated by the psychological, social and physical resources available to us. When we're in crisis the social capital richness of our networks determines how much help and support we can access (and how easily). Whiteford and colleagues (2005) suggest that those with less access to social capital are exposed to more psychosocial stressors and there's some evidence to support this theory. Researchers examining associations between community support, social support networks, sense of place and psychological stressors in a rural Australian community found that lower community support was associated with greater psychological distress among non-farm workers (Stain *et al.* 2008). A study which looked at the relationship between social capital and basic welfare in Russia (Rose 2000) found that measures of social integration explained almost 10% of the variance in emotional health.

---

* The *Diagnostic and Statistical Manual of Mental Disorders* (DSM), published by the American Psychiatric Association, is the standard classification of mental disorders used by mental health professionals in the United States.

IS SOCIAL CAPITAL ALWAYS HEALTHY?

Sociologist Nan Lin (2001) suggests that one of the reasons that social capital is so important is that our relationships give us a sense of recognition and reinforce our identity. This is crucial for our own self-esteem and for being perceived by the people around us as a worthy member of society (or some smaller social group, such as a family). The need for recognition and the role of those around us in forging our sense of identity can of course lead to negative consequences for individuals and society as a whole. One of the early criticisms of Putnam's work was that it idealised a period in American history when stronger community was maintained by exclusion of those whose face didn't fit and a repressive atmosphere in which there was little tolerance of individuality. Strongly bonded groups can become distrustful of those outside them and can spread negative behaviour just as easily as they can spread positive behaviour. The main advantage of small, well-established social circles is that they tend to contain strong levels of bonding social capital. The major disadvantage, however, is that access to this social capital is largely maintained by peer pressure. Sometimes this takes the form of one person openly pressuring another to conform, but often it's the unspoken threat and fear of disapproval if the norms of the group are not adhered to.

As young people seek greater autonomy and independence from their parents typically they increasingly transfer their allegiance to their peer group. The peer group, rather than the family, then supplies the means of resolving identity conflicts and dealing with uncertainties on the road to adulthood (Helve and Brynner 2007). This becomes problematic where the identity of the group is based on a rejection of positive mainstream values and unhealthy behaviour. Throughout our lives almost all of us are exposed to some degree of pressure to behave in certain ways by the people around us and to a degree this is necessary in order to hold society together. Negative peer pressure is at its worst when it becomes a source of stress for the individual, promotes attitudes and behaviours that are harmful to the individual and to society and holds social capital to ransom with the threat of rejection from the group or the weakening of ties as a response to non-conformity.

HOW DOES MEN'S SOCIAL CAPITAL DIFFER FROM WOMEN'S?

Studies have suggested that men's social support is generally inferior to that of women and that women report higher levels of social support than men (Mickelson and Kubzansky 2003; Turner and Marino 1994). A report by the HDA based on qualitative research concluded that men tend not to be involved in health-enhancing networks because of the constraints of playing out hegemonic masculinity (Swann and Morgan 2002). A study of 205 men in the US (Burda and Vaux 1987) found that the more they believed in traditional sex role values, the less they had access to social support.

Women and men rely on different types of relationships for support (Aukett *et al.* 1988; Fischer and Oliker 1983). Women tend to engage in more reciprocal and confiding relationships than men and rely more on wider family and friends for support.

Female family members are men's primary source of emotional support and in a time of crisis men tend to rely on their wives or partners (Burda and Vaux 1987; Sixsmith and Boneham 2002). A study by Kjerstad (2009) which looked at middle-aged men attending a health promotion intervention in the North-West of England found the prevalence of psychological distress to be more than double in those who weren't living with a partner compared to those who were.

In the case of gay and bisexual men, there's some evidence that they're less likely to live with a romantic partner and may have more distant relationships with their relatives than heterosexual men. The shortfall in bonding social capital that this creates may be compensated for by maintaining a stronger network of friends (see Strohm *et al.* 2007).

Sixsmith and Boneham (2002) conducted a case study of a socially deprived housing estate in Bolton in the North-West of England to investigate the relationship between social capital, health and gender. They found that while friendship networks were most important to young men (and family networks to older men), both younger and older men saw friendships as being about 'doing things together' rather than providing emotional support, even in times of great stress and sorrow. The idea of trusting people outside the family with personal problems was frowned upon and there was a tendency to see asking friends for emotional support or burdening them with your problems as amounting to using them in a way which could get you a bad reputation.

Trust is essential for social capital and does not typically come easily to men. We might assume that friends are trusted – that that's part of what makes them our friends – but the trust required to share a personal problem or anxiety is often too great and men choose instead to internalise their feelings for fear of being laughed at, talked about, or seen as weak. In some traditional masculine arenas, such as the armed forces, the emergency services or on the football field, trusting your fellow men is crucial for achieving success and is seen as part of the masculine role. In day-to-day life, however, this kind of team spirit is often conspicuously absent or only holds up when it serves in the performance of the hegemonic male persona. Indeed, Sixsmith and Boneham found that trusting people in itself could be seen by men as a sign of weakness. Trust had to be earned and could be taken away if it was deemed to be unwarranted at any stage in the future. For younger men, trust wasn't seen as either an appropriate or necessary element of the bond between a group of friends. Being trusting was equated with naiveté – a position built on experience of seeing others' trust casually betrayed. The generalised weak trust that is essential for Putnam's vision of the social capital-rich community was also strikingly absent among younger and older men – the older men being particularly mistrustful of the younger men in the neighbourhood.

WHAT ARE THE IMPLICATIONS FOR MEN'S MENTAL HEALTH PROMOTION?

It's argued that social capital, like public goods, will be under-produced if left to the market alone, i.e. the community (Conrad 2008). The men in Sixsmith and Boneham's study saw community involvement as a feminine pursuit, which both implies an under-production of social capital on their part and suggests that increasing men's participation in deprived communities will not be a small challenge. Boosting social connectedness should be seen as an essential element of health promotion rather than a separate fringe activity. The more limited access to social support that men experience and the reluctance which they typically demonstrate to building social capital-rich relationships beyond their close female family make it a particular issue for promoting men's mental health.

The building blocks of social capital are trust, norms of reciprocity and meaningful social interaction across networks which ideally incorporate a balance of strong bonding, bridging and linking connections. Our support networks can include the nuclear and extended family, friendships, work colleagues, neighbours, religious organisations, clubs and societies. In times of crisis we tend to help our immediate family first, then our extended family and then our friends and neighbours. As it is these basic social connections that are mostly looked to for emotional support, they have the greatest influence on mental health and the ability to recover from emotional stress and trauma throughout men's lives (Curry 1994). Although adolescent boys may look increasingly to the peer group for identity and validation, family relationships remain critical to the well-being and transitions of young people (Holland 2007). Interventions which help men and boys to strengthen and maintain these relationships are therefore the first line of attack in a strategy to boost their access to social capital. Work with 'dads and lads', anger management programmes and healthy sexuality education are examples of mental health promotion which ultimately help men to achieve more positive, trusting and stable close relationships with relatives and partners. These aren't referred to as social capital building interventions, or 'sold' to the clients on that basis, but they don't need to be in order to be effective.

Outside of the family, pubs and bars provide the traditional arenas for social bonding between men where interaction based on collective drinking facilitates support-giving without threatening the hegemonic masculine identity. Finding ways to get men who subscribe to traditional notions of masculinity to come together for the purpose of receiving and giving emotional support requires some innovative thinking though. The success of the It's A Goal programme described in Chapter 9, which is delivered at football grounds and uses football terminology to engage men with mental health issues, shows that it can be done. We also know that more informal men's groups that allow men a safe environment in which to openly discuss feelings, build meaningful relationships and provide each other with emotional support and advice do exist and should be applauded. In seeking to tackle the issue on a population wide basis, however, we have to accept that for the majority of men such a group would not be a sufficiently appealing proposition and the men's group will always be a minority sport.

Following on from *Bowling Alone*, Putnam published another book, called *Better Together* (Putnam and Feldstein 2003), which described a selection of projects that had successfully brought communities closer together and strengthened social capital networks. As the book's accompanying website* states, however, social capital is built through hundreds of everyday actions, some large and some small. Social capital building shouldn't be seen as a separate activity in itself, but rather an approach that underpins all health promotion programmes. Interventions that address the underlying causes of poor mental well-being can, in the process, improve access to social capital by creating channels of advice and support, developing social skills and confidence, and building trust. Whilst one-to-one work is the most appropriate for some service users, many initiatives that successfully tackle men's health issues are group-based and delivered in settings where men already come together and feel comfortable (see Conrad and White 2007). This could be, for example, a workplace, a barber shop in the South Asian community or a pub. The value of the social connections that are formed within these groups is not always fully recognised or utilised, however, because it's not an outcome against which the success of the project is measured.

Work to counter the negative mental health impact of unemployment provides a good example of how social capital can be improved, both during the intervention itself and in the longer term, while addressing mental well-being and an underlying cause of health inequalities. The workplace can provide a key network and potentially be a good source of both bonding and bridging social capital, the loss or absence of which can be particularly significant for the mental well-being of men who have few social-capital-rich connections in the community (Bolton and Oatley 1987). Unemployment has many negative impacts on mental health and the longer it continues, the more difficult it can be to rejoin the workforce (Cattan and Tilford 2006). Programmes based on coping resources theory using group sessions to increase social support, increase self-efficacy and develop skills for job searching and coping with set-backs have been shown to increase self-esteem, decrease psychological distress and reduce incidence and prevalence of severe depressive symptoms in the short and long term (Vinokur *et al.* 1991; van Ryn and Vinokur 1992).

Another example of successfully incorporating social capital building into a project with a more traditional primary focus is the Mental Health Guide Programme which began in East London in 2006 (*see* Whyte 2007; Atkinson *et al.* 2008). Mental Health Guides are service users, carers and concerned citizens who are trained and supported to act as health guides within their community, in their own language. The guides work in pairs, delivering sessions to groups of people in community and mental health settings, facilitating access to services by sharing information. They also listen to the concerns of local people and report them back to the local NHS senior management. All the Mental Health Guides trained in the first year of the

---

* www.bettertogether.org

programme and most of the session participants were African or African Caribbean, although no one was excluded from participating. As well as being an effective way to engage marginalised groups, increasing awareness of mental health issues and signposting services, this type of project helps to build trust and links between communities and public services. Through the course that the Guides attend and the sessions that they then go on to deliver, social connections are formed and valuable social capital is generated – bonding, bridging and linking.

CONCLUSION

Social capital is crucial for maintaining mental well-being and dealing with mental health problems when they arise. It's equally important for both genders, but we know that men typically have access to less social support than women and have few, if any, contacts with whom they feel able to share emotional crises. Improving men's access to social capital shouldn't be seen as a separate endeavour in itself but rather should be an underlying objective that's applied to all men's health promotion interventions. The various projects described in this book haven't been designed with the stated purpose of generating social capital and yet each involves the development of social skills and support-rich relationships, the sharing of advice, information and feelings, and requires a degree of trust to be built (both between service users and between service users and providers). By developing a greater 'social capital awareness' among practitioners, managers and policy-makers, the potential for giving men and boys greater access to social capital and helping them to develop social capital building skills through a whole range of interventions is enormous.

Once there is a greater appreciation of the potential benefits of the social experience that clients have while using a service, the door is open to designing and delivering services in ways which maximise those potential benefits. Incorporating this aspect of the client experience into service evaluations would be a crucial step forward. The role of all client-based health promotion interventions in improving mental well-being and building social capital, not just those that have 'mental health' in their brief, must be recognised and their successes reported. Only then can we put an end to the wasted opportunities that accumulate through the simplistic disconnected thinking that views needle exchanges as being just about the exchange of needles (*see* Chapter 21), or judges the value of weight management groups purely on the basis of a 'before and after' set of BMI scores.

REFERENCES

Atkinson A, Douglas C, Francis D, Laville M, Millin S, Pamfield J, Smith P and Smith R (2008) *Lifting Barriers*. London: Social Action for Health.

Aukett R, Ritchie J and Mill K (1988) Gender differences in friendship patterns. *Sex Roles.* **19**(1–2): 57–66.

Baker W (2000) *Achieving Success Through Social Capital: tapping the hidden resources in your personal and business networks*. San Francisco: Jossey-Bass.

Bolton W and Oatley K (1987) A longitudinal study of social support and depression in unemployed men. *Psychol Med.* **17**(2): 453–60.

Braunholtz S, Davidson S and King S (2004) *Well? What Do You Think? (2004): The Second National Scottish Survey of Public Attitudes to Mental Health, Mental Well-being and Mental Health Problems.* Edinburgh: Scottish Executive Social Research.

Briggs X (1998) Brown kids in white suburbs: housing mobility and the many faces of social capital. *Housing Policy Debate.* **9**(1): 177–221.

Burda PC and Vaux AC (1987) The social support process in men: overcoming sex-role obstacles. *Human Relations.* **40**(1): 31–43.

Burt RS (2000) The network structure of social capital. In RI Sutton and BM Staw, *Research In Organizational Behavior*, vol. 22. Greenwich CT: JAI Press, pp. 345–423.

Cattan M and Tilford S (2006) Adulthood: increasing responsibility and middle age (25–45 years and 45–65 years). In M Cattan and S Tilford (eds), *Mental Health Promotion: a lifespan approach.* Maidenhead: Open University Press, pp. 137–175.

Conrad D (2008) Defining social capital. In KR Gupta, GLH Svendson and P Maiti (eds), *Social capital*, vol. 1. New Delhi: Atlantic, pp. 53–59.

Conrad D, White A (eds) (2007) *Men's Health – How to Do It.* Oxford: Radcliffe Publishing.

Curry FC (1994) *Disasters and Development.* Dallas: Interact Press.

De Silva MJ, McKenzie K, Harpham T and Huttly SRA (2005) Social capital and mental illness: a systematic review. *J Epidemiol Community Health.* **59**: 619–627.

Fischer CS and Oliker SJ (1983) A research note on friendship, gender and the life cycle. *Social Forces.* **62**(1): 124–133.

Granovetter M (1973) The Strength of Weak Ties. *Am J Sociology.* **78**: 1360–1380.

Halpern D (2005) *Social Capital.* Cambridge: Polity Press.

Hanifan LJ (1916) The rural school community center. *Annals of the American Academy of Political and Social Science.* **67**:130–138.

Helliwell JF (2004) *Well-being and social capital: does suicide pose a puzzle?* National Bureau Of Economic Research. Working Paper 10896. Available at: www.nber.org/papers/w10896.pdf (Accessed 25 September 2009).

Helve H and Bynner J. (eds) (2007) *Youth and Social Capital.* London: The Tufnell Press.

Hendryx MS, Ahern MM, Lovrich NP, McCurdy AR (2002) Access to health care and community social capital. *Health Serv Res.* **31**(1): 85–101.

Hitt MA, Lee H and Yucel E (2002) The importance of social capital to the management of multinational enterprises: relational networks among Asian and Western firms. *Asian Pacific J Management.* **19**: 353–372.

Holland J (2007) Inventing adulthoods: making the most of what you have. In H Helve and J Bynner (eds). *Youth and Social Capital.* London: The Tufnell Press, pp. 11–28.

Kawachi I, Kim D, Coutts A and Subramanian SV (2004) Commentary: Reconciling the three accounts of social capital. *Int J Epidemiology.* **33**:1–9.

Kjerstad AG (2009) *Psychological distress in middle-aged men attending a health promotion project.* MPH Dissertation. Liverpool University.

Krishna A and Uphoff N (1999) *Mapping and measuring social capital through assessment of collective action to conserve and develop watersheds in Rajasthan, India.* Social Capital Initiative Working Paper No. 13, Washington, DC: The World Bank.

Leonard R and Onyx J (2004) *Social Capital and Community Building: spinning straw into gold.* London: Janus Publishing Co.

Lin N (2001) *Social Capital: a theory of social structure and action.* Cambridge: Cambridge University Press.

McKenzie K and Harpham T (eds) (2006) *Social Capital and Mental Health.* London: Jessica Kingsley Publishers.

Mickelson KD and Kubzansky LD (2003) Social distribution of social support: The mediating role of life events. *Am J Community Psychology.* **32**(3–4): 265–281.

Muntaner C, Lynch J, Davey Smith G (2001) Social capital, disorganized communities, and the third way: Understanding the retreat from structural inequalities in epidemiology and public health. *Int J Health Serv.* **31**: 213–37.

NICE (2008) *Occupational Therapy Interventions and Physical Activity Interventions to Promote the Mental Well-being of Older People in Primary Care and Residential Care.* London: NICE.

Pevalin DJ and Rose D (2003) *Social capital for health. Investigating the links between social capital and health using the British Household Panel Survey.* London: Health Development Agency.

Putnam R (1995) Bowling Alone: America's declining social capital. *J Democracy.* **6**(1): 65–78.

Putnam R (2000) *Bowling Alone: the collapse and revival of American community.* New York: Simon & Schuster.

Putnam R and Feldstein L (2003) *Better Together: restoring the American community.* New York: Simon and Schuster.

Rose R (2000) How much does social capital add to individual health? A survey study of Russians. *Social Science and Medicine.* **51**(9): 1421–1435.

Sixsmith J and Boneham M (2002) Men and masculinities: accounts of health and social capital. In C Swann and A Morgan (eds). *Social Capital for Health: Insights from Qualitative Research.* London: Health Development Agency.

Stain HJ, Kelly B, Lewin TJ, Higginbotham N, Beard J and Hourihan F (2008) Social networks and mental health among a farming population. *Social Psychiatry and Psychiatric Epidemiology.* **43**(10): 843–849.

Strohm CQ, Cochran S and Mays V (2007) *Gender and sexual orientation differences in social support from family, friends, and romantic relationships.* Paper presented at the annual meeting of the American Sociological Association, TBA, New York, New York City, Aug 11.

Swann C and Morgan A (eds) (2002) *Social Capital for Health: insights from qualitative research.* London: Health Development Agency.

Turner RJ and Marino F (1994) Social support and social structure: A descriptive epidemiology. *J Health and Social Behavior.* **35**(3): 193–212.

Twenge JM (2000) The age of anxiety? Birth cohort change in anxiety and neuroticism, 1952–1993. *J Personality and Social Psychology.* **79**: 1007–1021.

van der Linden J, Drukker M, Gunther N, Feron F, van Os J (2003) Children's mental health service use, neighbourhood socioeconomic deprivation, and social capital. *Soc Psychiatry Psychiatr Epidemiol.* **38**: 507–514.

van Ryn M. and Vinokur AD (1992) How did it work? An examination of the mechanism through which a community intervention influenced job-search behaviour among an unemployed sample. *Am J Community Psychology.* **20**: 577–599.

Vinokur AD, van Ryn M, Gramlich EM and Price RH (1991) Long-term follow-up and benefit-cost analysis of the jobs program: a preventive intervention for the unemployed. *J Appl Psychol.* **76**: 213–19.

Whiteford H, Cullen M and Baingana F (2005) *Social capital and mental health.* In H Hermann, S Sexana and R Moodie (eds), *Promoting mental health: concepts; emerging evidence; practice.* Geneva: WHO, pp. 70–80.

Whyte M (2007) Travelling companions: mental health guides and mentors. *Mental Health Today.* Nov 2007: 10–12.

Woolcock M (1998) Social capital and economic development: a critical review. *Theory and Society* **27**: 151–208.

CHAPTER 5

Urban distress and the mental health of men

April MW Young

INTRODUCTION

Working in distressed communities in the US, studying policies that affect these neighbourhoods and developing programmes to improve them, has highlighted for me the wider context in which mental well-being exists – the circumstances in which it is sustained or compromised. In forming a practical agenda to address the issue of poor men and mental health we have to consider:

➤ the importance of community context
➤ the influence of larger social phenomena and jeopardies relevant to poor men's lives (e.g. incarceration, migrant labour)
➤ the consequences of under-service.

And we must include:

➤ advice for reaching under-served poor men
➤ policy recommendations
➤ a plan for advocacy on the ground.

The following chapter is organised into sections accordingly. Offering examples from a wide variety of research, its aim is to provide readers with informative background, while convincing health practitioners and service providers that community context is an important and accessible part of their practice with men.

THE CASE FOR ATTENDING TO POOR MEN

There are many handbooks and much guidance on mental health for health practitioners and social service providers. In such well-populated territory, one might wonder whether anything worthwhile is yet unsaid. Nevertheless, with striking consistency throughout the world, men's mental health needs seem to remain under-served. In distressed or blighted urban settings in which the demands and strains of daily life are especially intense, poor men face particular pressures that can exact a high toll on their psychic well-being – pressures associated with the nature of their neighbourhoods and living conditions, the frequency with which they take the brunt of devastating social phenomena such as incarceration, and the lack of access to healthcare and mental health services.

While the discourse about needs in the mental health field often centres on the individual, it is critical to consider community context and larger social influences in order to address the needs of poor men in urban settings. To successfully reach poor men, it is important that mental health practitioners, social service providers, agents of community revitalisation and economic development, public and correc-tional health officials, health policy analysts and advocates for social justice recognise the relevance of poverty and urban distress.

There are data on excess morbidity and mortality among poor men that sug-gest that the health of poor men around the world is in particular jeopardy, with high rates of illness, injury, disability and premature death. In Latin American and Caribbean countries, for instance, there are strong associations between income and mortality risk. The probability of dying between 15 and 59 years of age is almost invariably at least double, occasionally nearly triple, for poor men compared to non-poor men (Casas *et al.* 2001). While on the other hand there is admittedly precious little information on poor men's mental health, it is important nevertheless to con-sider the relevance of poverty and its associated experiences to mental well-being. Continued under-service of poor men's mental health needs undermines families, civic infrastructure, peace and economic systems as well as the men themselves. As such, meeting these needs is a global priority we must articulate in a fashion to motivate local action.

WHY WE FAIL TO SERVE POOR MEN

Men in poor urban settings frequently suffer unaddressed mental health needs due to a range of structural, systemic, behavioural and attitudinal factors (*see* Box 5.1). We can point to social phenomena that may be common among residents of dis-tressed neighbourhoods, such as incarceration; victimisation and the witnessing of violence; economic hardship; under-education; racial, ethnic, linguistic, or cultural marginalisation; and disruption of household and community support networks. These issues pose mental health challenges for men and, at the same time, create obstacles to their accessing appropriate services. The mental health effects of living in poverty can constitute a troubling profile. However, identifying the predictable psychic imprint of urban distress upon men also enables good strategy to address poor men's mental health concerns.

BOX 5.1 Why do the mental health needs of men in distressed settings often go unaddressed?

Structural factors:

> ➤ lack of coverage for mental health services for poor men
> ➤ dearth of providers offering mental health services
> ➤ insufficient mental health awareness promotion
> ➤ frequency of highly traumatic events and high-stress circumstances.

Systemic factors:

> ➤ long waiting periods for mental health appointments
> ➤ low cultural competence among mental health practitioners
> ➤ limited treatment options (e.g. appropriate medications, detoxification for substance dependency)
> ➤ lack of familiarity with mental health discourse and health institutions.

Behavioural factors:

> ➤ tendency toward risk-taking
> ➤ lesser likelihood of help-seeking.

Attitudinal factors:

> ➤ anti-emotionalism and machismo
> ➤ mistrust of and lack of familiarity with health institutions
> ➤ exoticising stereotypes of toughness, insensitivity, nonchalance, simple-mindedness of and among racial and ethnic minorities.

THE IMPORTANCE OF COMMUNITY CONTEXT TO POOR MEN'S MENTAL HEALTH

Distressed settings

There are many indicators which can qualify an urban setting as blighted or distressed – the income level of its residents, the condition of its housing stock, the types of services and businesses that are available or not, rates of crime and the state of its civic infrastructure. Most of the world's large metropolises have blighted areas within their boundaries – Paris's Hain; Los Angeles's South Central and Miami's Overtown may come to mind. In other instances, poverty is not quite so geographically confined, but intersperses with apparent material privilege, as in Calcutta and Rio de Janeiro.

If we recognise that urban distress describes not only a condition of place, but also names an experience which residents abide day to day, its health implications beg attention. Coping daily with the circumstances of poverty amid the pressures and demands of urban life undeniably registers a psychological strain.

Given what we know of the obstacles to accessing healthcare among low-income groups and among men, we can expect that in distressed urban settings men will face particular jeopardy of unmet mental health needs.

Common features of poor urban settings are likely to impact strongly upon men's mental health. Income shortfalls and unreliable employment, along with tenuous lodging terms or substandard housing conditions can mean that utter financial ruin and homelessness are imminent and constant threats in the lives of poor men and their families. Proximity to illicit activity and illegal parallel markets – whether one is a participant or bystander – can mean heightened risk of violence and exposure to the criminal justice apparatus. While social networks in distressed settings are often of necessity strong and extensive, the nature of urban poverty can fracture central household structures, isolating men from their primary family units for long periods. In addition to facing their own difficulties, men may routinely witness the subjection and hopelessness of others around them. The results can be psychological and physiological stress; physical injury; self-medication with tobacco, alcohol, or illegal drugs; sexual risk-taking; and various forms of abusive or self-endangering acting out.

It is important that health practitioners and others in positions to be of assistance to men are aware of economic and social data on the areas in which their patients or clients may live. Perhaps knowing that more than 1 in 4 Central Harlem (New York City, US) residents smoke (Olson *et al.* 2006) may not yield much more insight about a man's asthma risk than would a personal health history. However, the fact that a study found two-thirds of adult men in Overtown (Miami, US) reported having been incarcerated (Young 2006) strongly suggests to a health practitioner – particularly to a mental health provider – that a man from this neighbourhood is quite likely to have psychological issues associated with extended confinement and the traumatic experiences typical in detention facilities.

The populations

What qualifies a person as poor is a relative measure that varies widely among cities. However, the common features would include difficulty meeting needs for food and shelter, marginal or no employment and uncertain access to education and healthcare.

Many of the realities that poverty visits upon men are also strikingly similar across cities. Lack of access to healthcare, disparate treatment experiences, and inadequate health-seeking behaviours further disadvantage poor men. For instance, Swedish researchers found that socioeconomic disadvantage and the perception of discrimination relate independently to the likelihood of refraining from seeking medical services (Wamala *et al.* 2007). Again, that which constitutes poverty is relative and highly variable from setting to setting. However, a population that may in many respects typify the US urban poor resides in the Overtown neighbourhood of Miami, Florida. A study of adult men in Overtown (Young 2006) found:

➤ 40% are employed
➤ 53% earned less than US$10,000 per year
➤ 55% have high school diplomas

➤ 2 in 3 have been in jail or prison
➤ more than 1 in 4 is a victim of police violence
➤ 28% have lived on the streets
➤ 1 in 4 has lived in a shelter for homeless persons.

In the Overtown example, the population's relatively low educational attainment, high rate of unemployment and incredibly high rate of incarceration are characteristics that mark and perhaps sustain men's poverty.

Jeopardies

It is important to call attention to some of the larger forces that disproportionately impact poor men throughout the world. Hazards in the social and physical environments that poor men often inhabit contribute to negative health outcomes and in nation after nation systematically undermine well-being. Incarceration, dangerous and under-regulated employment, labour-related displacement and migration (Calavita 2003), state-sponsored conflict and violent civil strife, pollution and substandard living conditions are a few examples of social phenomena that jeopardise men's well-being and may compromise their mental health.

Incarceration

Incarceration is a phenomenon of growing influence in so many countries and is arguably one of the most systematically crippling forces in poor communities worldwide. The existence of data is uneven, but in many countries incarceration and health disparities follow similar tracks along the social fault lines. Just as the poor are more likely to suffer negative health outcomes, socioeconomically disadvantaged persons have a greater likelihood of incarceration.

Imprisonment is a particularly deleterious part of the experience of social and economic marginalisation for men in many countries. In correctional settings and facilities of detention the well-being of already marginalised men is further jeopardised by exposure to a range of physiological and psychological risks that increase the likelihood of poor health outcomes. Those detained in correctional settings are frequently subject to communicable infections, injury by violence, sexual trauma and under-regulated clinical trials. Facilities' adherence to correctional healthcare standards is a matter of ongoing uncertainty and controversy around the world.

Concerning mental health particularly, psychological torment is a pervasive risk that inmates face. They are subjected to extreme custodial interventions such as 'close management', i.e. solitary confinement; injurious chemical, electrical and manual control techniques; strip searches and invasive body cavity searches; and documented physical torture in many countries. These experiences often have enduring effects in the form of post-traumatic stress disorder (PTSD), depression, anxiety, attachment and mood disorders, substance dependency to medicate psychic or physical pain (*see* Table 5.1) and anti-social or self-destructive acting out.

Strong evidence from many countries shows that it is socially marginalised men who have the greatest likelihood of incarceration. For example, more than a third of Italy's prison inmates are foreigners. Also, the nation's apprehension about its growing Romanian immigrant population would seem to be reflected in their disproportionate representation – nearly 6% – among Italy's incarcerated (Kimmelman 2008). In the US, correctional populations are less educated than the general population. The rate of failure to complete high school or its equivalent is more than double (40%) among US prisoners compared to the general population (18%) (US Department of Justice 2003).

Even after release from correctional facilities, the particular jeopardy of marginalised men remains in the form of sharply elevated risks of mortality. Elevated mortality was noted among a sample of male French prison releases (Verger *et al.* 2003). The French study findings resonate with US evidence. A Washington State study found that newly released prisoners were 12.7 times as likely to die in the two weeks following their release compared to other state residents in the same demographic groups (Binswanger *et al.* 2007). Drug overdose was the leading cause of death among former inmates in the Washington State study. It is reasonable to infer psychological vulnerability among newly released inmates and to hypothesise that a reaction to mental distress played a role in their demise.

Employment

Poor men's relationships to employment and the conditions under which they often must labour when they are able to work play an important role in their mental well-being. Lack of job security, low wages and dangerous working conditions frequently characterise the employment to which poor men have access. A lack of esteem, authority, or control on the job can lead to anxiety or depression. Humiliating circumstances at work or demeaning hierarchies can erode a man's sense of self-worth, diminish his social esteem as a breadwinner and provider, and thwart his ambitions for himself and his family. For migrant labourers, work often means separation from family and social network for extended periods.

Work or the lack of work can occasion stress-related addictive behaviours such as smoking, alcohol abuse and illicit drug use, all of which appear to occur more frequently among poor men. For instance, we see a higher prevalence of smoking in the world's poorer nations. Worldwide, 36% of men smoke tobacco (WHO 2008). However, 42% of men in India smoke. In 2003, the prevalence of tobacco smoking among Russian men 15 years of age and older was 56.7%. In China, the rate of smoking among men well exceeds half at 57.4%.

Similarly, health-compromising patterns of alcohol consumption are noted to occur among populations of poor men. The disease burden related to alcohol abuse by men is high across Europe (Rehm 2003a; 2003b), particularly in countries in the European part of the former Soviet Union. Pronounced socioeconomic differences have been noted in alcohol-related death in Russia and, perhaps quite predictably, unemployment is a strong correlate of heavy consumption (Ryan 1995; McKee 1999; Chenet *et al.* 1998). In the UK, one man in eight is dependent on alcohol and men are three times more likely than women to become alcohol dependent (White

2006). In the Ukraine, 38.7% of men are heavy alcohol users compared to 22% of the population overall (Webb *et al.* 2005).

Given the excessive rates of smoking among men, notable tendencies to dangerous alcohol consumption and the particularly class-laden nature of these phenomena, health practitioners and service providers should be mindful of their association with the difficult circumstances of poverty. These health-averse behaviours may indicate that men are straining under the burden of socioeconomic as well as personal stress.

Discrimination

While there are common physiological health and mental health issues affecting poor men globally, there are inflections among groups of poor men that are important to note. These variations often follow predictable courses, tracking the intricate social fault lines that divide and sub-divide the privileged in communities from their less-well-off counterparts. In addition to socioeconomic status, such inflections in the health jeopardy that poor men face can result from racial and ethnic discrimination (Read 2005), dynamics associated with immigration status (del Amo *et al.* 2003) and intolerance based on sexual orientation (Diaz *et al.* 2004). These phenomena can compound the jeopardy that poor men already confront.

A number of studies document racial and ethnic groups' subjection to excess mortality and morbidity (e.g. Gold *et al.* 2006; Tuan *et al.* 2007), although the complex interplay of associated risk factors can often make causality and clear correlation difficult to establish (Smaje 1995). Examining data from 12 countries with various growth rates, national income and population, researchers found economic disparity correlated with race and ethnicity throughout (Darity and Nembhard 2000). Because of the enduring significance of race and ethnicity in countries such as the US, having lower-class status and being of colour are often closely linked and it is difficult to separate the two issues. The findings of a study published in 2008, for example, indicate that young black men living in England and Wales are at higher risk of suicide than their white counterparts (Bhui and McKenzie 2008). It is also well established that poverty rates among black people in the UK exceed those of the other ethnic groups in the study.

Since 2000, findings of more than 100 studies documenting the damaging effects of racism on the body have supported recasting racism as a public health problem (e.g. Jackson *et al.* 1996; Clark 2001; Kwate *et al.* 2003). Experiences of racism have been found to act as a stressor, the impact of which is chronic and pervasive – elevating blood pressure, heart rate and cortisol levels; suppressing immune system response and inspiring health-averse behaviours such as overeating and smoking. Failure to acknowledge and address the mental health effects of discrimination arguably has contributed to the health disparities we observe today.

TABLE 5.1 Overtown Men's Health Study. Self-reported drug and alcohol use among the study population: Overtown neighbourhood in City of Miami, Florida USA, 2005; (n = 129)

	Number of respondents (n)	Percentage of respondents (%)
Drink alcoholic beverages	81	62.8
Use tobacco	61	47.3
Number of cigarettes per day		
≤ 1	2	3.3
2–10	38	62.3
11–20	16	26.2
> 20	4	6.6
Use illegal drugs or substances	52	40.3
Type of drug or substance		
Crack cocaine	12	23.1
Powder cocaine	15	28.9
Marijuana	39	75.0
Heroin	3	5.8
Ecstasy	1	1.9
Prescription drugs illegally obtained	1	1.9

While overall mortality and morbidity rates have improved in the US, men of colour are still more likely to die of cardiovascular disease, diabetes and cancer than their white counterparts. Life expectancy for African American men is 69.5 years, for Hispanic men is 73.7 years and for Native American men is 66.1 years. For men of colour, the life expectancy figures are an average of 7.8% lower than the 75.7 year lifetime that a white man in the US can anticipate.

In a longitudinal study of coronary heart disease incidence in Puerto Rican men, researchers concluded that skin colour – relative darkness or lightness – may be capturing dynamics in the social environment that influence mortality risk. While they found no association between skin colour and cardiovascular disease, skin colour did predict higher all-cause mortality among urban-dwelling men. Dark-skinned men living in urban areas in Puerto Rico have a higher risk of death than their lighter-skinned counterparts. Another notable finding was that dark-skinned Puerto Rican men were less educated than light-skinned men (Borrell *et al.* 2007).

These data suggest that other categories of social marginality, in addition to poverty, warrant identification, analysis and monitoring to account for disparities in health among various groups of men. Examining responses to discrimination and developing positive mental health strategies of coping with or countering its psychological and physiological assault is crucial.

REACHING UNDER-SERVED POOR MEN

Health practitioners should be vigilant for high-stress coping, dangerous periodic binging or substance dependency, physical injury and post-traumatic stress-related behaviours among men from poor urban settings. Gathering such information is made difficult by communication barriers that men themselves can erect. Bravado may mask depression and fear. Nonchalance could be a response to bewilderment and hopelessness. Silence may be practiced inarticulateness about difficult or sensitive topics.

Nevertheless, it is critical that we find ways to engage poor men, to support them and to treat them where there is the need. We must be successful at coaxing testimony from them and we must make a place for their voices. The mental health and well-being of poor men is a political issue for the men themselves and for communities. Connecting the issue of mental health explicitly to advocacy, understanding and presenting it as a cause, may be a way to enlist individual men as well as groups of men in programmes to improve their own health (*see* Box 5.2).

Outreach strategies

With successive conferences in 2006 and 2007 entitled 'Saving Men's Lives', the US programme 'Community Voices: Healthcare for the Underserved' kicked off an ambitious project – to launch a grass-roots movement of men dedicated to eliminating health disparities.

Men from distressed neighbourhoods around the eight Community Voices Learning Laboratory sites attended the conferences. They trained to serve as health advocates and agents of change in their local communities and beyond. Organisers carefully designed the conferences for men to whom policy and advocacy work was new. The conference activities prepared the men to represent themselves and their neighbours in local and national policy discussions about health.

BOX 5.2 Characteristics of successful mental health outreach to poor men in distressed communities

> - Neighbourhood-focused.
> - Bundled with other services.
> - Organised through peer groups and social networks.
> - Using holistic discourses to present mental health (mental health in context, to particular ends).
> - Culturally competent.
> - Age-appropriate.

They brought their concern about men's health and their local circumstances and teamed with Community Voices health policy researchers and advocates. It was clear that the stakes for the men were eminently personal. They recognised their demographic cohort, their neighbours and family members, their own bodies and spirits in the statistics and charts and graphs. They know that they are the ones to whom the jeopardy attaches: the cardiovascular and metabolic patterns of risk; the snare of public education failure and mass incarceration; the psychic strain of abiding on society's edge.

The conferences were an important step by Community Voices to extend its work deeper into vulnerable neighbourhoods. Male residents of the neighbourhoods empowered with knowledge about health issues and policies and with advocacy skills will be able supporters of health policy work going forward, as they disseminate the message and motivation among their neighbours.

The logic behind the approach was to transfer capacity directly into areas of need. Imparting information and giving broad exposure to members of communities enables them to expand locally upon their training when they return to their neighbourhoods. The men teamed with the policy staff from their local Community Voices Learning Laboratory to draft action plans for grass-roots men's health programmes targeting their neighbourhoods.

BOX 5.3 Journal entry from the author's 'Community Voices Men's Health Program' notes.

Through this work, we recognise the extent to which the everyday strivings and struggles of poor men go largely unnoticed along corridors of power in our country. The men on behalf of whom we fight are isolated in neglected and ignored communities. They are themselves civically disengaged, many prevented by law even from participating in the representative practices that shape their lives and determine their fate. And many are as yet unaware of the power of health as a discourse – as a means of talking about and addressing their various needs, needs that emerge from a range of difficult experiences like incarceration trauma, substandard housing, crime-burdened neighbourhoods, under-employment. So, the challenge of resisting and overcoming silence and voicelessness is a critical aspect of the work of Community Voices – aptly named.

We overcome the voicelessness of poor men by enlisting them directly as participants, to work on their own behalf, to speak up for themselves, and to tell their stories. We speak of 'capacity transfer,' meaning that through our multi-site structure, we engage men in distressed neighbourhoods on the ground, so to speak. Our sites have projects taking place in poor neighbourhoods from California to Michigan to Florida. They reach out to men directly, providing male-oriented health services in some instances, training in policy advocacy and neighbourhood research in others, and innovative collaborative programming in others still.

The notion is to build into neighbourhoods and into residents themselves the capacity to effectively pursue a men's health agenda – to pursue the agenda on a personal level as they take care of their health in their own individual lives, at a neighbourhood level as they become advocates for their fellow residents also in need of access to care and other services; and at a national level as they connect their experiences with those of other poor men in the US and give voice to the concerns of their class before federal legislators and policy-making bodies.

We're very happy about this aspect of our work. It is, of course, so very rewarding to see the transformation in a man – the confidence that emerges, the sense of community, and the empowerment – once he has spoken up for himself and testified in an informed manner on behalf of others who share his day-to-day struggles. We're happy to create opportunities such as these.

In addition, though, we recognise this transfer of capacity from our programs and staff people to the men in need and to their communities as a means of ensuring the long-term viability of the effort we've seeded.

By enlisting them as participants and partners in our men's health policy reform work, we've created a consciousness, a national network and a fire at the neighbourhood level . . .

Source: AMWY

The agendas for these grass-roots men's health conferences called upon policy leaders and analysts, clinicians, researchers, organisers, administrators, legal scholars and practitioners. The sessions ranged in nature from facilitated discussion to workshop to inspirational address. It was important to draw in the men – residents of distressed neighbourhoods who themselves live the experience of under-insurance and inadequate health service – to policy reform efforts, to enlist them to represent themselves in corridors in which their absence is remarkable in its typicality. Quite often, consequential policy discussions presume and can even enforce the silence of those in greatest need of consideration, those most entitled to a hearing. The agenda Community Voices set forward flew in the face of this paradox.

The programme armed the men with a language for their awareness, a productive idiom for their vulnerability and a mode and a venue for their legitimate indignation. The conferences sought to give them the opportunity to recognise that daily experiences and struggles, everyday realities, unite them with many others in categories that they could describe, analyse, object to, and try diligently to change (*see* Box 5.3).

Assessment approaches and tools

There are many challenges to finding poor men, effectively reaching out to them, connecting with them, determining their particular needs and issues, and ultimately meeting those needs. We enter complex territory in endeavouring to approach what is in effect a silenced community, unidentified and rendered largely invisible.

In light of the magnitude of the challenge and the complexity of the issues, an example may best suffice for insight. Turning again to the Overtown neighbourhood study conducted in a distressed quarter of Miami, US, researchers were able to render a rich picture of unmet and unarticulated needs by asking about well-being broadly and men's status on major life issues (Young 2006). The findings were based on lengthy interviews with men (usually of 40 minutes or more) during which they completed a questionnaire of 106 items with a survey administrator. The questionnaire probed a wide range of issues, from mental health, to police violence, to the relationship between social identity and health-related behaviours (*see* Box 5.4).

BOX 5.4 Overtown Men's Health Study Survey Instrument

---

106 items. Six primary sets of variables.

Demographic variables:

➤ racial and ethnic identity and first-language group

➤ annual income, educational attainment, employment status

➤ marital status

➤ parenthood.

Measures of subjective access to healthcare:

➤ availability of health services

➤ satisfaction with health services

➤ geographic accessibility of health services.

Measures of objective access to healthcare:

➤ having a primary care practitioner

➤ having visited a health practitioner within the previous 12 months

➤ having had dental care in the previous 12 months

➤ having received influenza vaccination in the previous 12 months

➤ having been tested for HIV.

Measures of physical well-being:

➤ ratings of physical health

➤ ratings of intensity and frequency of bodily pain.

Measures of mental well-being:

➤ frequency of feelings of sadness, restlessness, nervousness, hopelessness, and lack of motivation in the previous 30 days

➤ the degree of impact of the feelings on daily activity in the previous 30 days.

Behavioural and psychosocial health indicators:

➤ incarceration history

➤ housing status

➤ illegal drug use

➤ tobacco and alcohol use

➤ HIV risk factors.

Also part of the survey instrument were physical characteristics variables (height and weight); social identity variables measuring the associations between participants' social identity and health-promoting and -limiting behaviours and specific morbidity variables capturing diagnosed physiological and mental disorders.

Generally, there were apparent tensions and, sometimes, glaring inconsistencies in men's accounts and descriptions of their health status and behaviours. For instance, two in three (65.9%) of the men in the study described their health as 'good' or 'excellent' and 62% reported that compared to 12 months prior their health was 'about the same'. However, nearly 40% reported that they had physical health problems and 60.5% reported experiencing some degree of bodily pain in the previous 30 days. Similarly with mental health, while over half (53.5%) indicated feeling disabled to some degree by their mental health in the previous 30 days, only about 12% reported needing mental health care and even fewer (8.5%) had spoken to a mental health practitioner in the previous 30 days (*see* Table 5.2).

TABLE 5.2 Overtown Men's Health Study. Self-reported mental health status and mental health service patronage among the study population: Overtown neighbourhood in City of Miami, Florida, US, 2005 (n = 129)

	Number of respondents (n)	Percentage of respondents (%)
Report some degree of disability due to mental health	69	53.5
Report needing mental health care in previous 12 months	15	11.6
Have spoken to mental health practitioner in previous 12 months	11	8.5

So, these contradictions suggest that it matters greatly how one poses a health-related question to a man. A general question, 'How have you been feeling?' might return an equally general answer, 'Good'. A more specific probe such as 'How often do you feel worthless?' or 'Have you ever exchanged sex for money, drugs, food, shelter or other favours, even just one time?' might get us a bit closer to a more accurate self-assessment that paints a more detailed picture of a man's health needs.

But the contradictions are also quite probably symptomatic of a lack of reliable access to a healthcare resource to help men in Overtown to frame and address relevant health and mental health questions. It is critical to understand mental health in the context of various other experiences. While the point may be self-evident in theory, it can be missed in practice. Mental health exists – and is sustained or eroded – in a complex web of influences, experiences, capacities and realities (*see* Table 5.3 and Box 5.5). It is perhaps possible to anticipate some of the elements at play in the lives of poor men.

TABLE 5.3 Overtown Men's Health Study. Reported social experiences among the study population: Overtown neighbourhood in City of Miami, Florida, US, 2005 (n = 129)

	Number of respondents (n)	Percentage of respondents (%)
Victim of police violence	33	25.6
Immediate and enduring impacts		
Resulting injury physical	17	51.5
Resulting injury psychological or emotional	23	69.7

(*continued*)

	Number of respondents (n)	Percentage of respondents (%)
Suffer currently from resulting physical or psychological injury	13	39.4
Currently homeless	29	22.5
Have ever lived on the street	49	38.0
Have lived on the street in previous 12 months	28	21.7
Have lived on the street in previous 30 days	22	17.1
Have ever lived in a shelter	34	26.4
Have lived in a shelter in previous 12 months	12	9.3
Have lived in a shelter in previous 30 days	6	4.7
Ever incarcerated	85	65.9
Incarcerated in previous 12 months	24	18.6
Incarcerated in previous 30 days	5	3.9

In the Overtown study findings, several variables and features are quantifiably interconnected. It is apparent in the data, as it is on the ground in Overtown, how homelessness, for instance, is connected to incarceration, to psychological and physiological trauma, and to participation in the illegal drug trade. It is clear that the lack of provision for preventive care is linked to reliance on hospital emergency rooms for primary healthcare.

Taking as an example incarceration, it is indeed having measurable health impacts that researchers were able to capture in the men's health study. Among men who report having been incarcerated, there are statistically significant relationships to negative health outcomes. Men with a history of incarceration are more likely to report using illegal drugs, to report having less access to healthcare and to report a lesser sense of mental well-being.

The findings speak to a need for policy reform and for attention to community re-entry services. However, they also argue for considering community context and the influence on poor men of larger social jeopardies – not necessarily health-related in the immediate or strict sense.

BOX 5.5 Snapshot of a men's mental health crisis

Incarceration: Two in three self-reporting a history of incarceration

Under-education: Only 55% with high school diplomas

Under-employment: Only 40% working for pay at time of interview, and more than half report earning less than US$10 000 per year.

Under-housing: One in four reports having lived in a shelter and 28% have lived on the street.

Unreliable access to appropriate care: A startling 29% rely on the Emergency Room (ER) as a primary health facility and only 1 in 5 had received any dental care in the previous 12 months. While 54% reported some degree of disability due to the state of their mental health, only 8.5% had spoken to a mental health practitioner in the previous 12 months.

The point is not to pathologise poor men, according them some natural or essential dysfunction. It is instead to acknowledge the weight of poverty on their shoulders and psyches, and to anticipate that psychosocial costs register and accrue. It is to recognise that urban distress is not only the character of a poor metropolitan landscape, but also names an experience that its residents endure.

POLICY RECOMMENDATIONS
Public health and community redevelopment: a natural complement
Even from a community redevelopment perspective, given the data, improving men's health outcomes should be among the very highest priorities. Where community conditions cry out for social and economic reinvestment, where populations of women, children and men are disenfranchised, poor and distressed, it is imperative to empower men through health to participate fully in social revitalisation. Naturally, it is also imperative to reduce men's own suffering.

An important contribution of the Overtown Men's Health Study, for example, has been to expand local community revitalisation discourse to include a subjective account of urban distress and the experience of it. The approach to the collection of data, the consideration of men's experience as a subject of inquiry in Overtown, effectively enters people into the discussion of place.

Findings from this study and others make a strong argument for placing public health and community development in conversation. Too often distinct, more exchange between the two domains potentially offers much benefit to residents of distressed and transitioning neighbourhoods. The redesign of streetscapes, incorporation of public green spaces, and the relocation of certain businesses can be part of an aggressive health-promoting agenda that revitalises not only the economic and social life of a community, but its inhabitants as well.

Integrated health services
The findings of various studies concerning the health status and needs of poor men make a case for integrated physiological, mental and oral health services. Repeatedly, it is confirmed that men are not receiving what they need to support good health outcomes. The provision to men of an integrated package of health services, meeting and monitoring the range of their health needs, should be a policy priority for poor populations and areas.

Many health outreach efforts to poor men provide singular intervention – prostate screening, blood pressure or glucose testing, or a sports team qualifying physical exam. These are important methods to detect specific problems and they are often successful at gathering large numbers of men. However, these occasions are seldom used to their full advantage. They could more productively function as an entrée to integrated services. They also present the opportunity for training, so to speak, for men about how to think about and regularly seek the services they need, including mental health care. These occasions can also be a chance to 'transfer capacity', cultivating local knowledge and leadership, and seeding grass-roots health advocacy into poor communities.

Special care should be taken to instil mental well-being and psychological self-care-taking as natural and legitimate priorities for men. A successful outreach programme would impart this to men themselves and establish men's mental health as an explicit value in the wider community.

Global consciousness, local action

As yet, specific data are scarce that would allow us to precisely address the most pressing questions about how the world's poor men are faring health-wise and there is even less known about their mental health. However, indications gathered from a range of sources and phenomena suggest a troubling predicament – that male subjection to excess morbidity and mortality is magnified in poverty, even as poverty renders health structures and notions elusive.

Garnering political will within nation-states to provide access to care for poor men is a daunting undertaking. Providing systematic access to primary and preventive healthcare, mental and oral health services and, where appropriate, drug therapies, will enable employment, support of families and relief of the burden on states of male morbidity and early mortality. Advocacy and action both must proceed from above and below, with policy strategies bridging local realities and national means.

The Vienna Declaration on the Health of Men and Boys in Europe, ratified in 2005 and stating the principles and conditions necessary to improve male health outcomes, has been introduced to men in distressed urban neighbourhoods in the US. It has functioned as a tool to organise local men's advocacy for access to healthcare and male-appropriate approaches to outreach and provision. The Vienna Declaration insists upon men's health as a priority, but at the same time situates it within the context of family and community well-being.

Attendees of the October 2006 'Saving Men's Lives' conference participated in an innovative exercise entitled 'Conferring about Standards'. The focus of the two-part exercise was a document ratified the previous year in Vienna, Austria at the Fourth Biennial World Congress on Men's Health and Gender. Called 'the Vienna Declaration on the Health of Men and Boys in Europe', the document presents a list of lofty principles and standards.*

Part One of the exercise was called 'Write Back' and Part Two was called 'Talk Back'. For the Write Back portion, a large poster of the Vienna Declaration remained posted for the duration of the conference. Attendees were encouraged to write comments, anecdotes or edits directly onto the poster. For the Talk Back portion, attendees received the names of two other conference guests whom they were to 'interview' about the Vienna Declaration. They submitted their interviewees' responses to the exercise facilitator. The responses were the basis for a lunchtime discussion.

---

* For more information about the Vienna Declaration, please visit the website of the European Men's Health Forum at www.emhf.org

With a simple eloquence, the Vienna Declaration acknowledges the place of men's health in the broader agenda of disease prevention and public health. Its implications extend well beyond the realm of health in the strict sense, calling for greater mindfulness in school curricula and adequate integration of social policies with health concerns.

The conference delegates had an opportunity to closely consider the European declaration. Studying the document, they found that men's health issues – the disparities, the challenges with access to appropriate services, the quest to find ranking among other priorities – resonate across the Atlantic. They recognised in the Vienna Declaration's standards the global nature of their hopes for their own communities. In writing, 'This is what I want in my city,' on the poster, or in uttering, 'We need more "male-sensitive" stuff where I come from', they embraced the document's potential to anchor a movement.

REFERENCES

Bhui KS and McKenzie K (2008) Rates and risk factors by ethnic group for suicides within a year of contact with mental health services in England and Wales. *Psychiatr Serv.* **59**: 414–420.

Binswanger I, Stern MF, Deyo RA, Heagerty PJ, Cheadle A, Elmore JG and Koepsell TD (2007) Release from prison – a high risk of death for former inmates. *N Engl J Med.* **356**(5): 157–165.

Borrell LN, Crespo CJ and Garcia-Palmieri MR (2007) Skin color and mortality risk among men: the Puerto Rico Heart Health Program. *Ann Epidemiol.* **17**(5): 335–41.

Calavita KA (2003) 'Reserve army of delinquents': the criminalization and economic punishment of immigrants in Spain. *Punishment & Society.* **5**(4): 399–413.

Casas JA, Dachs JN and Bambas A (2001) Health disparities in Latin America and the Caribbean: the role of social and economic determinants. In *Equity and health: Views from the Pan American Sanitary Bureau.* Occasional publication No. 8. Washington, DC: Pan American Health Organization, pp. 22–49.

Chenet L, Leon D, McKee M and Vassin S (1998) Death from alcohol and violence in Moscow: socioeconomic determinants. *European J Population.* **14**: 19–37.

Clark VR (2001) The perilous effects of racism on blacks. *Ethn Dis.* **11**(4): 769–72.

Darity Jr W and Nembhard JG (2000) Racial and ethnic economic inequality: the international record. *Am Econ Rev.* **90**(2): 308–11.

del Amo J, Broring G and Fenton K (2003) HIV health experiences among migrant Africans in Europe: how are we doing? *AIDS.* **17**: 2261–3.

Diaz RM, Ayala G and Bein E (2004) Sexual risk as an outcome of social oppression: data from a probability sample in Latino gay men in three U.S. cities. *Cultural Diversity and Ethnic Minority Psychology.* **10**(3): 255–67.

Gold R, Michael YL, Whitlock EP, Hubbell FA, Mason ED, Rodriguez BL, Safford MM and Sarto GE (2006) Race/ethnicity, socioeconomic status, and lifetime morbidity burden in the women's health initiative: a cross-sectional analysis. *J Womens Health (Larchmt).* **15**(10):1161–73.

Jackson JS, Brown TN, Williams DR, Torres M, Sellers SL and Brown K (1996) Racism and the physical and mental health status of African Americans: a thirteen year national panel study. *Ethn Dis.* 6(1–2): 132–47.

Kwate NO, Valdimarsdottir HB, Guevarra JS and Bovbjerg DH (2003) Experiences of racist events are associated with negative health consequences for African American women. *J Natl Med Assoc.* 95(6):450–60.

Kimmelman M (2008) Italy gives cultural diversity a lukewarm embrace. *New York Times,* 25 June.

McKee M (1999) Alcohol in Russia. *Alcohol & Alcoholism.* 34 (6): 824–829.

Olson EC, Van Wye G, Kerker B, Thorpe L and Frieden TR (2006) *Take Care Central Harlem.* NYC Community Health Profiles 2nd ed. 20(42): 1–16.

Read JG (2005) Racial context, black immigration and the U.S. black/white health disparity. *Social Forces.* 84(1): 181–99.

Rehm J (2003a). The relationship of average volume of alcohol consumption and drinking patterns of drinking to burden of disease – an overview. *Addiction.* 98: 1209–1228.

Rehm J (2003b). The global distribution of average volume of alcohol consumption and patterns of drinking. *European Addiction Research.* 9: 147–156.

Ryan M (1995) Russian report: alcoholism and rising mortality in the Russian Federation. *BMJ.* 310: 648–50.

Smaje C (1995) *Health, 'Race' and Ethnicity: making sense of the evidence.* London: King's Fund Institute.

Tuan WJ, Hatfield P, Bhattacharya A, Sarto GE and Kling PJ (2007) Possible factors illuminating increased disparities in neonatal mortality in Wisconsin from 1991-2005. *WMJ.* 106(3): 130-6.

U.S. Department of Justice (2003) *Bureau of Justice Statistics Special Report: education and correctional populations.* Catalog No. 01/03 NCJ 195670. Washington, DC: US Department of Justice.

Verger P, Rotily M, Prudhomme J and Bird S (2003) High mortality rates among inmates during the year following their discharge from a French prison. *J Forensic Sciences.* 48(3): 614–6.

Wamala S, Merlo J, Bostrom G and Hogstedt C (2007) Perceived discrimination, socioeconomic disadvantage and refraining from seeking medical treatment in Sweden. *J Epidemiol Community Health.* 61: 409–15.

Webb CPM, Bromet EJ, Gluzman S, Tintle Nl, Schwartz JE, Kostyuchenko S and Havenaar JM (2005) Epidemiology of heavy alcohol use in Ukraine: findings from the world mental health survey. *Alcohol & Alcoholism.* 40(4): 327–335.

White A (2006) Men and mental well-being – encouraging gender sensitivity. *The Mental Health Review.* 11(4): 3–6.

Wolf Harlow C (2003) Bureau of Justice Statistics Special Report: Education and Correctional Populations. NCJ 195670. US Department of Justice. Available at: www.ojp.usdoj.gov/bjs/pub/pdf/ecp.pdf (Accessed 20 September 2009).

World Health Organization (WHO), (2008) The World Health Statistics 2008. Geneva: World Health Organization. Available at: www.who.int/whosis/whostat/EN_WHS08_Full.pdf (Accessed 1 May 2008).

Young AMW (2006) *Overtown: Men's Health Study.* Miami: Collins Center for Public Policy.

CHAPTER 6

Rural men's mental health

Steve Robertson, Keith Elder and Ruth Coombs

INTRODUCTION

The importance of paying attention to both community context and social capital in relation to men's mental health has been highlighted elsewhere in this book (*see* Chapters 4 and 5). Nowhere is this more apparent than when considering the mental health of men in rural settings. This chapter starts by providing some general background to the rural context in the UK before progressing to consider what we currently know about rural mental health and specifically that of rural men. We then move on to look at how the issue of 'rural masculinities' might impact on rural men's mental well-being.

BACKGROUND

In the UK, one-fifth of the population live in rural areas – though definitions of what counts as 'rural' have until recently often remained unclear, with measures such as population density, complex indices and arbitrary judgement all being used at various times and in different ways (Gregoire and Thornicroft 1998). Hill's (2003) report on rural data and rural statistics pointed to the strong contrast between the statistical provision for agriculture as an economic activity and user of resources, and rural policy. He suggested that the inadequacy of rural data to service scientific enquiry and inform policy had been a longstanding concern and that an agri-centric view of the rural world in statistics was demonstrably inadequate and potentially misleading. This is because, whilst agriculture and forestry remain predominant users of rural land and the agricultural landscape remains an important feature of many rural areas, the proportion of people living in the countryside who work in these sectors is now only 2% of the population in England and 3% in Wales. The statistical provision for rural policy as a result has until recently been weak and fragmented because statistics which separate the rural from the non-rural are not available.

In 2004, the Department for Environment, Food and Rural Affairs (Defra) and the Countryside Agency began to introduce some clarity with the publication of new definitions for 'rural' and 'urban'. The new rural definition differed from its predecessors by focussing exclusively on land use, derived in such a way as to identify patterns of rural settlement (i.e. small rural towns, villages, hamlets and scattered dwellings) and was developed for use by funders, policy-makers and the Office for National Statistics. Defra admits that defining an area as either rural or urban may conflict with the 'look' or 'feel' of that area from the perspectives of local people (Countryside Agency *et al.* 2004). The new definitions were also developed to encompass the diversity of rural England and Wales in the 21st century, e.g. 'honey pot villages' that depend heavily on tourism, urban fringe commuter villages and former coal mining communities, and be applied to help target policy to those groups, communities and businesses that most required support.

RURALITY, HEALTH AND WELL-BEING

In general, rural communities enjoy better health and well-being than their urban counterparts. On standard measures of health (such as life expectancy and infant mortality) rural communities consistently score better. Evidence suggests that levels of the most common mental health problems are lower in rural areas (Weich *et al.* 2006). Generally, rural residents make less use of health services and have a more positive view of the state of their own health (Commission for Rural Communities 2005).

Urban and rural communities agree on the main factors that make the countryside a healthier and more pleasant place to live – peace and quiet, the predominantly natural or agricultural environment, lower crime rates and close-knit communities. These perceptions are reflected in the fact that more people living in rural areas wish to stay in their community for the long-term compared to people living in urban areas. Moving from towns and cities to the countryside is a growing trend in England and Wales (Commission for Rural Communities 2005).

Unfortunately, the widely recognised benefits of life in the countryside have led to the concept of the 'rural idyll' – an idealised stereotype of country life that ignores the real difficulties faced by many rural communities. Such difficulties include poverty, lack of services, poor public transport and traumatic social or economic change at a local level.

THE IMPACT OF POVERTY

Poverty is a reality across rural UK, especially in the most remote areas. The proportion of men and women in rural areas who earn low wages is greater than in the rest of the UK population and one in three individuals in rural Britain experienced at least one period of poverty during 1991–1996 (Shucksmith 2003). Furthermore, there have been big shifts in farming income in the UK – a steady decline since the 1960s reached a low point in 2000, with average Net Farm Income for all types of farm at just £8700, before rising to £38 600 by 2007/8. Farming incomes have been particularly affected by specific crises (such as foot-and-mouth and BSE) as well as more usual problems, such as falls in wheat prices and poor harvests (Gregoire 2002).

Those living on low incomes, however, may be dispersed over large, sparsely populated districts. They are often as geographically near to more affluent members of the community as they are to others on low incomes. This means that their poverty is less visible to community planners and policy-makers, who use 'indicators of deprivation' that are more suited to the higher concentrations of poverty found in towns and cities. This 'hidden' poverty has a major impact on the health of individuals and families. People who are more vulnerable to mental distress are also less likely to enjoy the same level of health and well-being as the rest of the population.

MENTAL HEALTH IN RURAL AREAS – THE ISSUES

There are difficulties with access to services, low levels of health and social care service provision, isolation, higher product costs (for food, clothes etc) and lack of choice or quality of these products, all of which contribute to health and social care problems (Craig and Manthorpe 2000). Although rural England and Wales have social, economic and cultural differences, they do share some issues that are likely to affect the mental health of both their populations.

Provision of care and support services

Economies of scale mean that most services are located in urban areas, which are more highly populated. This is especially true of specialist services, such as care and support services for people with mental health problems.

Not only are there fewer specialist services in rural areas, but those that exist are likely to be many miles from a patient's home (British Medical Association Board of Science 2005). This has a serious effect on access to services in urgent or crisis situations, the availability of outreach services for those who cannot leave their homes and response times for on-call doctors who serve large, sparsely populated areas. The right of all NHS patients to choose between service providers (Department of Health 2004) means little if there is only one specialist provider across a large geographical area.

The time, money and effort required to travel to specialist services can impede the recovery and good management of mental health problems.

Access to transport

The quality of available transport is a major factor in whether urban-based care and support services are accessible to people who live in rural areas. People in rural areas usually find that public transport does not meet their daily mobility needs. Only 50% of the rural population have an hourly bus service within ten minutes walk from their home (Commission for Rural Communities 2005). The frequency, reliability and timing of rural public transport can make travelling to mental health services difficult or impossible. In many cases, a day return journey from home to a service outlet cannot be made using public transport (Swindlehurst 2005).

Due to inadequate public transport, most people living in rural areas find that owning a car is essential to their daily life. Frequently, people who are already in financial hardship get further into poverty from the costs of buying, insuring and maintaining a vehicle. People in rural areas who do not own cars are often reliant on private or voluntary arrangements such as taxis or lifts from family members and neighbours. However, these arrangements can be expensive or dependent on the willingness and ability of a small number of volunteers. The Institute of Rural Health has found examples of taxi fares (between £40 and £70 for a round trip) preventing patients in rural areas from accessing mental health services (Swindlehurst 2005).

Those who suffer from a lack of access to transport are often those most in need of accessing services. In some localities the NHS services provide a transport service to patients and elsewhere voluntary 'social car' transport schemes may operate. The availability of voluntary transport schemes will vary from one community to the next, with the Rural Community Council (England),* a branch of the Community Transport Association,† the Council for Voluntary Action,‡ the Women's Royal Voluntary Service§ or the British Red Cross¶ being good sources of local information about what might be available in a particular locality.

Access to information

Access to reliable, high quality information has a profound effect on mental health and well-being. It enables people to make the most of their lives, fully aware of their rights and the resources available to them. This applies to local and national community information in general, as well as to information specifically about health.

In rural areas it may be more difficult to obtain information about mental health issues locally due to a lack of infrastructure. Often shops, post offices, libraries and GP surgeries are widely dispersed or run services that do not meet an individual's needs (for example, shop opening hours may clash with an individual's working hours).

Some information services do have coverage of the countryside. The Post Office was until recently required by central Government to maintain its rural network.

---

* Rural Community Councils: the Rural Community Action Network is the collective name for the 38 Rural Community Councils throughout England, their eight regional bodies and their national umbrella, ACRE. RCCs are charitable local development agencies, generally based at county level, which support and enable initiatives in rural communities. www.acre.org.uk

† Community Transport Association: the CTA supports a wide range of organisations delivering innovative and flexible transport solutions to achieve social change in their communities. www.ctauk.org

‡ Councils for Voluntary Action: NAVCA is the national voice of local third sector infrastructure in England. www.navca.org.uk See also Wales Council for Voluntary Action (www.wcva.org.uk) Scottish Council for Voluntary Action (www.scvo.org.uk) and Northern Ireland Council for Voluntary Action (www.nicva.org)

§ Women's Royal Voluntary Services: an age-positive charity that offers a range of practical services to help and support older people to live well, maintain their independence and play a part in their local community. www.wrvs.org.uk

¶ British Red Cross: a volunteer-led humanitarian organisation that helps people in crisis, whoever and wherever they are. www.redcross.org.uk

However, despite recent closures in its rural network the Post Office still has an important presence in some rural communities. All public library services have mobile facilities for remote parts of their catchment areas and organise visits to housebound library users. Citizens Advice,* through its network of local bureaux, may have a small outlet in a rural area, often in a small market town which is linked to a main bureau in a nearby urban centre.

Although the coverage of information outlets is inadequate, especially in rural areas, most organisations now use a range of media (print resources, telephone, email and internet) to communicate. Mind runs its Infoline[†] through both telephone and email and maintains a comprehensive website that is updated daily. Other national organisations involved in health and well-being, such as the Samaritans[‡] and Age Concern,[§] also provide information by telephone, email and internet. These methods reduce the need for 'physical' information outlets but do not replace them.

The barriers to accessing information faced by many people with physical disabilities can be greater in rural areas. Travelling long distances to information outlets can be difficult or impossible. Where small, local outlets do exist, they may be less likely to have had the 'reasonable adjustments' made that are laid down by the Disability Discrimination Acts (1995 and 2005) to make buildings accessible to disabled people.

People who do not have English as their first language may find it more difficult to find information on mental health in their 'mother tongue' in rural areas. Information on mental health in a range of languages can be accessed through Mindinfoline, which offers the Language Line service. Language Line is an organisation that provides interpretation services for non-English speakers and plays a 'third party' role between caller and a member of the Mindinfoline staff. Mental health information booklets in a range of languages are also available from Mind.[¶] The Welsh-based information and advice service Community Advice and Listening Line[**] provides web-based and telephone services in English and Welsh.

WHAT DO WE KNOW ABOUT RURAL MENTAL HEALTH?

Given this background, these difficulties and concerns with major aspects of life in rural settings, what do we know about the impact this has on the mental health of those in rural communities and specifically on men in those communities?

---

* The Citizens Advice service helps people resolve their legal, money and other problems by providing free, independent and confidential advice, through a network of local bureaux. www.citizensadvice.org.uk

† Mindinfoline is Mind's mental health information service. www.mind.org.uk

‡ Samaritans provides confidential non-judgemental emotional support, 24 hours a day for people who are experiencing feelings of distress or despair, including those which could lead to suicide. www.samaritans.org

§ Age Concern/Help the Aged: the four national Age Concerns in the UK have joined together with Help the Aged to improve the lives of older people. www.ageconcern.org.uk

¶ Mind Publications: www.mind.org.uk

** CALL is the mental health helpline for Wales. www.callhelpline.org.uk

Despite the apparent stresses that such difficulties might suggest, there is evidence of lower rates of depression, anxiety disorder, panic, alcohol and drug dependency, and psychosis (Meltzer *et al.* 1995; Paykel *et al.* 2000) and schizophrenia (McCreadie *et al.* 1997) among rural populations in the UK. Yet such work may not present a full picture. For example, the reasons for apparently lower rates of various mental health diagnoses could be due to reticence to recognise or label symptoms as those relating to 'mental health' conditions – by both the rural population themselves and the health professionals that serve them. In turn, this has been suggested to be linked to a greater sensitivity to the stigma of mental health and to greater concerns about confidentiality in small rural communities (Sherlock 1994; Lobley *et al.* 2004). These issues of stigma and confidentiality may be of particular concern for rural men through links to notions of 'rural masculinity' and related stoicism and we shall look at this further shortly. For example, one study showed that despite a lower prevalence of psychiatric morbidity than the general population in Britain, male farmers were more likely to report thinking that 'life is not worth living'. The conclusion being that the relation between depression and suicidal thoughts appears different amongst male farmers than in the general population (Thomas *et al.* 2003).

These apparently lower rates of mental health problems may also partly be attributable to 'resource drift' where service accessibility is easier in urban locations. For example, in one study it was found that there was less specialist psychiatric (and more GP) treatment, lower psychotropic drug use and administration and later presentation for mental health symptoms in rural settings (Gregoire and Thornicroft 1998; Gregoire 2002). Therefore, as others have previously identified, such figures around lower rates of mental health need to be treated with caution as there may be evidence of greater hidden morbidity and higher thresholds for reporting symptoms in rural areas (Gregoire and Thornicroft 1998).

Men and young men feature significantly amongst those high risk groups which are particularly vulnerable to developing a mental health problem. For farmers, the difficulties and concerns associated with rural poverty outlined earlier cause stress through particular processes, with farmers showing higher levels of stress than the general population (Booth and Lloyd 1999). Farmers' stress has been shown to be related to new legislation and associated paperwork, financial pressures, media criticism and isolation (Booth and Lloyd 1999; Raine 1999). These issues have been compounded in the last decade by the outbreak of BSE and foot-and-mouth (Raine 1999) with a postal survey study showing farmers in affected rural areas having significantly higher levels of psychological morbidity than those in unaffected rural areas (Peck *et al.* 2002).

This being the case, it is no surprise that rates of suicide are of particular concern, with farmers being one of the professional groups at highest risk, accounting for 1% of all suicides in England and Wales (Booth *et al.* 2000). Likewise, in Scotland, 307 male farmers and farm workers died by suicide or undetermined cause between 1981 and 1999 (Stark *et al.* 2006). Factors associated with suicide in farmers are similar to those that cause stress outlined above. They include not having a confidant, work, finance, legal problems, physical health and relationships. However, the most common single factor is the presence of mental health problems (mainly depression) which is found in 82% of farmer suicides (Hawton *et al.* 1998). Interestingly, male farmers who commit suicide are no more or less likely than men who committed suicide in the general population to have consulted a GP or mental health practitioner in the three months before their death. However, farmers are more likely to have presented with exclusively physical symptoms, suggesting differences in help-seeking behaviours. They are also significantly less likely to have left a suicide note and more likely to use violent methods, particularly firearms, in committing suicide (Booth *et al.* 2000; Stark *et al.* 2006). There is also some evidence that farmers have experienced mental health problems as a result of exposure to organophosphate chemicals found in sheep dip and other products that farmers use in their work (Health and Safety Executive 2000; Myhill 2003).

One positive outcome of the BSE and foot-and-mouth crises, however, is that public attention has been drawn to the experiences of affected communities, including the impact of these experiences on farmers' mental health. In addition, farming communities have generated self-help and mutual-aid organisations to support people in crisis. The Farm Crisis Network[*] recruits volunteers from the farming community (farmers, people from farming families, agricultural chaplains) who understand the practical difficulties that farmers face. Volunteers offer technical and pastoral support and respond quickly and confidentially to requests for help. They suggest the use of other services where necessary and provide support while farmers resolve their own problems. Many counties now have Farm Crisis Network support groups. Other national organisations involved in health, well-being or personal finance have gained a deeper understanding of the issues facing farmers over recent years.

Currently, and for the foreseeable future, farmers face the stresses of conforming to UK and European legislation, including complex bureaucratic procedures and financial uncertainty. Farmers who develop mental health problems rarely approach mental health services due to the stigma attached to mental health problems and the shame of being seen as 'not coping'. Due to their geographical location, farmers are often at a distance from mental health services, which makes them difficult to reach. In addition, farmers work long hours and may not be able to take time off during 'office hours' to use mental health services.

SUICIDE IN RURAL SETTINGS

It is not only farmers that commit suicide in rural settings. There is evidence that since the 1960s suicide rates in rural areas, in both men and women, have risen disproportionately compared to overall rates for England and Wales (Hill *et al.* 2005) leading some to suggest that the mental health of young adults, which influences

---

[*]   Farm Crisis Network provides pastoral and practical support to farming people during periods of anxiety, stress and problems relating to both the farm household and the farm business. www. farmcrisisnetwork.org.uk.

suicide risk, may have deteriorated more in rural than urban areas in recent years (Middleton *et al.* 2003). Despite this rise in both men and women, rurality has a bigger impact on men's suicide than women's and the greatest risk of male suicide is in remote rural locations (Levin and Leyland 2005).

MINORITY GROUPS

Black and minority ethnic (BME) populations and lesbian, gay and bisexual and transgender (LGBT) populations make up minorities in many parts of the UK. They make up even smaller minorities in the countryside. Negative attitudes towards BME and LGBT people, reported across rural England and Wales (Hastings 2004), are not tackled effectively, mainly because the groups affected are so small that they cannot easily build strong local support networks.

Often, those who plan services believe that members of BME or LGBT populations do not live in rural areas (Mind 2003). This is not the case. As these populations tend to be small and isolated, individuals can suffer doubly from being visible within their local community but invisible to those who plan services. This situation can lead to culturally inappropriate services, expressions of racism and homophobia, and consequent mental distress.

Work in tackling negative attitudes towards BME and LGBT groups has been undertaken in rural England and Wales at national and local levels. For example, the Countryside Agency's Diversity Review (2005)* researched the diversity-awareness of service providers in rural England and the perceptions of groups who are under-represented in their use of rural services; Mind Out Cymru† provides an all-Wales support and information network for lesbian, gay and bisexual people who either have, or have had, contact with mental health services and Intercom‡ in the South West of England is an umbrella organisation for LGB communities that are dispersed across rural areas.

CHILDREN AND YOUNG PEOPLE

A series of Joseph Rowntree Foundation studies, that form part of their 'Action in Rural Areas' programme (Rugg and Jones 1999; Storey and Brannen 2000; Cartmel and Furlong 2000; Shucksmith 2004), show that issues around employment, housing, education and transport are of particular concern to young people in rural settings. However, there are clear social and environmental benefits for children and young people who live in rural England and Wales. In comparison with their urban counterparts, rural children and young people are generally in better health, living in higher income households and have higher levels of educational achievement (Defra 2005). However, these generalisations hide huge disparities within and between rural communities. Children and young people in lower income families or

---

* www.naturalengland.org.uk/ourwork/enjoying/outdoorsforall/diversityreview
† www.mind.org.uk
‡ www.intercomtrust.org.uk

in the most sparsely populated rural areas are more vulnerable to the full range of social problems that are likely to affect their mental health.

Children and young people in rural areas have the same rights to health services as those based in urban and suburban areas. Details of these rights for those aged 16 and under are described in the Department of Health's and the Welsh Assembly Government's National Service Frameworks for Children and Young People. All children and young people have the right to specialist, age-appropriate mental health services, flexibility as to the location at which they are seen by health professionals and, if necessary, emergency referrals within 24 hours. In practice, many services are less available in rural areas. Access to specialist services may involve out-of-area referrals which will mean longer waiting times for appointments and longer travelling times to service providers.

YoungMinds[*] run an information service for parents and carers, and another for children and young people. The service covers all aspects of mental health including diagnoses and conditions, NHS services and legal issues. Many mental health charities run telephone and email support services for children and young people. Examples include Samaritans, Childline[†] and the Eating Disorders Association.[‡] Such services are particularly important for young people in rural areas who do not have access to face-to-face support services.

OLDER PEOPLE

A higher proportion of people aged over 65 live in rural areas. Evidence shows that this proportion is continuing to grow (Commission for Rural Communities 2005; Davies *et al.* 2008). Mental health problems affect a significant minority of older people (Mind 2005) and older men are a high risk-group for suicide. People over 75 are 16 times less likely to be asked about suicide by their GP and five times less likely to be asked about depression (Mind 2009). Older people in rural areas are less likely than their urban counterparts to have relatives nearby to support them and are more likely to live alone. These factors can lead to feelings of isolation. Studies have also shown that older people make up the largest group of people living in poverty in rural areas which, combined with the higher cost of living in the countryside, can cause considerable stress (Mind 2003).

Despite their numbers, older people in rural areas are disadvantaged in terms of health service provision compared with their urban counterparts. Mental health problems experienced by older people are more likely to be misdiagnosed and neglected at primary care level and are less likely to be referred to mental health services.

---

[*] YoungMinds is committed to improving the emotional well-being of children and young people by providing expert knowledge, online resources, training, development and outreach. www.young-minds.org.uk

[†] Childline provides a free and confidential helpline for children and young adults in the UK. www.childline.org.uk

[‡] Eating Disorders Association provides information and help on all aspects of eating disorders, including anorexia nervosa, bulimia nervosa, binge-eating disorder and related eating disorders. www.b-eat.co.uk

Contrary to the stigmatising view of older people as 'dependent', evidence shows that older people make a significant contribution to community life in rural areas. They are more likely than other age groups to participate in organisations such as parish councils, village hall committees and religious groups and to use community facilities such as shops and post offices. Older people are also most likely to provide unpaid care to others, including those with physical or mental health problems (Mesurier 2004).

Of the various networks and services that may be of interest to older people living in the countryside, Age Concern is the largest and best known. Age Concern is active in all parts of the country, with many groups located in rural areas.

TRAVELLERS

Travellers have been part of rural communities since the 14th century, when the first Romany Gypsies arrived in England and Wales. Since the 19th century Irish Travellers have joined this population, as well as former house dwellers who have adopted the Traveller life through choice or circumstance. Although economic change has forced many to seek work and accommodation in urban areas, Travellers still make up part of the migrant worker population that takes seasonal employment in the countryside.

Historically, friction has occurred between settled and Traveller populations and this is often the case today. Tensions are further fuelled by the shortage of well-run, authorised sites for Travellers and the negative representation of Travellers in the mass media. This takes its toll on Travellers' mental health and well-being.

Travellers face huge barriers in their access to health and related services, such as social care and education. This is largely because they are subject to frequent evictions from unauthorised sites. As temporary residents in a health authority's catchment area and lacking a fixed abode, it can be difficult for Travellers to register with a GP. This can also make it difficult for them to receive long-term treatment provided by the NHS. There are two main sources of information on Travellers' issues that are relevant to mental health. The Travellers Times[*] magazine and the Friends, Families and Travellers[†] website, which gives information on law, planning and evictions as well as health, education and community information.

Traveller communities identify with a holistic concept of health as opposed to medical models that are rooted in concepts of disease and medication. The holistic approach emphasises social and environmental factors as 'key determinants' of health. Using research and outreach into Traveller health undertaken over the past decade, the Department of Health has worked with Traveller communities to establish a model of Traveller participation in the promotion of health and to assist in

---

[*] TT Online brings news, pictures, video, opinion and resources from within the Gypsy, Roma and Traveller communities. www.travellerstimes.org.uk

[†] FFT seeks to end racism and discrimination against Gypsies and Travellers, whatever their ethnicity, culture or background, whether settled or mobile, and to protect the right to pursue a nomadic way of life. www.gypsy-traveller.org

the dialogue between Travellers and Health service professionals, e.g. through the Sussex Travellers Health Project, 2003–2006.[*]

MIGRANT WORKERS

British farmers depend on migrant workers to perform a range of seasonal tasks. The many thousands of migrant workers who work on British farms and in other agri-culture-related businesses are drawn from Eastern Europe, from Asia and the Middle East as well as from Traveller and Gypsy communities.

The mental health of migrant workers, and especially illegal migrant workers, presents particular challenges to service providers. Workers may speak little or no English (nor any of the languages spoken by groups established over a longer period in the UK). They may find British mental health services difficult to understand and even threatening, particularly if they have received hostile treatment from settled local communities. If employed in seasonal work, a migrant worker may not be res-ident in a NHS Trust catchment area long enough to receive the treatment they need.

Over the past few years, organisations involved with health and well-being have begun working with rural migrant workers. The Citizens' Advice[†] has undertaken many outreach projects with migrant workers through its Rural Bureau Network. The Arthur Rank Centre, the national focus for rural churches in England, has identified migrant workers as a priority group for pastoral care and has published a leaflet on this issue in partnership with Defra.

Migrant workers' language needs can sometimes be met by a local or national organisation that offers information and support services to a particular national or cultural group, for example, the Chinese Mental Health Association.[‡]

STIGMA

People with mental health problems are often stigmatised in our society; labelled as violent, unpredictable or dangerous. These negative images and ideas are often caused by confusion about what 'mental distress' actually is. Stigma is particularly associated with regard to mental health issues in rural areas, with high levels of con-cern around lack of anonymity and confidentiality (Buchan and Deaville 2005). The fear around anonymity is particularly noted by young people living in the most rural parts of Wales (Mind Cymru 2008)

In many rural communities, the stigma can be especially strong – caused in part by social structure. The mental health service user movement is weak owing to popu-lation sparsity and consequent lack of group support for those who speak out. This is often compounded by the lack of anonymity or confidentiality found in many

---

[*]   www.gypsy-traveller.org/health/health-project

[†]   www.citizensadvice.org.uk/index/publications/assisting_migrant_workers

[‡]   The Chinese Mental Health Association (CMHA) specialises in providing community-based mental health assistance and support to the Chinese community, in an attempt to assist those in need. www.cmha.org.uk

small, close-knit rural communities. In a wider sense, many rural communities have a deeply ingrained culture of stoicism and self-reliance. This can apply to all aspects of a person's life, including their health. Stoicism and self-reliance have proved great strengths in the countryside, enabling individuals and families to survive major financial and personal difficulties, to persevere and even prosper. However, stoicism and self-reliance can sometimes have a negative effect on mental health. Where these qualities are highly valued, external intervention – especially from public, urban-based health services – is likely to be rejected in favour of trying to cope alone.

The consequences of stigma can have a serious effect on a person's willingness to access mental health services or confide in potentially supportive individuals and agencies. In this atmosphere, mental health problems are more likely to develop and recovery is more difficult. This can lead to chronic poor mental health.

Fortunately, attitudes to mental health have improved across the countryside over the past decade. High profile crises in agriculture, such as BSE and foot-and-mouth disease, have brought public attention to the stresses in farming communities that can lead to mental health problems. Rural organisations which have a mental health remit, such as the Farm Crisis Network, the Arthur Rank Centre* and Farming Help[†] have been active across England and Wales.

Having outlined some of the issues around rural mental health and drawn some attention to the specific concerns for rural men, it is important now to explore how this relates to notions of masculinity; that is, to how it relates to ideas about what it is to 'be a man' in the rural context.

RURAL MASCULINITIES AND MENTAL HEALTH

Several chapters in this book highlight how traditional, stereotypical images of men are built on notions of strength, rationality, self-control/sufficiency and stoicism. These are the very same values, what some have termed 'agrarian values', which are suggested as shaping rural and particularly male rural identities (Campbell and Bell 2000; Judd *et al.* 2006). The stereotyped image of the rural man therefore almost constitutes a hyper-masculinity. It combines notions of (often extreme) physical action (labour) and endurance with a rational mind that can overcome adversity through the ability to adapt and be decisive (Liepins 2000). Changes in wider socio-economic circumstances clearly affect the way that these ideals become expressed, with some suggesting a shift from rural men as dirty, manual workers to organised businessmen willing and able to diversify in order to maximise family income (Brandth 1995; Bryant 1999). The shift in the way these ideals are expressed may be even more profound when viewed through the perspective of the new rural definition with less than

---

* The Rural Stress Helpline at the Arthur Rank Centre provides a confidential, non-judgemental listening services to anyone in a rural area feeling troubled, isolated, anxious, worried, stressed or needing information. www.arthurrankcentre.org.uk.

† Farming Help brings together three national charities which work to benefit the farming community. Each charity provides different but complementary forms of help and support to meet a wide range of needs. www.farminghelp.org.uk.

1.5% of the UK working population employed in agriculture. Most likely though, these seemingly contradictory masculine identities often continue to sit beside one another with rural men choosing to, and also having to, shift between them at various times (Evans 2000; Little 2002; Coldwell 2007).

In terms of mental health, these stereotyped (and often idealised) images of rural masculinities create a double bind for rural men. The pressure of living up to these images can readily take its toll in terms of increased stress and anxiety that becomes internalised when notions of showing weakness are seen as unacceptable.* Work on understanding suicide in farmers confirmed this, with farmers identifying that they had limited capacity to acknowledge or express the stressors they experienced and that this was related to specific attitudes the men held around 'maleness' and help-seeking (Judd *et al.* 2006a). On the other hand, not living up to these stereotypes, through circumstance or choice, may also generate significant stress, depression and suicidal ideation. The current stressful context for farmers, outlined above, of new legislation, increasing paperwork, financial pressures and media criticism can overwhelm individual men. This can create feelings of hopelessness, entrapment, isolation and loss of control, which are significant factors in suicide associated with men living in rural locations (Ni Laoire 2001). As Coldwell (2006) identifies, failing as a farmer means being seen to have failed to live up to the expectations of family and community members. Farming masculinities therefore entail a constant struggle to perform in order to survive and maintain one's identity in a culture where to fail as a farmer means to fail as a man.

This rural 'hyper-masculinity' is also linked to heterosexuality (Little 2003) and for those specifically choosing to reject these rural male stereotypes, such as rural gay men, there may be specific concerns about the impact on mental well-being when structural difficulties are experienced (Bell and Valentine 1995). The mental health impact of life events may be compounded by the stigmatisation attached to others, homophobic attitudes (Ross 1990) and these attitudes may be more apparent in hyper-masculine rural contexts.

Factors affecting men's mental health and well-being often have higher impacts on the mental health and well-being of men in rural areas, due to such factors as isolation, lack of alternatives, the stigma surrounding mental health and the issue of socialisation theory. The theory may explain why some men find it very difficult to articulate their feelings and seek help (Mind 2009). Men are also more likely to get angry when worried and often 'act out', whereas women are more likely to 'act in'. As the principles for diagnosing depression are more focussed on 'acting in' behaviours they can be seen as feminised (Kilmartin 2005). This may make engagement with men much more difficult, particularly in rural areas, given the additional barriers referred to here.

---

*   It can also take its toll physically with some research showing farmers to be a 'high risk' group in
    terms of health and safety (Gerrard 1998).

CONCLUSION

Rural environments bring with them particular challenges in relation to a range of issues such as employment, housing, transport, access to education and healthcare. These can be compounded in times of economic hardship and specific crises (such as foot-and-mouth, BSE, etc.). There is no doubt that these hardships create particular concerns and outcomes in relation to mental well-being for those in rural settings. Despite some evidence of lower psychiatric morbidity, it is likely that rural identities and 'resource drift' to urban locations hide the reality of the levels of mental health concerns in these settings. In addition, such concerns, particularly stress, depression and suicide, are experienced differently by men and women in rural contexts. The links between the values attached to stereotypes of 'masculinity' and those attached to stereotypes of 'rural' identity – strength, rationality, self-control/sufficiency and stoicism – can create a 'hyper-masculine' rural identity. In turn, this creates challenges for rural men's mental well-being in terms of the stresses involved in living up to such idealised stereotypes or the disappointment and hopelessness that can come of being unable (or unwilling) to live up to them.

REFERENCES

Bell D and Valentine G (1995) Queer country: rural lesbian and gay lives. *J Rural Studies*. **11**(2): 113–122.

Booth NJ and Lloyd K (1999) Stress in farmers. *Int J Social Psychiatry*. **46**(1): 67–73.

Booth NJ, Briscoe M and Powell R (2000) Suicide in the farming community: methods used and contact with health services. *Occup Environ Med*. **57**: 642–644.

Brandth B (1995) Rural masculinity in transition: gender images in tractor advertisements. *J Rural Studies*. **11**(2): 123–133.

British Medical Association Board of Science (2005) *Healthcare in a Rural Setting*. London: BMA.

Bryant L (1999) The detraditionalisation of occupational identities in farming in South Australia. *Sociologia Ruralis*. **39**: 236–261.

Buchan T and Deaville J (2005) *Contemporary Rural Health Issues: intelligence from Wales and beyond*. Rural Health Research Report Series Issue 8.

Campbell H and Bell MM (2000) The question of rural masculinities. *Rural Sociology*. **65**(4): 532–546.

Cartmel F and Furlong A (2000) *Youth Unemployment in Rural Areas*. York: York Publishing.

Coldwell I (2006) *Traditional masculinities: obstacles in the turn towards sustainable farming practices*. In RJ Petheram and RC Johnson (eds), *Practice Change for Sustainable Communities: Exploring Footprints, Pathways and Possibilities*: APEN 2006 International Conference, Latrobe University, Beechworth, Victoria, Australia, 6–8 March 2006. Available at: www. regional.org.au/au/apen/2006.

Coldwell I (2007) New farming masculinities: 'more than just shit-kickers', we're 'switched-on' farmers wanting to 'balance lifestyle, sustainability and coin'. *J Sociology*. **43**(1): 87–103.

Commission for Rural Communities (2005) *Rural Proofing Report 2004–2005*. London:

Commission for Rural Communities.

Countryside Agency (2004) Rural and Urban Area Classification 2004: An Introductory Guide. Available at www.defra.gov.uk/evidence/statistics/rural/documents/rural-defn/Rural_ Urban_Introductory_Guide.pdf (Accessed 29 September 2009).

Craig G, Manthorpe J (2000) *Social Care in Rural Areas: developing an agenda for research, policy and practice*. Joseph Rowntree Foundation.

Davies P, Deaville J and Randell-Smith J (2008) *Health in Rural Wales: a research report to support the development of the Rural Health Plan for Wales*. Institute of Rural Health. Available at: www.irh.ac.uk/pdfs/publications/RuralHealthPlanFullVersion.pdf (Accessed 29 September 2009).

Defra (2004) *Rural Strategy*. London: Defra.

Defra (2005) *The State of the Countryside 2005*. London: Defra.

Department of Health (2004) *Choose & Book – Patients Choice of Hospital and Booked Appointment*. London: DH.

Evans R (2000) *You questioning my manhood, boy? Masculine identity, work performance and performativity in a rural staples economy*. The Arkleton Centre for Rural Development Research, Arkleton Research Paper, Number 4, Scotland: University of Aberdeen.

Gerrard CE (1998) Farmers' occupational health: cause for concern, cause for action. *J Advanced Learning*. **27**: 683–691.

Gregoire A (2002) The mental health of farmers. *Occupational Medicine*. **52**(8): 471–476.

Gregoire A and Thornicroft G (1998) Rural mental health. *Psychiatric Bulletin*. **22**: 273–277.

Hastings S (2004) Homophobia. *Times Educational Supplement*, 28 May, pp. 11–14.

Hawton K, Simkin S and Malmberg A (1998) *Suicide and Stress in Farmers*. London: The Stationary Office.

Health and Safety Executive (2000) *Medical aspects of work-related exposure to organophosphates*, MS17 Medical Guidance Note for doctors and other health care professionals. HSE.

Hill B (2003) *Rural Data and Rural Statistics*. Swindon: Economic and Social Research Council.

Hill SA, Pritchard C, Laugharne R and Gunnell D (2005) Changing patterns of suicide in a poor, rural county over the 20th century: a comparison with national trends. *Social Psychiatry and Psychiatric Epidemiology*. **40**: 601–604.

Judd F, Jackson H, Komiti A, Murray C, Fraser A, Greave A and Gomez R (2006) Help-seeking by rural residents for mental health problems: the importance of agrarian values. *Aus and NZ J Psychiatry*. **40**(9): 769–776.

Judd F, Jackson H, Fraser C, Murray G, Robins G and Komiti A (2006a) Understanding suicide in Australian farmers. *Social Psychiatry and Psychiatric Epidemiology*. **41**: 1–10.

Kilmartin C (2005) Depression in men: communication, diagnosis and therapy. *J Men's Health and Gender*. **2**(1): 95–9.

Levin KA and Leyland AH (2005) Urban/rural inequalities in suicide in Scotland 1981–1999. *Social Science & Medicine*. **60**: 2877–2890.

Liepins R (2000) Making men: the constructions and representation of agriculture-based masculinities in Australia and New Zealand. *Rural Sociology*. **65**(4): 605–620.

Little J (2002) Rural geography: rural gender identity and the performance of masculinity and femininity in the countryside. *Progress in Human Geography*. **26**(5): 665–370.

Little J (2003) Riding the rural love train: heterosexuality and the rural community. *Sociologia*

Ruralis. **43**(4): 401–417.

Lobley M, Johnson G, Reed M, Winter M and Little J (2004) *Rural Stress Review: Research Report No.7.* Exeter: Centre for Rural Research, University of Exeter.

McCreadie RG, Leese M and Tiak-Singh D (1997) Nithsdale, Nunhead and Norwood: similarities and differences in prevalence of schizophrenia and utilisation of services in rural and urban areas. *Br J Psychiatry.* **170**: 31–36.

Meltzer H, Gill B and Petticrew M (1995) *The prevalence of psychiatric morbidity among adults living in private households.* London: Office of Population Censuses and Surveys.

Mesurier N (2004) *Older People's Involvement in Rural Communities.* London: Age Concern.

Middleton N, Gunnell D, Frankel S, Whitley E and Dorling D (2003) Urban-rural differences in suicide trends in young adults: England and Wales, 1981–1998. *Social Science & Medicine* **57**: 1183–1194.

Mind (2003) *Rural Policy Toolkit.* London: Mind.

Mind (2005) *Access all Ages.* London: Mind.

Mind (2009) *Men and Mental Health: get it off your chest.* London: Mind.

Mind Cymru (2008) *More Than a Number: A study into young people's experiences of mental health services in Wales.* Big Lottery Fund. Available at: www.biglotteryfund.org.uk/er_res_morethannumber-full.pdf (Accessed 30 September 2009).

Myhill S (2003) *Organophosphate Poisoning: systems and treatment.* Available at: www.drmyhill.co.uk/article.cfm?id=291 (Accessed 29 September 2009).

Ni Laoire C (2001) A matter of life and death? Men, masculinities and staying behind in rural Ireland. *Sociologia Ruralis.* **41**(2): 220–236.

Paykel ES, Abbott R, Jenkins R, Brugha TS and Meltzer H (2000) Urban-rural mental health differences in Great Britain: findings from the National Morbidity Survey. *Psychol Med.* **30**(2): 269–280.

Peck DF, Grant S, McArthur W and Godden D (2002) Psychological impact of foot and mouth disease on farmers. *J Mental Health.* **11**(5): 523–531.

Raine G (1999) Causes and effects of stress on farmers: a qualitative study. *Health Education J.* **58**(3): 259–270.

Ross MW (1990) The relationship between life events and mental health in homosexual men. *J Clinical Psychology.* **46**(4): 402–411.

Rugg J and Jones A (1999) *Getting a job, finding a home: rural youth transitions.* Bristol: Policy Press.

Shucksmith M (2003) *Social Exclusion in Rural Areas: a review of recent research.* Aberdeen: Arkleton Centre.

Shucksmith M (2004) Young people and social exclusion in rural areas. *Sociologia Ruralis.* **44**(1): 43–59.

Sherlock J (1994) *Through the Rural Magnifying Glass.* London: Good Practices in Mental Health.

Stark C, Gibbs D, Hopkins P, Belbin A, Hay A and Selvaraj S (2006) Suicide in farmers in Scotland. *Rural and Remote Health.* **6**(509): 1–9.

Storey P and Brannen J (2000) *Young people and transport in rural communities: access and opportunity.* York: York publishing services.

Swindlehurst H (2005) *Rural Proofing for Health: a toolkit for primary care organisations.*

Newtown, Wales: Institute of Rural Health.

Thomas HV, Lewis G, Thomas DR, Salmon RL, Chalmers RM, Coleman TJ, Kench SM, Morgan-Capner P, Meadows D, Sillis M and Softley P (2003) Mental health of British farmers. *Occupational and Environmental Medicine.* **60**: 181-185.

Weich S, Twigg l and Lewis G (2006) Rural/non-rural differences in rates of common mental disorders in Britain: prospective multilevel cohort study. *Br J Psychiatry.* **188**: 51–57.

CHAPTER 7

Fatherhood and mental health difficulties in the postnatal period

Svend Aage Madsen and Adrienne Burgess

INTRODUCTION

Traditionally, the literature addressing parental psychiatric disorders has reported only, or mainly, on mothers (e.g. Gopfert *et al.* 2004). This is becoming increasingly unacceptable as fathers' impact on their children (Jaffee *et al.* 2001; Flouri 2005; Sarkadi *et al.* 2008) and on their partner's mothering (Eiden and Leonard 1996; Guterman and Lee 2005) is now established. Furthermore, fathers and fathering are rising up public policy agendas for other important reasons, which include gender equity, mothers' participation in the paid workforce, fathers' increasing participation in the direct care of children and the design of parental leave systems; concerns about teenage pregnancy, anti-social behaviour and boys' underachievement; awareness of the impact of the quality of the parental relationship and of the parenting alliance on children's adjustment, as well as the related issues of child support and father-child contact after separation and divorce.

The perinatal period has been described as the 'golden opportunity moment' for intervention with fathers (Cowan 1988). During this transition almost all fathers are in touch with services (Kiernan and Smith 2003; TNS System Three 2005) and most parents are still in a close relationship – in England 90% are married, cohabiting or regard themselves as 'a couple who live separately' at the time of their baby's birth (Kiernan and Smith 2003); and most of the rest are in contact and remain so for some time afterward (Dex and Ward 2007).

In women, emotional distress in the post-natal period has been well studied. Usually, however, post-natal/post-partum depression in mothers is now defined as a measurable non-psychotic depression linked to adjustment to becoming a parent and developing attachment to the infant(s). The incidence for women of post-partum depression is 10–14% measured with the Edinburgh Post-natal Depression Scale (EPDS) (Cox *et al.* 1982; 2003). From work supporting fathers at hospital

(Madsen 2009) and in other settings, it has become clear that, as with mothers, the processes of becoming a parent and developing attachment to an infant can render males vulnerable to developing depression (Madsen 1996). This is why both men and women can suffer from post-natal/post-partum depression.

An increasing number of researchers are studying men's psychological reactions to fatherhood, including pre-natally (Fletcher *et al.* 2008) and post-natally (Condon *et al.* 2004; Deater-Deckard *et al.* 1998; Goodman 2004; Matthey *et al.* 2001). During 2005 a study was conducted in Denmark at Rigshospitalet (Copenhagen University Hospital) (Madsen and Juhl 2007) which explored not only the incidence of traditional symptoms of depression, as represented in the EPDS, but also the incidence of the so-called male symptoms of depression, labelled 'male depressive syndrome' by Winkler and colleagues (2005) and 'masked depression' by Cochran and Rabinowitz (2000). The conditions indicated in this are: outbursts of anger, emotional rigidity, exaggerated self-criticism, alcohol and drug abuse, withdrawal from relationships, over-involvement in work, denial of pain and rigid demands for autonomy. Among others, Walinder and Rutz (2001), Winkler and colleagues (2004), Cochran and Rabinowitz (2000) and Piccinelli and Wilkinson (2000) have found that the incidence of such symptoms is greater for men. The Danish study used the only existing validated scale at the time, the Gotland Male Depression Scale (GMDS) (Rutz *et al.* 2002) in combination with the EPDS (*see* Box 7.1).

When the findings from the two scales were combined, approximately 7% of new fathers were found to have post-partum depression (Madsen and Juhl 2007). These included both first-time fathers and men who had previously had children. This was the first time that 'male symptoms' had been included in assessing post-partum depression. The 5% prevalence rate for men's post-partum depression found in this study from the application of EPDS alone (with its traditionally accepted symptoms of depression) very much accords with Matthey and colleagues' (2001) validation study. Including the GMDS with its male depression symptoms detected a further 2% of men, with the overall prevalence rate still within the range established in earlier studies using only the EPDS. However, this study found that among the 5% of the participants scoring above cut-off on the EPDS, 40.7% of the men also scored above cut-off on the GMDS while 20.6% of the at-risk men had a score above cut-off only on the 'male symptoms' and a score under cut-off on the 'traditional' symptoms of depression. Thus, a considerable number were detected only with the male symptoms scale. Consideration of male depression symptoms when investigating men for post-partum depression would therefore seem to be important. The findings of this study accord with the hypothesis of male-specific symptoms and indicate that among non-clinical samples of men more individuals with depression, including post-partum depression, will be identified by using assessments which include male-specific symptoms.*

---

* In the UK, a draft assessment tool to review the emotional health of fathers in the post-natal period which builds extensively on a framework of ante and post-natal interviews with mothers (Davis *et al.* 2000), has been developed by the Fatherhood Institute and Surrey Parenting Education and Support. Funding is not yet available to validate the tool. www.dcsf.gov.uk/everychildmatters/strategy/parents/pip/PIPrkfatherinclusiveservices/PIPfatherinclusiveservices/

BOX 7.1

EPDS ('traditional' depression):

> ➤ unable to laugh or see funny side of things

> ➤ cannot look forward with enjoyment to things

> ➤ blamed myself unnecessarily when things went wrong

> ➤ have been anxious or worried for no good reason

> ➤ have felt scared or panicky for no good reason

> ➤ felt things have been getting on top of me

> ➤ have been so unhappy that i have had difficulty sleeping

> ➤ cried because i was unhappy

> ➤ had thoughts of hurting myself.

The Gotland scale ('male' depression):

> ➤ lower stress threshold/more stressed

> ➤ aggressive, acting out, difficulty with self-control

> ➤ burnout and emptiness

> ➤ unexplainable fatigue

> ➤ irritable, restless and frustrated

> ➤ difficulty in making everyday decisions

> ➤ sleeping too much/too little/restlessly

> ➤ difficulty in falling asleep/waking early

> ➤ feelings of unrest/anxiety/discomfort

> ➤ excessive consumption of alcohol and pills

> ➤ hyperactive/works hard and is restless, jogs, etc.

> ➤ behaviour changed so you are difficult to deal with

> ➤ feel yourself/others regard you as gloomy, negative

> ➤ feel yourself/others see you as self-pitying, complaining.

The finding that around 7% of men are at risk of post-partum depression is important, as very little attention has been paid to this problem in health services or among health professionals. There are at present approximately 65 000 births every year in Denmark. Nationally this suggests that about 4500 fathers annually suffer from post-partum depression. There are strong reasons to believe that the incidence of post-partum depression in men will be at the same level in most countries. In

England and Wales, where approximately 700 000 births are registered each year, the figure for male post-partum depression is therefore likely to be about 49 000 individuals. Very few of the affected men in either Denmark or the UK are identified or receive professional support or treatment, despite the importance of locating and supporting men who require help during such a vulnerable period in their own life – and in the lives of their children and their children's mothers.

In evaluating these results it is important to take into consideration that just as research on women's post-partum depression took a long time to become established, research into men's post-partum depression still has a long way to go until there is agreement on definitions and until usable scales have been developed and validated. It is especially important to be able to identify different kinds of depression among men who become fathers and clear correlates, as families tend to suffer from multiple stressors at this time which may independently cause, or contribute to, a negative emotional state. Partner factors have substantial impact on mothers' depression (see Fisher *et al.* 2006) and fathers' depression puts the quality of the relationship between the parents at risk (Phares 1997). Moreover, as shown by such researchers as Ramchandani and colleagues (2005; 2008), Paulson and colleagues (2006; 2007) and Huang and Warner (2005), fathers' depression (like mothers') tends to limit their ability to parent effectively and children (particularly sons) of fathers with post-partum depression may exhibit emotional and behavioral problems which can still be in evidence, or be impacting on their functioning, many years later.

Future research should focus on the development of more exact assessments of the male-specific symptoms of both general and post-partum depression. One goal should be the development of screening instruments that can assess both men and women with post-partum depression, since 'male symptoms' may occur in women and many men exhibit 'traditional' symptoms of depression. Although there is a need for further research, it has been shown that it is possible to identify men with post-partum depression using the two scales mentioned here. The use of both of these scales is therefore recommended in work with fathers of newborns. Where possible depression is identified the father should be referred to a mental health specialist.

MEN'S EXPERIENCES OF POSTPARTUM DEPRESSION

By 2009 more than 150 fathers and expectant fathers suffering from depression had received psychotherapeutic intervention at Copenhagen University Hospital. The fathers are referred to the clinic before, during and after childbirth. The distribution of these referrals is approximately 25% during pregnancy/fertility treatment, 25% at the time of the birth and during the first four weeks, and the remaining 50% more than one month after birth. From this therapeutic work (Madsen 2009) and with the background knowledge from the Fatherhood Research Programme (Madsen *et al.* 2002), the following symptoms have been identified:

➤ withdrawal
➤ feelings of abandonment in relation to own parents
➤ difficulties in the relationship with the infant and with attachment;

➤ major problems in the couple relationship, often associated with aggressive behaviour
➤ anger
➤ confusion about what it means to be a father and a man.

Other researchers have reported the following correlations with male postpartum depression:
➤ a general lack of support, with the quality of the couple relationship including disagreement about the pregnancy and perceived lack of supportiveness from the mother particularly central (Huang and Warner 2005; Dudley *et al.* 2001; Matthey *et al.* 2000)
➤ infant-related problems (Dudley *et al.* 2001)
➤ the father's neuroticism and substance abuse/dependence (Huang and Warner 2005)
➤ the mother's personality difficulties, unresolved past events in her life and her current mental health status (Huang and Warner 2005), most particularly her depression. A review of 20 research studies found 24–50% of new fathers with depressed partners affected by depression themselves (Goodman 2004).*

It is worth noting that, like young mothers, young fathers are likely to be particularly vulnerable to depression in the postnatal period, seemingly due to interacting factors. For example, in a low-income African American sample, 56% of new (young) fathers were found to have 'depressive symptoms indicating cause for clinical concern'. Correlates included resource challenges, transportation and permanent housing difficulties, problems with alcohol and drugs, health problems/disability and a criminal conviction history (Anderson *et al.* 2005). While these factors are not uniquely symptomatic of the relational disorder described in the Danish model, they might influence its development. Similar factors are found as correlates with postnatal depression in mothers. Interacting factors and selection effects would seem to explain this in part, but the circumstances of the pregnancy might also be relevant, as may difficulties seeing or maintaining contact with the child. Rates of paternal depression in one recent US study were 6.6% (married fathers), 8.7% (cohabiting), 11.9% (romantically involved but not living together); and among the fathers who were described as 'not involved' with the mother, 19.9% were depressed (Huang and Warner 2005).

---

* A recent study not only recorded more depressive symptoms among such men, but also more aggression and non-specific psychological impairment, as well as higher rates of depressive disorder, non-specific psychological problems and problem fatigue. New fathers whose partners were depressed were also more likely to have three or more co-morbid psychological disturbances. On measures of anxiety and alcohol use there was no difference between men whose partners were depressed and men whose partners weren't (Roberts *et al.* 2006).

TREATING MEN WITH POSTPARTUM DEPRESSION

In the psychotherapeutic treatment of men with post-partum depression, the Danish experience suggests that there are two key issues to address simultaneously. The first, as in all treatments for emotional distress, is to look at improving the depressed father's mood. The extent to which this is being achieved can be measured, for example, by the absence of symptoms in EPDS and GMDS. The second important issue involves the man's relationship with his infant(s) and his perceptions of fatherhood. Post-partum depression is a relational disorder, that is to say it concerns a relational situation (parenthood and attachment to the child) and is rooted in relational psychological material (one's own experiences of care and attachment while growing up and currently). Psychotherapeutic treatment must be attentive to both these issues and results should be measured in both areas. Where partner factors are significant, the couple relationship and/or the mother's mental health and the father's experience of this, should also be addressed.

As shown by Madsen (2009), a mentalisation[*] approach (Allen *et al.* 2008) in working psychotherapeutically with men suffering from post-partum depression is indicated in the following four areas:
➤ working with the men's states of anger and withdrawal
➤ a 'two-pronged approach' which draws together the man's past and present relationships with caregivers and his current situation as his infant's caregiver;
➤ the man's ambivalence about attachment/independence
➤ the man's images of masculinity brought face to face with the child's need for care.

Given the co-occurrence in male postpartum depression of maternal depression and of issues such as resource challenges mentioned earlier identified by researchers engaging with perhaps more challenging samples, practical support and referral of the man and/or his partner to other services may also be indicated.

In the absence of a universal screening programme for post-partum depression in men, it would seem at the very least that professionals should be made aware of its correlates. A checklist, which would contain the key factors listed above, as well as other known correlates, such as previous mental health disorders, multiple births or hostility by the father towards the pregnancy, may help professionals identify at-risk men before the births of their children and use scarce resources to best effect.

Since, in Denmark, it is only two years since the first scientific article on the prevalence of post-partum depression in men was published (Madsen and Juhl 2007), interventions in that country are sparse. Indeed, throughout the world there are few systemised interventions which have sought to treat men with this disorder and evaluations of processes and outcomes in treatment have yet to be carried out. In the UK, a local hospital briefly set up a post-natal depression helpline for men, but funding for this was not sustained and the intervention was not evaluated. Also, Britain's

---

[*] 'Mentalisation' refers to the ability to recognise one's own and others' mental states, and to see these mental states as separate from behaviour.

Association for Post-natal Illness (www.apni.org), which provides a helpline, does not acknowledge the existence of post-natal depression in males, refusing calls from them or from individuals phoning on their behalf.

Given the paucity of evidence relating to effective treatments, the recommendations from the psychotherapeutic treatment model presented here have limitations. They are, however, consonant with the most recent research concerning men and depression in general (Cochran 2005; Winkler *et al.* 2006); men and psychotherapy in general (Pollack and Levant 1998; Good and Brooks 2005); the understanding of parent-child relationships, especially attachment; and the concept of mentalisation therapy. Furthermore, the understanding of the psychological dynamics of fatherhood (which forms the basis for the understanding of psychological disturbances in fatherhood) upon which the Danish model is based is solidly scientifically anchored (Madsen *et al.* 2002). There is, therefore, theoretically, experimentally and clinically-good justification for the suggested treatment model for fathers with post-natal depression.

REFERENCES

Allen J, Fonagy P and Bateman A (2008) *Mentalizing in Clinical Practice*. Arlington: American Psychiatric Publishing.

Anderson EA, Kohler JK and Letiecq BL (2005) Predictors of depression among low-income, nonresidential fathers. *J Family Issues*. **26**(5): 547–567.

Cochran S (2005) Assessing and treating depression in men. In G Good and G Brooks (eds), *The New Handbook of Psychotherapy and Counseling with Men*. San Francisco: Wiley, pp. 229–245.

Cochran S and Rabinowitz F (2000) *Men and Depression: clinical and empirical perspectives*. San Diego, California: Academic Press.

Condon JT, Boyce P and Corkindale CJ (2004) The First-Time Fathers Study: a prospective study of the mental health and well-being of men during the transition to parenthood. *Aust N Z J Psychiatry*. **38**: 56–64.

Cowan PA (1988) Becoming a father: a time of change, an opportunity for development. In P Bronstein and CP Cowan (eds), *Fatherhood Today: men's changing role in the family*. New York: Wiley, pp. 13–35.

Cox J and Holden J (2003) *Perinatal Mental Health: A guide to the Edinburgh Postnatal Depression Scale*. London: Gaskell.

Cox JL, Connor Y and Kendell RE (1982) Prospective study of the psychiatric disorders of childbirth. *Br J Psychiatry*. **140**: 111–117.

Davis H, Cox A, Day C, Roberts R, Loxton R, Ispanovic-Radojkovic V, Tsiantis J, Layiou-Lignos E, Puura K, Tamminen T, Turunen M, Paradisiotou A, Hadjipanayi Y and Pandeli P (eds) (2000) *Primary Health Care Worker Training Manual*. Belgrade: Institute of Mental Health.

Deater-Deckard K, Pickering K, Dunn JF and Golding J (1998) Family structure and depressive symptoms in men preceding and following the birth of a child. *Am J Psychiatry*. **155**(6): 818–823.

Dex S and Ward K (2007) *Parental care and employment in early childhood*. Analysis of the

Millennium Cohort Study (MCS) Sweeps 1 and 2. London: Equal Opportunities Commission.

Dudley M, Roy K, Kelk N and Bernard D (2001) Psychological correlates of depression in fathers and mothers in the first postnatal year. *J Reproductive and Infant Psychology.* **19**(3): 187–202.

Eiden RD and Leonard KE (1996) Paternal alcohol use and the mother-infant relationship. *Development & Psychopathology.* **8**: 307–323.

Fisher JRW, Cabral de Mello M, Patel V and Rahman A (2006) Maternal depression and newborn health. Newsletter for the Partnership of Maternal, Newborn & Child Health. **2**: 13. Available at www.who.int/pmnch/media/lives/lives_newsletter_2006_2_english.pdf (Accessed 20 September 2009).

Fletcher R, Vimpani G, Russell G and Sibritt D (2008) Psychosocial assessment of expectant fathers. *Archives of Women's Mental Health.* **11**(1): 27–32.

Flouri E (2005) *Fathering and Child Outcomes.* Chichester, West Sussex: John Wiley & Sons.

Good G and Brooks G (2005) *The New Handbook of Psychotherapy and Counselling with Men.* San Francisco: Jossey-Bass.

Goodman J (2004) Correlates of postnatal depression in mothers and fathers. *J Advanced Nursing.* **45**(1): 26–35.

Goodman JH (2004) Paternal postpartum depression, its relationship to maternal postpartum depression, and implications for family health. *J Advanced Nursing.* **45**(1): 26–35.

Gopfert M, Webster J and Seeman MV (eds.) (2004) *Parental Psychiatric Disorder: distressed parents and their families* (2nd ed). Cambridge: Cambridge University Press.

Guterman NB and Lee Y (2005) The role of fathers in risk for physical child abuse and neglect: possible pathways and unanswered questions. *Child Maltreatment.* **10**(2): 136–149.

Huang CC and Warner LA (2005) Relationship characteristics & depression among fathers with newborns. *Social Service Review.* **79**: 95–118.

Jaffee SR, Caspi A, Moffitt TE, Taylor A and Dickson N (2001) Predicting early fatherhood and whether young fathers live with their children: prospective findings and policy reconsiderations. *J Child Psychology and Psychiatry.* **42**: 803–815.

Kiernan K and Smith K (2003) Unmarried parenthood: new insights from the Millennium Cohort Study. *Population Trends.* **114**: 23–33.

Madsen SA (1996) *Bånd der Brister – Bånd der Knyttes* [Breaking bonds – Tying bonds). Copenhagen: Hans Reitzels Forlag.

Madsen SA and Juhl T (2007) Paternal depression in the postnatal period. *J Men's Health & Gender.* **4**(1): 26–31.

Madsen SA, Lind D and Munck H (2002) *Fædres Tilknytning til Spædbørn* [Fathers' Attachment to Infants). Copenhagen: Hans Reitzels Forlag.

Madsen SA (2009) Men's mental health: fatherhood and psychotherapy. *J Men's Studies.* **17**(1): 15–30.

Matthey S, Barnett B, Ungerer J and Waters B (2000) Paternal and maternal depressed mood during the transition to parenthood. *J Affective Disorders.* **60**: 75–85.

Matthey S, Barnett B, Kavanagh DJ and Howie P (2001) Validation of the Edinburgh Postnatal Depression Scale for men and comparison of item endorsement with their partners. *J Affective Disorders.* **64**: 175–184.

Paulson J, Dauber S and Leiferman J (2006) Individual and combined effects of postpartum depression in mothers and fathers on parenting behaviour. *Pediatrics*. **118**: 659–668.

Paulson JF, Keefe HA and Leiferman JA (2007) *Negative effects of maternal and paternal depression on early language*. Paper presented at the 2007 Annual Conference of the American Psychological Association.

Phares V (1997) Psychological adjustment, maladjustment and father-child relationships. In ME Lamb (ed.), *The Role of the Father in Child Development* (3rd ed.). New York: Wiley, pp. 261–283

Piccinelli M and Wilkinson G (2000) Gender differences in depression. Critical review. *Br J Psychiatry*, **111**: 486–492.

Pollack W and Levant R (1998) *New Psychotherapy for Men*. NY: Wiely.

Ramchandani P, Stein A, Evans J and O'Connor T (2005) Paternal depression in the postnatal period and child development: A prospective population study. *Lancet*. **365**: 2201–2205.

Ramchandani PG and Stein A (2008) Depression in men in the postnatal period and later child psychopathology: a population cohort study. *J American Academy of Child Adolescent Psychiatry*. **47**(4): 390–398.

Roberts SL, Bushnell JA, Collings SC and Purdie GL (2006) Psychological health of men with partners who have post-partum depression. *Aus and NZ J Psychiatry*. **40**(8): 704–711.

Rutz W, Rihmer Z and Dalteg A (2002) The Gotland Scale for assessing male depression. *Nord J Psychiatry*. **56**(4): 265–71.

Sarkadi A, Kristiansson R, Oberklaid F and Bremberg S (2008) Fathers' involvement and children's developmental outcomes: a systematic review of longitudinal studies. *Acta Paediatrica*. **97**(2): 153–158.

TNS System Three (2005) *NHS Maternity Services Quantitative Research*. Edinburgh: TNS System Three.

Walinder J and Rutz W (2001) Male depression and suicide. *Int Clin Psychopharmacol*. 1(Supplement 2): 21–24.

Winkler D, Pjrek E and Heiden A (2004) Gender differences in the psychopathology of depressed inpatients. *European Archives of Psychiatry and Clinical Neuroscience*. **254**(4): 209–214.

Winkler D, Pjrek E and Kasper S (2005) Anger attacks in depression – evidence for a male depressive syndrome. *Psychotherapy and Psychosomatics*. **74**: 303–307.

Winkler D, Pjrek E and Kasper S (2006) Gender-specific symptoms of depression and anger attacks. *J Men's Health and Gender*. **3**: 19–24.

CHAPTER 8

Marketing masculinities: a social marketing approach to promoting men's mental health

Paul Hopkins and Jeremy Voaden

'SOCIAL MARKETING'?

Can brotherhood be sold like soap? The psychologist GD Wiebe sought an answer to this question as long ago as 1951. His evaluation of four social change campaigns concluded that commercial marketing had much to offer behavioural change interventions.

The phrase 'social marketing' and the application of its theoretical frameworks to practice have become increasingly familiar to people working in public health during the last decade. However, among some practitioners in disciplines involved in work with men social marketing has been seen to be associated with images of social engineering, advertising, a lack of honesty and integrity, 'the nanny state', 'big business' and 'big brother'. As a consequence, it is perceived as lacking ethical validity. But what does social marketing mean? What place does it have in the delivery of mental health work with men? How have social marketing theoretical frameworks informed current practice? How can we apply it to our future practice?

Social marketing is not a new concept. The term 'social marketing' was first used by Kotler and Zaltman in 1971 to describe 'the systematic application of marketing concepts and techniques to achieve specific behavioural goals relevant to a social good'. Health-related social marketing is the systemic application of marketing concepts and techniques to achieve specific behavioural goals to improve health and reduce health inequalities. Social marketing thinking has informed health-related behavioural change interventions for a decade in the US, Australia and Canada.

In the UK, strategic endorsement was demonstrated in the Department of Health White Paper Choosing Health (DH 2004). This highlighted social marketing as an important and under-utilised approach with potential to enhance and make a significant contribution to both national and local work. In Scotland, NHS Health Scotland and the Scottish Executive commissioned the Institute of Social Marketing at Stirling University* to undertake research aimed at developing a more sophisticated understanding of previous achievements in marketing and communications on health improvement and reducing inequalities. This was carried out with a view to developing an integrated marketing strategy for health improvement and published as Research to Inform the Development of a Social Marketing Strategy for Health Improvement in Scotland. It concluded that health improvement needed to shift its focus to the consumer: 'to move away from unexciting piecemeal propositions – eat less fat, walk more – to an aspirational vision selling satisfied and healthy lives, integrating physical health with mental and emotional well-being' (Stead *et al.* 2007: 4).

HOW DOES SOCIAL MARKETING WORK?

Social marketing works by directly tailoring interventions to a particular audience; it is not a theory in itself. Social marketing integrates public health, health promotion, and health communication's practice and is inclusive of a wide range of theories – biology, psychology, sociology, anthropology and environment and ecology (MacFadyen *et al.* 2003). It enables the targeting of identified populations with initiatives designed to affect health-behavioural change, but goes beyond targeting approaches based on epidemiology or demographics to incorporate a deeper understanding of how people react to issues and what motivates their behaviours. It enables people to take control rather than act as passive recipients. In a practical sense, social marketing segments populations or cultures so that marketing theory can then be applied to that population, or segment, using the marketing techniques most likely to succeed with that segment.

Social marketing is based on a commercial marketing concept called the 4 'P's; these are:

➤ *Product:* The information, service, physical or emotional product you wish to deliver, that may effect behavioural change. What are you offering the potential consumer that will persuade them to invest in it?

➤ *Price:* The financial, physical, emotional or social cost of the product. What must the segment of the population you are aiming the product at do to engage and invest in it? If the cost is likely to be too high, whether financially, socially, culturally or emotionally, then members of the segment may be deterred from engaging with it.

➤ *Place:* Where will the product that will effect behavioural change be delivered? Key opportunities involve securing the most effective distribution, accessibility and appropriate outlets for the delivery of the product. How accessible is the product to the population you wish to engage with?

---

* www.ism.stir.ac.uk

➤ *Promotion:* How is the product delivered? Methods used include advertising, public relations, promotions, media, entertainment, personal selling; what are the familiar vehicles that the segment of the population is comfortable with and responds to that will provide an incentive for the consumer to engage?

Social marketing has built on the commercial marketing approach and added other 'P's; these include:

➤ *Participation:* The input a target audience has in the development and implementation of an intervention; if the product is not wanted by its intended user and has not been tested with them it will be of little value to the 'producer' or to the intended user.

➤ *Policy:* A shared and clearly understood aspirational vision is required and this needs to be underpinned by national, regional and local strategic commitment. Strategic timeframes can be generational and require long-term political endorsement.

➤ *Partnerships:* The evidence is clear that single initiatives do not result in sustained behavioural change. Work with partners must focus on monitoring and achieving outcomes, but we must not lose sight of the importance of the process. The process of partnership work is the glue that holds the work together.

➤ *Purse-strings:* Strategic commitment requires funding to fuel the operational engine!

The application of these in the design of a health intervention creates a 'marketing mix'. To apply social marketing to initiate behavioural change around men's health issues, consideration of a mix of theories and methodologies appropriate to this segment of people is required. People are the most significant 'P' of all.

GENDER SENSITIVITY: MASCULINITIES AND MASCULINE CULTURAL SEGMENTS

Gender sensitivity provides a starting point for the development of a social marketing initiative with men. In health terms, this is a recognition that the manner in which men experience their health, the concept of 'health' and healthcare systems, the way in which men react to healthcare, how their needs are met and how they respond to health information, can be different to that experienced by women. If we consider a gender sensitive approach to work with men, then it is also vital that within a gender sensitive context we recognise that all men are not the same. In recognising this, heed must be taken of the concept of 'masculinities' – that there is not one defined masculinity but that there are many masculinities.

The concept of masculinities arises from Marxist Feminist theory. Being aware of 'what works' with men can create awareness of a schism in critical theory in the field of work with men. The Marxist Feminist camp considers masculinity as a social construction via a critique of gender power relations. They argue that each masculinity is seeking a dominant or 'hegemonic' position over other masculinities. The 'men's studies' camp (Lohan 2007) maintains that there are physiological and psychological explanations for men's actions. For practitioners, the debate may be intellectually stimulating and useful for our own 'internal supervision' and reflective practice. However, the polarisation of political thinking and the expectation that the practitioner will adhere to one camp or the other, with resultant consequences for any health-related activity, ultimately means a loss of focus on the customer. Practitioners need to deal with the situation as they find it, not debate the casus belli. Practitioners need to make use of 'what works'.

Social marketing provides a framework with which to piece together theoretical approaches from different disciplines in order to initiate practical behavioural change; it is a strength of social marketing that it is accepting and inclusive of many theoretical approaches and disciplines. The inclusion of the concept of different and diverse masculinities thus provides a basis for segmentation of masculinities and the application of a social marketing approach to health improvement work with men. From some theoretical perspectives, it may appear simplistic to identify specific male cultures; from a social marketing perspective, recognition that men of different cultural backgrounds have different experiences of masculinity – that being a man means different things to different men, in different cultures, that there are many different masculinities – allows for the proposal of segmentation into masculine cultural groups or segments.

Case study: MEN-tal

Some boys can't talk about it – this is why musicians are so successful. They articulate it for them – films and music. So many people get so shy and nervous when it comes to their problems. There shouldn't be one path only set out for you – then you feel a failure. There should be different paths you could try.

18-year-old man – Samaritans report *Young Men Speak Out* (Katz 1999)

The Gloucestershire Boys and Young Men Network (www.gbymn.org.uk) is a multi-agency network formed in 2001 to develop coordinated responses to address the needs of boys and young men. A significant early concern for the Network was the vulnerable emotional health of young men. Specifically, the Network identified the lack of culturally appropriate resources to encourage young men to consider aspects of their own emotional health, take positive steps to improve it, build resilience and signpost to mental health promoting services and opportunities. The strategic context for this focus included the National Service Framework for Mental Health (Department of Health 1999) with its Standard One requirement for a local mental health promotion strategy and the National Suicide Prevention Strategy for England (Department of Health 2002). This unmet need led to work on the MEN-tal initiative by the Network.

MEN-tal is a comic-book style resource aimed at a defined masculine cultural segment. These were young men who were remote from the mainstream, who were considered by some as 'hard-to-reach', but who had their own sub-cultural media, language and terminology. A team of Network members drawn from the county youth service, Primary Care Trusts (including school nurses and health promotion professionals) and the Mental Health Trust established a partnership with the Gloucestershire Association of Mental Health to develop the resource.

In order to establish 'what worked' with the young men whose behaviour we wanted to influence, a Network youth worker developed a working relationship with a group of young men to identify their concerns and issues with them. The chosen method of communication was to be a comic book. Fanzines and comics, as means of sub-cultural expression associated with youth cultures, provide an 'authentic' media with which ideas and messages can be conveyed to young men.

A cartoon narrative with positive and negative outcomes of risk-taking behaviours for the characters involved provided the main focus of the comic. Sections containing positive messages about realistic and segment-acceptable activities which young men could do to improve their mental health, along with information on websites, helplines and local mental health services, were threaded throughout its pages. A young comic book artist, of a similar age to the young men, was found via the internet to illustrate the comic. The artist's material was then piloted with the young men and the material adapted as the young men directed in order that it gave the best incentive for the target segment to engage with it.

Following piloting and subsequent printing of the resource (paid for via the partnership member organisations) the resulting product was then made available via youth services in the county, within Gloucester Prison (a male remand establishment) and the youth criminal justice infrastructure. Following work with the Military Men's Health Symposium, it was also distributed within the armed forces. Due to concerns expressed by Primary Care Trust management about some of the language used in the resource, the product was branded with the GBYMN logo rather than a statutory NHS one. Piloting with some young men had already identified the importance of a recognised and credible 'brand' and that an NHS logo may be a deterrent to engagement with a product as it is not deemed to be 'authentic'.

MEN-tal: applying the 4 'P's

Having ascertained the most effective approach to deliver information to the targeted masculine cultural segment, the 4 'P's of social marketing were then applied:

- *Product:* The product's purpose is to raise awareness of culturally acceptable and accessible things the targeted masculine cultural segment could do to improve their coping strategies around emotional concerns, build resilience and to signpost to services, via a culturally specific comic.

- *Price:* Will the resource give them a culturally acceptable incentive to consider behavioural change? In other words, is the behaviour change a price worth paying?

- *Place:* The comic is available via the local youth service, the youth criminal justice infrastructure and within HMP Gloucester. Future dissemination of MEN-tal resources will include outlets and environments specific to the masculine cultural segment; e.g. record and comic stores, clothing outlets, gigs, festivals.

- *Promotion:* Information is delivered to the targeted segment via application of the cultural codes, customs, idioms and media, i.e. via a micro-media comic – a medium popular with the masculine cultural segment.

MEN-tal had been considered as the umbrella term for a larger initiative around young men and mental health in Gloucestershire, but this was not realised due to financial and target-driven boundaries. If you are planning a social marketing campaign ensure you are working within your financial limits. Knowing your people is a priority, but retain a focus on your purse-strings.

SOCIAL MARKETING – THE EVIDENCE FOR PROMOTING THE MENTAL AND EMOTIONAL HEALTH OF MEN

Making It Possible: Improving Mental Health and Well-being in England (National Institute for Mental Health In England 2005) summarises the evidence base for the improvement of mental and emotional health. Good mental health, a valid outcome in itself, is linked with improved outcomes for relationships, parenting, employment, education and physical health. A systematic review of mental health interventions by the World Health Organization identified a wide range of evidence-based preventive programmes that have been found to reduce risk factors, strengthen protective factors and decrease psychiatric symptoms and the onset of some mental disorders (WHO 2004).

The key areas to target in addressing these risk and protective factors with boys and men include employment, workplace health, schools and education, nutrition, substance misuse, housing, parenting, relationships, spirituality and economic security. Following a review of the evidence of effectiveness, *Making It Possible* lists nine priorities for action, the first of which is 'marketing mental health and well-being'.

NHS Health Scotland commissioned Mental Health Improvement: evidence-based messages to promote mental well-being (Friedli *et al.* 2007). This concluded that there is good evidence to support the effectiveness of 'positive steps messages' for the promotion of positive mental health. These messages addressed the issues of keeping physically active; eating well; drinking alcohol in moderation; learning new skills; creativity; spirituality; relaxing; valuing yourself and others; talking about your feelings; social networks; caring; making a contribution and asking for help.

BEST PRACTICE IN SOCIAL MARKETING FOR MENTAL HEALTH PROMOTION WITH MEN

The following best practice criteria have been identified from a range of work looking at effective social marketing and communication initiatives with men (see Men's Health Forum 2002; Men's Health Forum 2006; Stead *et al.* 2007):

Participation and people

At the heart of all effective social marketing work promoting the mental health of boys and men is stakeholder involvement. Always start with the consumer.

The male target group should be properly defined. Research amongst the men that the initiative is targeted at is essential to provide insight into their perception of the defined problem, perceived benefits or barriers to behaviour change and opportunities for acceptable intervention methods. Professionals need to synthesise and take seriously what young men tell them about their beliefs, ideas and experiences of mental health.

Product

It is essential that there is a clear definition of the specific problem that the initiative is addressing. Clearly stated objectives provide a focus for activity planning and support effective evaluation. Social marketing allows for the selling of positive, aspirational 'can do' messages promoting resilience – developing skills and coping strategies, rather than focus on negative 'don't do that' messages that have been the focus of many previous initiatives.

Generic initiatives on a one-size-fits-all basis are not effective. Men are not a socially homogenous group. Class, culture, race and age are key factors that should inform the product. Younger men are more challenging to engage for mental health promoting organisations. More research is required with younger men to improve insight into their interests, cognitive capacities and frameworks and peer group cultures. Social disadvantage, including unemployment, crime, gang involvement, social isolation and poor housing conditions are important areas for future social marketing research.

Effective social marketing recognises male-specific indicators of mental health and mental distress. The product must speak to men as they are, not as we might wish them to be. Some men have to celebrate traditional positive badges of masculinity such as strength or 'facing the challenge' to maximise their mental health. Effective social marketing will maximise the potential of this badging. Alternative terms to 'mental health' such as 'well-being', 'stress management' or 'emotional health' are more effective in securing the engagement of men.

Price

Competition and conflicting messages must be identified in advance and addressed. For example, contacting a health professional about an emotional health issue might be seen as 'soft' and men may regard high levels of emotional stamina and stress tolerance within the workplace as a wholly positive attribute.

Some groups of men take a perverse pride in poor mental health and behaviours that promote it. Conversely, good mental health is perceived as conforming, boring or unexciting. Effective social marketing initiatives address these perceptions.

Place

Community-based locations, including youth centres, street work, pubs, cafes and youth-oriented services, are the most successful places for marketing with young men as their perceptions of statutory services are a significant barrier to their use as a marketing conduit.

Promotion

Credible branding of initiatives is essential to establish a long-term emotional connection with the consumer.

Partnerships

A marketing mix is required. An over-reliance on a 'campaign' delivered solely through communications is unlikely to result in sustained behaviour change. A joined-up approach is required locally.

Mental health promotion activity should be integrated into the everyday work of non-health service organisations such as Connexions, local authority leisure and community services, learning providers and workplaces.

Policy

Future policy developments should acknowledge the important role played by non-statutory and health-oriented organisations in promoting the mental health of men. Social marketing initiatives to promote mental health will take place within a wider context that influences individual and community ability to adopt positive behavioural changes. Social marketing is not a panacea and the achievement of mental health promoting objectives must be supported by national, regional and local strategic frameworks enabling access to physical activity, mental health promoting employment practice, affordable fresh food and adult learning opportunities. Social marketing needs political commitment to secure success in promoting the mental health of men.

Purse-strings

Sustained financial support is required if organisations (and in particular non-statutory organisations) are to maintain involvement. Securing behavioural change through effective social marketing initiatives can be generational.

PRACTICAL TIPS FOR MARKETING MESSAGES AT MEN

The following provides guidance on the application of social marketing principles to projects targeted at men:

➤ *Gender sensitivity and masculinities:* First, consider gender sensitivity in relation to men. In doing so, consider masculinities. All men are different, therefore consider which segment of masculinity (i.e. group of men) you wish to target your initiative at and ensure that your material is acceptable and accessible to this segment.

➤ *Research and piloting:* Research your segment. Work with members of the masculine cultural segment in order to establish an understanding of what will work with them. Pilot your material with them. Ask them about 'what works' and what language, terminology and culture they affiliate with. What will make it culturally easy for them to invest in your project and consider behavioural change? What is the price they have to pay? Will they pay it? Build these considerations into your project. Consider whether your organisation is best placed to work alongside and pilot material with masculine cultural groups. For example, it may be more appropriate for a youth worker who has established a rapport with a group of young men to pilot material. Alternatively, you may be fortunate enough to find men who wish to do this themselves or with members of their peer group. Understanding of the cultures that men inhabit is a prerequisite to a marketing initiative.

➤ *Don't be blinkered:* Look beyond your own field of work for examples of practice that have worked with the masculine cultural segment that you wish to work with. The Terence Higgins Trust publications on sexual health provide a good example of social marketing work with a masculine cultural segment of young gay men. The language and style of their publications mean that they are culturally acceptable to a specific segment and hence for that segment to invest in them; however, whilst some gay men engage with the publications, as with any masculine segment, others will not, hence it is important that you get your market research about 'what works' correct before you further develop an initiative.

The field of substance use also provides examples of a social marketing approach popular with some groups of young men, e.g. the Peanut Pete Lifeline Publications series and CALM, the Campaign Against Living Miserably, which applies social marketing to communicate with young men by harnessing youth, music and sports cultures (*see* Chapter 25).

An approach designed to appeal to another masculine cultural segment is that of the Haynes Men's Manuals, produced in association with the Men's Health Forum. The series includes a 'Brain Manual' (Banks 2006), which covers men and mental well-being, and is sold in branches of the car maintenance shop Halfords, as well as in bookstores and via the internet. The manuals are set out in a similar fashion to the well-known Haynes car manuals and are packed full of appropriate health information delivered in a humorous fashion. There has been some academic criticism of these manuals, pointing out that they are only speaking to one masculine cultural segment. This criticism, however, fails to recognise that this is the strength of the manuals and renders them an effective mechanism for securing behavioural change amongst a group of men traditionally regarded as hard to reach. Take a look at the media popular with your target group and consider adapting it to your own project. Thus the maintenance manual for a Ford Focus car informs a Brain Manual promoting emotional health.

➤ *Beyond boundaries:* While masculine cultural segments will differ on a global scale, don't dismiss interventions that have been successful in other countries. Ideas can be adapted. For example, the Gloucestershire Boys and Young Men Network publication MEN-tal drew inspiration from SPIN, a New Zealand comic-style resource produced to engage young men in discussion as part of a suicide prevention strategy. SPIN is available to download from the Suicide Prevention Information New Zealand website at www.spinz.org.nz

➤ *Authenticity:* The cultures of our target groups may be remote from the mainstream, yet they are authentic to our target masculine cultural segments. As professionals, both we, and our organisations, are likely to also be culturally remote from their lives. It may be easy to dismiss them as ephemeral or without meaning; yet to the men who inhabit these cultures they are authentic. It is important if you wish to engage with those labelled 'hard to reach' that you consider whether what you are doing in terms of media, messages and language used is authentic to the segment you have targeted.

Branding is paramount. A local authority or Connexions logo will not carry as much currency with some young men as, for example, logos associated with lifestyle statements, music, or endorsements by individuals and organisations popular with the segment. The credibility 'cost' of engaging in behavioural change associated with a non-authentic brand may be too great for the men concerned. The 'hard to reach' can be described as such because we are not using the correct marketing method to engage with them. No masculine cultural segment should be hard to reach if we get the 4 'P's right.

➤ *Ethics – your own:* We all have our own moral codes about what is acceptable and what is not. However, your ethical stance may not be the same as that of the masculine cultural segment that you are trying to reach. You may even be offended by the culture, the language or the humour that a segment uses. Whilst you would not wish to use or endorse oppressive or discriminatory language and behaviour, the mere fact that certain things may be offensive to you should not necessarily be a barrier to their use. Rather, their use as an effective social marketing tool for engagement should be assessed as part of a wider, holistic impact assessment. Understand where your segment is coming from. Is your social marketing initiative a health one, or a social engineering one?

➤ *Ethics – your organisation's:* Is your organisation ideally placed to deliver an initiative informed by social marketing principles with the masculine cultural segment you are targeting? If you work for a statutory organisation you may find that some masculine cultural segments identify more closely with 'authority' than others. It may be that the philosophy of your organisation does not condone aspects of the segment you wish to work with. There may be organisational challenges in the production and endorsement of specific media. For example, members of the Gloucestershire Boys and Young Men's Network were unable to obtain Primary Care Trust endorsement of a fanzine. A culturally specific website will not sit easily within a portal and one-size fits all template of a local authority website.

Consider other agencies in your local community who you may be able to work in partnership with to deliver your product. IT students in local education establishments, third sector organisations and umbrella networks and partnerships may be able to help. Is it possible to establish your initiative as a social enterprise and involve your target segment in establishing and running the organisation? The extent to which people are 'hard to reach' depends where you start from.

➤ *A community approach:* The success of a social marketing initiative will depend upon where your initiative is delivered. For example, if you're trying to reach a segment of young men that affiliate themselves with a distinct youth culture then your product will not only need to reflect the values of that culture and make use of the codes and idioms of that culture to deliver your message, it will also need the correct placement within that culture. Where does your segment gather? Festivals, gigs, raves, football matches, web-based locations, computer game road-shows, public spaces? You may also wish to establish a working relationship with someone from within the masculine cultural segment who is willing to promote your material and work with you to develop an emotional connection (Friedli *et al.* 2007) with your target audience – a community champion or inspirational figure that a segment affiliates itself with.

➤ *Media:* Establishing a communications pathway means using the media. Which media outlets does your masculine cultural segment affiliate with? Fanzines and comics, for example, are known media of sub-cultural expression with some young men. Football and rugby match-day programmes are popular collectors' items with men attending sports events; some programmes have community pages where you can place material. Don't dismiss opportunities – a regional gardening publication or parish magazine may provide an opportunity for engagement with a segment who may have no interest in communal events.

The internet is often quoted as being a source of information for many men. If you are designing a website ensure it connects with the segment you wish to work with in terms of access and acceptability, especially in terms of design. Web design can be financially expensive or prohibitive, therefore consider one of the many blogging platforms out there that are free to use and are popular with some male segments.

Statements, slogans and endorsements on clothing, badges and cultural paraphernalia (for example, skateboards or DJ-ing boxes) can help to promote behavioural change messages and engender an ethos of acceptability of health-related behaviours as part of an initiative. Think about long-term campaigns by groups that have previously been considered 'leftfield' but are now very much mainstream. Some effective health-related social marketing interventions need to be generational to truly embed behaviour change.

➤ *Innovation:* Think beyond the one-size-fits-all approach. Target specifically. Some segments will not affiliate with or will even dismiss your approach, but providing it is targeted and culturally acceptable to the segment it is aimed at, you will be able to deliver your product and hence contribute towards health behavioural change.

➤ *Measure the impact:* How successful has your intervention been? You may be pleased with the results of your intervention, or it may not have been as effective as desired. Go back and consider the 4 'P's. Has your product worked? Was the price of the product such that your intended segment was easily able to engage and invest in it – are the behavioural change goals something that can be part of the lifestyle of the segment? Has it been marketed in the place most likely to succeed with the masculine cultural segment? Have you incorporated the values of the masculine cultural segment into your product so that promotion of it is optimised? The experts by experience and the prime source of primary research material are your target group themselves.

CONCLUSION

Social marketing is not the province of a privileged elite. Whether you work for a statutory, third sector or private sector organisation there is a robust evidence base that the application of social marketing principles to your work with men will be a major factor in securing desired behavioural change. Integrating social marketing principles into our work to promote mental health can secure health improvement outcomes through improved coping strategies, increased resilience through enhanced protective factors and a reduction in the impact of risk factors in our lives.

To check whether or not your current activity embraces social marketing principles, audit your work against the National Social Marketing Centre's 10-point Checklist for Assessing Social Marketing Programmes (*see* www.nsmcentre.org.uk). For an independent perspective, if you are part of a network of organisations promoting the health of men, work as reciprocal 'Critical Friends' to audit each other.

As a counter-balance to the concerns about coercion and state or social control outlined at the start of this chapter, let us close with a quartet of positive key features for any social marketing initiative. Effective social marketing work with men will involve:

➤ *voluntary change:* social marketing is about voluntary, willing and informed behaviour change
➤ *reciprocity:* behavioural change will only take place if there is an exchange and a clear benefit to the men concerned
➤ *use of a marketing mix:* customer-oriented research informing targeted work with segments of male cultural identity
➤ *improved individual and social welfare:* our priority is to promote the mental health of men. This is what differentiates our use of social marketing from commercial marketing.

REFERENCES

Banks I (2006) *Brain Manual: the step by step guide for men to achieving and maintaining mental well-being.* Sparkford: Haynes Publishing.

Department of Health (1999) *National Service Framework for Mental Health.* London: DH.

Department of Health (2002) *National Suicide Prevention Strategy for England.* London: DH.

Department of Health (2004) *White Paper: Choosing Health.* London: DH.

Friedli L, Oliver C, Tidyman M and Ward G (2007) *Mental Health Improvement: evidence based messages to promote mental well-being.* Edinburgh: NHS Health Scotland.

Katz A (1999) *Young Men Speak Out.* London: Samaritans.

Kotler P and Zaltman G (1971) Social Marketing: an approach to planned social change. *J Marketing.* **35**: 3–12.

Lohan M (2007) How might we understand men's health better? Integrating explanations from critical studies on men and inequalities in health. *Social Science & Medicine.* **65**: 493–504.

MacFadyen L, Stead M and Hastings GB (2003) Social marketing. In MJ Baker (ed). *The Marketing Book* (5th ed.) Oxford: Butterworth Heinemann. Chapter 27.

Men's Health Forum (2002) *Soldier It! Young Men and Suicide.* London: Men's Health Forum.

Men's Health Forum (2006) *Mind Your Head.* London: Men's Health Forum.

National Institute for Mental Health In England (2005) *Making It Possible: improving mental health and well-being in England.* London: NIMHE.

Stead M, McDermott L, Hastings G, Lawther S, Angus K and Lowry R (2007) *Research to Inform the Development of a Social Marketing Health Improvement Strategy for Scotland.* Edinburgh: The Scottish Executive.

WHO (2004) *Prevention of Mental Disorders: effective interventions and policy options – summary report.* WHO: Geneva.

Wiebe GD (1951) Merchandising commodities and citizenship on television. *Public Opinion Quarterly.* **15**(4): 679–691.

CHAPTER 9

Men and suicide

Pete Sayers

INTRODUCTION

Despite some recent welcome falls in the rate for male suicide, it remains a major cause of death of men aged 25–34, with young men almost four times more likely to take their own life than women (Alexander 2001). The extent of the problem can be seen in the fact that most families in the UK will directly know of a man in their community who has taken his own life. This is somewhat at odds with the statistics for people suffering with depression, where approximately twice as many women are diagnosed with the condition as men. This anomaly is mostly explained by the fact that men's reluctance to acknowledge problems or seek help is as prominent in emotional or mental health situations as it is in other areas of men's health.

Steward and Harmon (2004) suggest that men will often define themselves as mentally healthy when they can produce behaviours resonant with concepts such as stoicism, self-reliance, strength, work, status and aggression. A state of mental health is also thought to be shown, conversely, by denying any vulnerability and by avoiding any overt displays of emotionality. Rees *et al.* (2005) acknowledge some movement away from this view within the male population but suggest that there are still many who cling to the gender stereotypes, with the macho image of a man represented as dominant, competitive, strong, fit, healthy and providing for the family. This perceived need to present as invulnerable and in control is one that has potentially damaging, even fatal, consequences for men as the internalisation of emotion and the physical, social and emotional withdrawal from potential help often serves only to exacerbate feelings of failure, hopelessness and despair.

This chapter is informed by my work as a Community Psychiatric Nurse (CPN) and with the It's A Goal! project, which I founded in 2004. It's A Goal! is a mental health intervention delivered at football grounds and aimed at tackling depression and suicide amongst young men between the ages of 16 and 35. The project began at Macclesfield Town Football Club, funded by the Laureus Sport for Good Foundation and now also runs at Manchester United's Old Trafford stadium, at Stockport County FC and at Plymouth Argyle FC. The service users, or 'players', can be referred by GPs, education authorities, social workers and health professionals, as well as family, friends, colleagues or themselves. The programme, or 'season', is based around football metaphors and comprises eleven sessions, or 'matches', covering a range of aspects of mental well-being. Follow up groups, or 'supporters clubs', provide extra support once the season is over and also take place within the football club (Pringle and Sayers 2004; 2006). Perhaps the most significant comment in the review of the process was the observation by one participant that the process was 'therapy in disguise' (Pringle and Sayers 2004).

WHY SHOULD SUICIDE PREVENTION BE AIMED SPECIFICALLY AT YOUNG MEN?

Emslie *et al.* (2007) propose that men and women actually experience depression in a similar way, but have different methods of manifesting and expressing their distress. They go on to describe the findings of Brownhill *et al.* (2005), who suggest that although both men and women tried to avoid emotional distress by attempting to block out negative thoughts, men were more likely to be overwhelmed after a longer period of time and release the emotion in the form of anger or violence. This is in contrast to women, who were more prepared to release emotions early by crying and seeking help. Wilhelm *et al.* (2002) suggest, however, that once a diagnosis is made and men are actively treated there are few gender differences in the severity, course or outcome of major depression. Real (1997) suggests that depression may also be a factor behind several of the problems we think of as being typically male, such as alcohol and drug abuse, domestic violence and failures in intimacy. The fact that women often access help and use services whereas men often do not is reflected in the statistics for suicide in this group.

STATISTICS

The statistics for men and suicide, especially young men, make for poignant reading. Men accounted for three-quarters of the suicides in 2007, with a rate of 16.8 per 100 000 population (peaking at 21.1 per 100 000 in 1998) compared to a rate of 5.0 per 100 000 population for women. Since 1997 the highest suicide rates have been in men aged 15–44 (17.6 per 100 000 population in 2007). Female suicide rates have been consistently much lower than males (Office for National Statistics 2009).

➤ *Age:* Suicide in men peaks in the 20s and again in the 60s and 70s.
➤ *Unemployment:* The suicide rate has been shown to rise and fall with the unemployment rate in a number of countries – half of the record 33 000 people who committed suicide in Japan in 1999 were unemployed.
➤ *Alcoholism* leads to suicide in 10% of affected people. Alcoholism is much more common in men (though it is increasing rapidly among women).
➤ *Schizophrenia* leads to suicide in up to 10% of affected people.

➤ *Social isolation:* Those who kill themselves often live alone and have little contact with others; they may have been recently widowed or have never married.

➤ *Chronic illness:* Any chronic illness increases the risk of suicide.

➤ *Certain occupations:* People with certain occupations are more likely to die by suicide; for example, farmers (who usually work alone and have access to the means of suicide, such as a shotgun or poisonous weed killer).

➤ *Imprisonment:* Men make up approximately 96% of the prison population in the UK and a large proportion of prisoners have mental health problems. A study for the Office of National Statistics (Singleton *et al.* 1998) showed 58% of male remand prisoners, for example, were assessed as having significant neurotic symptoms and over 20% of male prisoners stated that they had made a serious attempt at suicide at some point in their lives.

When I was working as a CPN, just prior to starting with the It's a Goal! project, I undertook a review of my caseload at that time. It revealed, surprisingly to me then, that 86% of the people I was seeing were women. When I looked at their presentation there were some interesting differences too. Women in the main were very keen to talk about things that were happening in their life at that moment and got into the personal stuff very quickly. Men on the other hand were generally more diffident, saying things like, 'I probably should have come here years ago', or 'this has been building up inside me for ages'. Women, I found, had often shared their problems previously with family, friends or workmates. Men, on the other hand, had almost never spoken about their issues before, many saying 'This is the first time I have ever talked about this stuff.'

In my current clinical practice, the above key indicators with regard to suicide are borne out. The average age of my client group is 29, 71% are unemployed and a high proportion of these young men report feeling suicidal, thinking about suicide or have previously made serious attempts to end their own lives. A massive 80% are living on their own and again, a huge number are seen to be socially isolated, drinking heavily and using illicit drugs.

WHY DO MEN KILL THEMSELVES?

The inability to provide for themselves and their family is seen by many men as a testament to their failure as a person. Over the last 40 years there have been dramatic changes in patterns of employment in the UK. Mining, steel manufacturing, shipbuilding and other heavy industries which traditionally employed men have closed, while the newly created jobs have tended to be in the service sector, often seen in the traditional view as 'women's work'. Experiencing satisfaction at work is an important predisposing factor for positive mental health in men; one of the reasons for this being the importance of 'breadwinning' as a cultural indicator of the 'male role'.

Unemployment is high amongst those labelled as mentally ill and a diagnosis can in some cases make people feel almost unemployable.

In considering the whole question of suicide in men in the UK, Gunnell *et al.* (2003) draw the conclusion that the increases in suicide amongst young males in England and Wales in the last 30 years have paralleled rises in a number of risk factors for suicide in this age group, namely unemployment, divorce, alcohol and drug abuse, and declines in marriage. Mortality data for the UK show a link between deprivation and suicide in men – those considered the most deprived (deprivation twentieth) having significantly higher mortality from suicide than any other deprivation group (Uren and Fitzpatrick 2001). The extent of the gradient various in different parts of the UK, with the greatest difference between the least deprived and most deprived being in Scotland.

Extreme and traumatic events, such as physical and sexual abuse, have been shown to distinguish suicidal adolescents from those who are depressed but experience no self destructive thoughts or behaviours (Kienhorst *et al.* 1995). Violence plays an extensive role in the lives of those young people that are suicidal when compared with the non-suicidal. This could be through bullying or violence from an adult. It might also involve their own violent attitude to others (Katz *et al.* 1999; Kaltiala-Heino *et al.* 1999).

My experience working as a CPN and with It's a Goal! has thrown up wide and varying reasons why men kill themselves, or consider doing so. Perhaps the most common presentation is loneliness and a feeling of low self-esteem for whatever reason. I have worked with guys who have had their perceptions altered by drink or drugs, who have lived with issues of abuse from childhood days and more recently, and being on the receiving end of bullying. I see men whose marriages and relationships have crumbled, men who have lost jobs or have never worked, who live in squalid conditions and have little or no money. In these days where we are often shown that money and the ability to use it is paramount, not having any reflects poorly on individuals and engenders feelings of failure and not being good enough. An increasingly materialistic and competitive world would seem to build up these feelings of inadequacy and 'not feeling part of it all'.

The young men referred to It's a Goal! are often facing all sorts of challenges and difficulties, but the uniting factor is always one of poor self-esteem or how they view themselves and this, to me, seems to be a key factor when we are looking at reasons for suicide combined with an isolation from society and a feeling of not belonging.

HOW DO MEN KILL THEMSELVES?

The method chosen to attempt suicide has a definite gender influence with men predominantly choosing hanging and firearms over the female preference for self poisoning. With firearms, shotguns are used in over three-quarters of cases, with handguns and other firearms making up the rest (ONS 2008). These suicides are mostly enacted by people who have legitimate ownership of a weapon, through sport and occupational use. Approximately one in three adolescents who die by suicide is alcohol intoxicated at the time of death and a further number are under the influence of drugs (Brent *et al.* 1986).

TREATMENTS

The effective treatments available for depression range from talking treatments through pharmacological interventions and electroconvulsive therapy (ECT) and these appear to have as much efficacy in men as in women. As Emslie and colleagues (2007) point out, however, the actual symptoms of depression contribute to problems in accessing help; for example, lack of confidence and assertiveness, low self-worth and feelings of lack of entitlement to GP time and resources. Perhaps the most worrying aspect for those involved with mental health care is the outcome for those who actively avoid treatment.

As mentioned earlier, it appears men have always been more reluctant to come forward and speak openly, to 'own', if you like, their problems and difficulties. Garnering referrals for the project has consistently been tough. It seems that men don't like to talk, or perhaps that should read 'they think they don't like to talk'. What has been overwhelmingly clear to me is that once men break through that barrier they can be as articulate and use talking therapies just as effectively as women. Of course, there is a place for medication and in more severe cases even ECT, but working with the mild to moderate mentally ill group, it can be seen that it is as much about empowerment and control than anything else. If someone feels in control of their situation and that they themselves have reached their goals and targets rather than 'the doctor' or a pill, it is at this point that the longest lasting positive effects can be seen and self-belief begins to emerge.

APPROACHES TO SUICIDE

In response to concern around suicide a specified target in the Government's White Paper, *Our Healthier Nation* (DH 1999) was a reduction in suicides by at least 20% in the ten years following the 1999 baseline. This was followed in 2002 by the National Suicide Prevention strategy (DH 2002). The strategy document for England noted that factors associated with suicide include social circumstances, biological vulnerability, mental ill-health, life events and access to means, while risk factors include being male, living alone, unemployment, alcohol and drug misuse, and mental illness. Such factors lead to considerable socio-economic and geographical variations in suicide rates. Key measures in the strategy included reducing the suicide risk of men under 35 who are most likely to take their own lives; for example, by improving the treatment of alcohol and drug misuse among young men who self-harm.

Prevention strategies have also been launched in recent years in Scotland and Northern Ireland. In 2002, the Scottish Executive launched 'Choose Life' (Scottish Executive 2002), a national strategy and action plan to prevent suicide in Scotland with the goal of reducing suicide rates by 20% by 2013. The 'Protect Life' (DHSSPS 2006) draft strategy in Northern Ireland particularly focuses on males and those most at risk, with part of the work being to investigate if there is any link between suicide/attempted suicide and civil unrest in Northern Ireland.

THE SETTINGS FOR ENGAGEMENT

Conrad and White (2007) describe how traditionally men have been seen as reluctant to access health services, but also how getting men to engage with their health is not an impossible task once you are equipped with a few tricks of the trade. One of the tricks is to make services and health promotional activities more appealing to men by locating them outside of the traditional GP/hospital setting. Football facilities offer just one example of 'traditional male-friendly settings', where projects like It's a Goal! can engage men over a sustained period in a place that's convenient for them to access and where they feel comfortable. Another way of using football to engage men with mental health problems is in playing the game. Evans and colleagues (2008) describe how the CSIP league in Manchester brings together over 200 service users, many with serious depressive illnesses, to play at the JJB Soccer Dome in Trafford Park and how this process can help impact positively on depression. Other work in this field is seen in the development of close working relationships between the Derbyshire mental health trust and a range of clubs in the county from the largest, Derby County, to the small, non-league Belper Town. This process includes the creation of mental health drop-in centres in the clubs.

Other examples of promoting health to men in innovative ways include the successful Hayes Manual-style health promotion books from the Men's Health Forum (e.g. Banks 2006) and similarly Jo McCullagh's creation of a set of comic strip characters like 'Colin the Cabbie' to put messages across in an innovative and engaging way at Sefton Primary Care Trust.

WHO SHOULD DELIVER THE WORK?

Key to the success of this work is having the right people in place. Ideally, workers who live locally and have a good understanding of local mental health politics and issues would be front runners for these jobs. Also some experience of working in therapeutic groups and understanding the dynamics that lie within are advantageous too. Perhaps this goes without saying but to ably run the It's a Goal! programme, for example, the worker would need to have a good understanding of football and football-related matters.

Four years ago when the project was in its infancy, I was minded to think that other qualities were required, such as the need for the worker to be professionally qualified and even that they needed to be male. I have revised this opinion somewhat and now feel that the person's personal attributes are far more important. The ability to relate to their clients on a non clinical level, talking their language, if you like, is a special skill and is not the sole preserve of qualified mental health workers. A great advantage of being local, however, and particularly a worker already in the field, will be knowledge of potential referrers, something that would give the programme leader a head start. Hard headedness, stubbornness and a passion for the work are other benefits that the potential worker should have, as well as the ability to self-start and work independently. Much of the job of starting up It's a Goal! required seemingly endless foot slogging around town putting up posters, handing out leaflets and giving presentations. Fine when you have the statistics and the anecdotes to back it all up, but not so easy when all you are doing really is selling your dream and trying to infect others with your enthusiasm.

I never envisaged, when passing on the torch, as it were, that it would be to some-one who had passed through the programme himself, but nonetheless this is what is happening. In June 2008 I moved on to other things within the project, and the 'coalface' work with the clients was passed on. In many ways, it is a complete vin-dication of the project that a user can develop to become a worker and demonstrates how a courageous approach, openness and flexibility can be used to positive effect in a therapeutic area.

IS THE NATIONAL SUICIDE STRATEGY WORKING?

Since the introduction of the National Suicide Strategy there has been a drop in the rate of suicide among young men. A progress report published by the National Institute for Mental Health in England acknowledged that good progress was being made towards meeting the Government target to reduce suicide by 20% by the year 2010. Despite this welcome development, suicide remains the major cause of death of men aged 25–34, with young men almost four times more likely to take their life through suicide than women (Davidson and Lloyd 2001).

THE NEXT STEP?

Although suicides represent only 1% of the total number of deaths in the UK, they have long been recognised as a major public health concern, especially in young men. Clearly some thought has to continue to go into creating services that address the differing needs of men and women in mental health care. Services should acknow-ledge that men may seek 'masculine' solutions to problems of emotional distress while approaches to improving mental health that rely on messages perceived as 'feminine', such as preparedness to open up or admitting to vulnerability, fail to engage them (Wilkins 2006). The failure of men to access services has resulted in them often being blamed for being poor consumers of health services and so being seen to be victims of their own behaviour (Courtenay 2000). Addressing the chal-lenges of improving men's uptake of services may well require service providers to focus on education, attitudes and environment.

Men are seen as having a poor uptake of educational material around health but it may be that men simply have a different approach to seeking information. Tudiver and Talbot (1999) suggest that the initial approach by men seeking help for health-related issues tends to be indirect and that they tend to view their partners and friends as a primary resource for help.

Emslie *et al.* (2007) claim that while both men and women valued good com-munication skills in health professionals, men tended to value skills which helped them to talk, while women valued listening skills. Good and Wood (1995) suggest that one way to increase men's use of counselling services would be to focus less on emotional expressiveness and more on instrumental changes and control.

In terms of the environment, we know that some men often feel unwelcome in what they see as 'feminised' premises in terms of decor and display material, and perceive a gender bias in the provision of some services (Newland 2006).

CONCLUSION

The National Service Framework for Mental Health (DH 1999) put an emphasis on mental health promotion and outlined standards for care focusing on the mental health needs of working-age adults up to 65. The document set out seven standards around health promotion, access to services, caring about carers, and suicide, describing them as realistic but challenging. If these goals are to be achieved for men with mental health issues then services and initiatives must recognise the specific needs of men as a distinct group. Initiatives are needed to raise the awareness of the prevalence of depression, combined with a better understanding of the illness and promotion of good mental health. McKenzie (2006) emphasises the importance of educating men about the symptoms of psychiatric disorders, reducing the stigma of mental ill-health and making services more accessible to working men, utilising language and approaches that are relevant and comprehensible.

Banks (2007) optimistically suggested that developing services that genuinely address these issues may be helped in the UK by the 2007 'Gender Equality Duty Act' which, for the first time, has made it a legal requirement to deliver all services in the public sector on a gender equitable basis by outcome rather than process. Although there is much that health services can do to target and improve men's health, we must realise that men's health is not a medical issue but a societal one and that as such a much broader approach needs to be taken (White 2001). Co-operative working between not just health and social agencies, but also community facilities, support groups, retail and food outlets, health facilities and even football clubs, holds out hope for a more integrated approach that can help address men's health issues.

REFERENCES

Alexander J (2001) Depressed men: an exploratory study of close relationships. *J Psychiatric and Mental Health Nursing.* **8**(1): 67–75.

Banks I (2006) *Brain Manual: the step by step guide for men to achieving and maintaining mental well-being.* Sparkford: Haynes Publishing.

Banks I (2007) The Vienna Declaration: just one more thing? *J Men's Health & Gender.* **4**(3): 220–221.

Brent D, Perper J, Goldsteing CE, Kolko D, Allan MS, Allman C and Zelenak J (1986) Risk factors for adolescent suicide. A comparison of adolescent suicide victims with suicidal inpatients. *Archives of General Psychiatry.* **45**: 581–8.

Brownhill S, Wilhelm K, Barclay L and Schmied V (2005) 'Big build': hidden depression in men. *Aus & NZ J Psychiatry.* **39**: 921–931.

Conrad D and White A (eds) (2007) *Men's Health – How to Do It*. Oxford: Radcliffe Publishing.

Courtenay W (2000) Behavioural factors associated with disease, injury, and death among men: evidence and implications of prevention. *J Men's Studies*. **9**: 81–142.

Davidson N and Lloyd T (eds) (2001) *Promoting Men's Health: a guide for practitioners*. London: Harcourt Publishers Limited.

Department of Health (DH) (1999) *National Service Framework for Mental Health*. London: DH.

Department of Health (DH) (1999) *Saving Lives – Our Healthier Nation*. London: DH.

Department of Health (DH) (2002) *National Suicide Prevention Strategy for England*. London: DH.

Department for Health, Social Services and Public Safety (DHSSPS) (2006) *Protect Life: A Shared Vision: The Northern Ireland Suicide Prevention Strategy & Action Plan 2006 – 2011*. Dublin: DHSSPS.

Emslie C, Ridge D, Zieblands S and Hunt K (2007) Exploring men's and women's experiences of depression and engagement with health professionals: more similarities than differences? A qualitative interview study. *BMC Family Practice*. **8**: 43.

Evans P, McElroy P and Pringle A (2008) Sick as a parrot or over the moon: an evaluation of the impact of playing regular matches in a football league on mental health service users. *Practice Development in Health Care*. **7**(1): 40–48.

Good GE and Wood PK (1995) Male gender role conflict, depression and help seeking: do college men face double jeopardy? *J Counselling and Development*. **74**(1): 70–75.

Gunnell D, Middleton N, Whitley E, Dorling D and Frankel S (2003) Why are suicide rates rising in young men but falling in the elderly? A time-series analysis of trends in England and Wales 1950–1998. *Social Science & Medicine*. **57**: 595–611.

Kaltiala-Heino R, Rimpela M, Marttunen M, Rimpela A and Rantanen P (1999) Bullying, depression, and suicidal ideation in Finnish adolescents: schools survey. *BMJ*. **319**: 348–351.

Katz A, Buchanan A and McCoy A (1999) *Young Men Speak Out*. Ewell, Surrey: Samaritans.

Kienhorst IWM, De Wilde EJ and Diekstra RFW (1995) Suicidal behaviour in adolescents. *Archives of Suicide Research*. **1**: 185–209.

McKenzie S (2006) The strong silent type. *Public Health News*. 5 Jun: 14–5.

Newland J (2006) Not going for checkups: is it a guy thing? *Nurse Practitioner*. **31**(9): 6.

Office for National Statistics (ONS) (2009) Suicides. Available at: www.statistics.gov.uk/cci/nugget.asp?id=1092 (Accessed 20 September 2009).

Pringle A and Sayers P (2004) It's a Goal!: basing a community psychiatric nursing service in a local football stadium. *J Royal Society for the Promotion of Health*. **124**(4): 234-238.

Pringle A and Sayers P (2006) It's a Goal!: the half time score. *Mental Health Nursing*. **26**(3): 14–17.

Real T (1997) *I Don't Want to Talk About It: overcoming the secret legacy of male depression*. New York: Scribner.

Rees C, Jones M and Scott T (2005) *Exploring men's health in a men-only group*. Nursing Standard. **9**(43): 38–40.

Singleton N, Meltzer H, Gatward R, Coid J and Deasy D (1998) *Psychiatric Morbidity Among Prisoners: summary report*. London: Office for National Statistics.

Stewart D and Harmon K (2004) Mental health services responding to men and their anger. *Int J Mental Health Nursing*. **13**(4): 249–254.

Scottish Executive (2002) *Choose life: a national strategy and action plan to prevent suicide in scotland*. Edinburgh: Scottish Executive.

Tudiver F and Talbot Y (1999) Why don't men seek help? Family physicians' perspectives on help-seeking behaviour in men. *J Family Practice*. 48: 47–52.

Uren Z and Fitzpatrick J (2001) Chapter 11: Analysis of mortality by deprivation and cause of death. In C Griffiths J Fitzpatrick (eds), *Geographic Variations in Health* (DS No 16). TSO: London.

White AK (2001) *Report on the Scoping Study on Men's Health*. London: Department of Health.

Wilhelm K, Roy K, Mitchell P, Brownhill S, Parker G (2002) Gender differences in depression risk and coping factors in a clinical sample. *Acta Psychiatrica Scandinavica*. 106(1): 45–53.

Wilkins D (2006) *Mind Your Head: men, boys and mental well-being*. London: Men's Health Forum.

CHAPTER 10

Men bereaved through suicide

Mike Bush

INTRODUCTION

In Britain there is a suicide every 85 minutes. The true figure could be far higher than this, however, as coroners often return verdicts of misadventure or open verdicts. Studies have shown that most open verdicts are in fact suicides (Linsley *et al.* 2001). The highest incidence of suicide is amongst young men. Male macho culture, the concept that 'big boys don't cry', alcohol and drug misuse, feelings of being disenfranchised from society and men's general difficulty in articulating and venting emotional problems are issues discussed elsewhere in this book which may partly contribute to the difference in suicide rates between men and women. As well as making depressed men more likely to kill themselves than depressed women, for those left behind these kinds of issues also impact on men's ability to deal with bereavement in a healthy way.

All bereavement is hard but suicide bereavement is different – even to a murder or a sudden accident. The sense of rejection from knowing that a loved one has chosen not only to leave the world but to leave you too can be crushing. People bereaved through suicide have a particularly hard path to tread as they try to make sense of what appears to be a very senseless act, typically struggling with feelings of guilt and constant self-searching reflections. Losing someone you love through suicide has been described as a personal holocaust. The replaying in the mind of countless permutations of possible scenarios of what may have been, the crushing sense of rejection, a sense of frustration that the person was 'let down' by health services and the guilt of 'if only I'd done this or that' can all add to the underlying grief. On average, six to eight people around the person will be deeply affected by their suicide and those bereaved by suicide will be at increased risk of suicide themselves. There are around 5000–6000 suicides a year in the UK. Multiplied by 6–8 that's a lot of people deeply affected by suicide each year. As coroners often return misadventure or open verdicts, the true figure is not known.

I was 15 when my father took his own life. All I got was some antidepressants from the GP. There was no counselling, no bereavement organisation. The only support my sister and I had was the support we could provide to each other. Most people are simply too embarrassed to talk to you about suicide bereavement. My sister became depressed and I went with her to see a psychiatrist who basically told her to take tablets. There was no referral for her to a counsellor to whom she could vent her feelings. The tablets had all sorts of nasty side effects and she gave up taking them. As a consequence, she became more depressed and suffered with depression for many more years.

As a man I felt that I couldn't be seen to be letting my feelings get the better of me. I did what a lot of men do and buried myself in my work – something which being a mental health social worker offered ample opportunity for. Talking about personal feelings is enough of a challenge in itself for many men, in addition to living in a society where suicide is stigmatised, talking about death is largely taboo and cultural representations of bereavement have made it largely a feminised concept (how often do we talk about the grieving widower as opposed to the grieving widow?) Having lost my father through suicide, I didn't want to get too close to people. I didn't want friendships that were too demanding. Although I was lonely, I didn't want to run the risk of having a relationship, it breaking down and then having to deal with another abandonment. Professional relationships were OK, but I needed to maintain emotional distance.

SUICIDE BEREAVEMENT SUPPORT GROUPS

In 1993, I became involved with a newly formed group which was set up to help support people who had been bereaved through suicide. The LOSS group (Leeds Organisation for Survivors of Suicide) met twice a month and was run by people who had themselves been bereaved through suicide, so they knew first hand what it was like and that was very important to the people who came to the group. Often one of the first things that new members asked was, 'Have you lost someone through suicide?' We saw people individually first and then if they didn't want to come to the group we'd continue to see them individually. One man who attended said that he'd gained more from one session talking to others in the same situation than he had from two years of talking to a psychologist. However, only a handful of men came to the group; it was almost all wives, girlfriends and mothers. Some men find it easier to talk to women, of course, but for those that find it harder it would be better to have the option of attending a men-only suicide bereavement support group. Ideally there would be dedicated groups for young people, men, and women.

It's easy to think that men will be too reluctant to talk about any kind of mental health issue in a group but, as with most men's health work, if it's framed and presented in the right way, you find that they are willing to engage. You have to reassure people that grief is a natural process (although it can make you feel like you're going mad) and do that in a way that doesn't threaten their masculinity. It's about getting people to see that it takes strength to admit a problem. Weakness is bottling it up and not wanting to discuss it with other men. When I first did a session on mental health for a men's health group their initial reaction was very dismissive, with a general tone of 'oh no we're going to be talking about nutters'. Their perception was that men with health issues must be particularly weak guys but when I told them that I'd had a breakdown myself they really started to listen and what was meant to be a 10–20 minute session went on over an hour and half. At the end two or three came up and said that they also had issues which they hadn't wanted to mention in front of the group. From being very dismissive of the idea of men's mental health they ended up asking for a weekly session.

A NATIONAL RESPONSE

Bereavement is a normal process and not something that should be medicalised, but there should be support available for people who need help to get through it, especially when it has come about through particularly traumatic circumstances. As well as dealing with the immediate effects on mental well-being of suicide bereavement this type of work plays a role in preventing further suicides. Suicide bereavement and prevention are opposite sides of the same coin. People bereaved through suicide are at greater risk of suicide themselves (Qin *et al.* 2002). This was apparent through my work with the LOSS group, where people would often have experienced more than one suicide in the family.

Suicide bereavement services in the UK are currently all delivered by voluntary organisations with limited resources. With an estimated 30 000–48 000 people in the UK severely affected by suicide each year, however, there is a need for a coordinated national programme with proper government funding. People bereaved through suicide are a badly neglected group whose acute needs and problems are very considerable and warrant a compassionate, well-organised systematic response.

The approach which has been adopted in Australia provides an excellent example of what can be done in this area if there is proper recognition of the scale of the issue and sufficient political will to tackle it. In 2005, as a result of the first National Annual Suicide Prevention Planning Forum, hosted by the National Advisory Council on Suicide Prevention (NACSP), the Australian Prime Minister announced a range of initiatives to address the issue which included funding to progress national activities targeting people bereaved by suicide. The National Bereavement Reference Group (NBRG) was established to oversee the development of a nationally coordinated approach to suicide bereavement interventions.

The Australian approach recognised that it is not enough simply to have services offering suicide bereavement support; there have to be national standards or benchmarks based on best practice. Where suicide bereavement support services are provided by a range of voluntary organisations they can be based on very different models with little guidance or evidence to help ensure that they achieve their objectives. Some are 'support groups', some offer a psycho-educational component, some are self-help groups and others are guided by professionals. The 'Lifeline Australia – Suicide Bereavement Support Group Standards and Practice' project was set up to inform the development of best practice guidance and training tools for facilitators of SBS groups to be rolled out nationally to other organisations following trials to evaluate their effectiveness.*

Australia's move to deliver more proactive and targeted support for high-risk groups includes funding men's networks, strengthening mental health promotion programmes for secondary school children, and providing funding for suicide bereavement support services, including indigenous-specific services. The need for addressing suicide on a community basis is also recognised in Australia, with locally tailored projects to support those local populations which have been particularly affected by or at particular risk of suicide. Countries with large indigenous populations require services targeted at these groups, not least because of the high rates of suicide which often occur in indigenous populations relative to the rest of the population (Hunter and Harvey 2002). In Canada, for example, European models of grief counselling have been adapted for programmes tailored for indigenous people. The Suicide Bereavement Programme in Australia developed a community assessment framework to identify history of loss in a particular community, the impact of those losses on that community as they perceived them and the community's preferred bereavement practices (Swan and Raphael 1995).

Survivors of Suicide

Lifeline Australia publish a pamphlet for people dealing with suicide bereavement. The pamphlet describes the stages of grief, based around first-hand accounts by people who themselves have lost someone to suicide (Dunne and Wilbur 2005).

You can download a copy of *Survivors of Suicide: coping with the suicide of a loved one* from: www. readthesigns.com.au

---

A national coordinated response to suicide bereavement is still a long way off in the UK. We need to develop a national network of coordinated suicide bereavement services, working in partnership with other bereavement services and incorporating tailored provision for men, women, young people, ethnic minorities and the gay and lesbian community (which has a higher suicide rate). The development of a suicide bereavement information pack has been an important milestone. The pack, entitled 'Help is at hand', is available from the Department of Health (2008), although its existence does not currently appear to be widely known among professionals.

Being proactive is essential to implementing an effective suicide bereavement strategy. Because death and especially suicide are largely taboo subjects, the natural tendency is not to seek professional support, especially when combined with the traditional male reluctance to acknowledge emotional problems and access health services. Simply setting up a disconnected service and waiting for people to come to it therefore isn't enough. A common policy needs to be adopted by all health and social welfare agencies, with a central body developing working relationships with the coroner, police, prison service, Samaritans, colleges, universities and schools

---

* See www.lifeline.org.au

to support suicide bereavement work, signpost those affected and help implement anti-suicide strategies.

Mental health promotion in general should be a key priority in tackling bereavement issues. There is a need for much more work to teach men and boys coping strategies for dealing with life's difficulties and emotional problems and ensure that they have the knowledge, skills and confidence to access support services when needed. Suicide bereavement brings with it a particularly strong and complex range of emotions which can lead to serious mental health problems in the future if not adequately dealt with in a healthy way. This is an area where the classic male reluctance or inability to express emotions in a way that counters the hegemonic masculine identity simply won't get you through. The kind of health promotion projects which are described in this book are an essential part of the work that needs to be done to change men's attitudes to mental health and emotional issues. At the same time as working to equip men and the next generation of men to deal better with emotional crises, we also need to meet the needs of men who are already in crisis.

REFERENCES

Department of Health (DH) (2008) *Help is at Hand: a resource for people bereaved by suicide and other sudden, traumatic death*. London: DH.

Dunne E and Wilbur MM (2005) *Survivors of Suicide: coping with the suicide of a loved one*. Deakin, ACT: Lifeline Australia.

Hunter E and Harvey D (2002) Indigenous suicide in Australia, New Zealand, Canada and the United States. *Emergency Medicine Australasia*. **14**(1):14–23.

Linsley KR, Schapira K and Kelly TP (2001) Open verdict v. suicide – importance to research. *British Journal of Psychiatry*. **178**: 465–468.

Qin P, Agerbo E and Mortensen PB (2002) Suicide risk in relation to family history of completed suicide and psychiatric disorders: a nested case-control study based on longitudinal registers. *Lancet*. **360**:1126–1130.

Swan P and Raphael B (1995) *National Aboriginal and Torres Strait Islander Mental Health Policy National Consultancy Report*. Canberr-a: Australian Government Publishing Service.

CHAPTER 11

Grumpy Old Men? Older men's mental health and emotional well-being

Toby Williamson

INTRODUCTION

'Grumpy Old Men' was the name given to a popular TV series featuring a number of male celebrities in their 50s and 60s bemoaning the state of the world, from people speaking 'bad' English to shopping in Ikea. While it has a sister series, 'Grumpy Old Women', it is the men who caught most of the attention. They seemed to confirm that the Victor Meldrew-type character from another popular TV series, 'One Foot in the Grave', really did exist in reality, and that grumpiness was a defining characteristic of older men. Clearly the mental health of older men is a lot more complex than this pejorative and stereotypical view suggests. Furthermore, with the numbers of older men increasing as the population ages in general, it is essential to get a better understanding of specific issues relating to their health and well-being and to reconsider some of the perceptions that exist of who they are and how they relate to the world. Nowhere is this more important than in relation to their emotional health and well-being. This chapter aims to do that. Part I looks at some of these issues and uses depression as an example of how a particularly common mental health problem affects older men. Part II uses research evidence and practical examples to describe a number of factors to incorporate into everyday practice when working with older men to promote their mental health and emotional well-being.*

---

* References in this chapter to official policy and guidance usually relate to England only because responsibility for health policy has in the main been handed over to the devolved administrations in the UK. However, the more general points about promoting older men's mental health are likely to be as relevant to people working in Scotland, Wales, or Northern Ireland as they are to those in England.

PART I – CHALLENGES

Age, mental health and mental well-being – definitions, policy and guidance

Age

People in 'old age' or 'older people' are often defined as those over retirement age – 65 and over. In some ways it is understandable to have this as a threshold, although with more people living longer and healthier lives increasing numbers of people over the age of 65 challenge having the label of 'old' applied to them, especially if they still have their own parents or other older relatives still alive. On the other hand, there is the view that the years after turning 50 are a time when many people may experience significant changes in their lives, including early retirement and changes occurring in their physical health. Organisations such as Age Concern* and Saga have 50 as their threshold, partly for these reasons. For the same reasons, this chapter uses 50+ as its threshold. Any age threshold, however, runs the risk of being some-what arbitrary and age thresholds relating to older people may in part contribute to ageism and age discrimination that continues to exist in society. We should, there-fore, be mindful of Standard 1 of the National Service Framework (NSF) for Older People in England (DH 2001), which seeks to root out age discrimination, and the forthcoming Equality Bill, which is likely to outlaw discrimination in the provision of goods and services based upon age.

Equality Bill

The Equality Bill is of particular significance for people working in the field of mental health because historically mental health services have used an age threshold of 65 to differentiate between services for younger and older adults. Services for people above and below that age have developed quite separately and there are a number of very significant differences and inconsistencies between the two. There is considerable debate about the merits and drawbacks of retaining this threshold but already a number of NHS mental health trusts have decided to integrate services, partly in anticipation of the Equality Bill making this a requirement.

Mental health and well-being

It is only in the last ten years or so that there has been significant attention paid to the concept of 'mental health' or 'mental well-being' as distinct from mental health problems or mental illness. Unfortunately, 'mental health' has often been used or interpreted to mean 'mental illness' or 'mental health problems' and the term 'men-tal' is a somewhat tainted word, frequently used pejoratively. This is a point that we shall return to later but 'emotional well-being' is, therefore, an alternative term which may be more helpful, particularly in relation to groups such as older men, who may be more reluctant to seek help because of issues of embarrassment or stigma. What is important is that good mental health or emotional well-being is not sim-ply an *absence* of mental health problems, but a *positive* state of being for a person,

---

* Please note that in 2009 Age Concern and Help the Aged came together to form a new national older people's charity called Age UK.

involving a combination of internal and external factors, that enable the person to function in society, to their own satisfaction and broadly speaking, the satisfaction of others.

Standard 1 of the NSF for Mental Health in England (DH 1999) focused on mental health promotion, although it only referred to people up to the age of 65.* Unfortunately, the Government's 2004 policy document on public mental health failed to take the mental health promotion agenda forward (DH 2004) and the following year the Mental Health Foundation published its own public mental health document, *Choosing Mental Health*, to try to remedy this (Mental Health Foundation 2005), though even this latter said little about older people's mental health.

In 2006, however, Age Concern and the Mental Health Foundation published *Promoting Mental Health and Well-being in Later Life* (2006), the first report from the UK Inquiry into Mental Health and Well-being in Later Life.† The Inquiry heard evidence from nearly 900 older people and 150 organisations and professionals. This established five main areas (*see* Box 11.1) that influence mental health and well-being in later life and, though not gender-specific, these should underpin any work that is done with older men to promote their mental health and emotional well-being.

BOX 11.1 What are the five key influences on mental health and well-being in later life?

> ➤ Discrimination on the basis of age is commonly experienced by older people and has a negative impact on their mental health.
> ➤ Participation in meaningful activity and having a sense of purpose are vital for good mental health and well-being.
> ➤ Relationships that are secure and supportive are important for good mental health and well-being.
> ➤ Good physical health is inextricably linked with good mental health – and vice versa.
> ➤ Poverty is a risk factor for poor mental health.

Source: Age Concern and the Mental Health Foundation (2006)

2006 also saw the Men's Health Forum focus its National Men's Health Week on mental health and the publication of 'Mind Your Head', their policy report on men, boys and mental well-being (Wilkins 2006). This report made several important recommendations about how men's mental health and well-being could be enhanced but made little reference to issues facing older men specifically. However, in its discussion of depression among men it made several useful observations about the

---

* The NSF for mental health is 10 years old in 2009 and work is currently underway both by the Department of Health and by seven national mental health organisations (Future Vision Coalition) to build on the successes of the NSF and take this work forward into the next decade. It is not clear whether anything similar may occur for the NSF for older people when it is 10 years old in 2011.

† The Inquiry, supported by Age Concern, published a second report in 2007, *Improving Services and Support for Older People with Mental Health Problems*.

effect of 'traditional' masculinity and possible variations in symptomology for men as compared to women.

More recently, as the public policy agenda around older people has grown, it has almost run parallel with the 'well-being' agenda that Lord Layard has been so influential in promoting (Layard 2005). This has stimulated further influential reports that have focused on (or included a significant focus on) older people's well-being (e.g. Allen 2008; Foresight 2008), yet these also have said little about gender differences among older people in relation to mental health.

In 2008 the Department of Health also published *The Gender and Access to Health Services Study* (Wilkins *et al.* 2008). This contains a useful chapter on mental health and gender differences, although it focuses primarily on mental health problems and looks across all age ranges. It is a significant acknowledgment by the Government that gender differences are of importance in people's mental health and use of mental health services, though its main recommendation relating to older men's mental health simply re-emphasises the need for more research into the needs of this group.

Older men, mental health, and mental health problems

In the UK there are currently more than 4 million men over the age of 65. There are a further 5–6 million men aged between 50 and 65. As the UK population grows older, and people live for longer, these numbers are set to rise – between now and 2018 the numbers of people aged over 50 will increase by 17%. By 2028 the over-50s will have increased by 30%, with a staggering increase of 79% among people over the age of 80 (Age Concern 2008).

Although women continue to outnumber men within older age ranges in the UK population, the gap is steadily reducing and in 2003 stood at 85 men aged 50 and over per 100 women (Age Concern and Mental Health Foundation 2006). Older men are more likely to be married than older women and fewer live on their own or in institutions – where necessary, spouses are usually the primary source of care. Although older men have fewer social relationships, older women experience more social exclusion because they are likely to experience more years of poor health and have fewer material and financial resources, including communication and transport (though there are significant differences between social classes).

It is also important to recognise that older men represent an increasingly heterogeneous group compared to previous generations. Because older men are living longer* it may well be the case that a man aged 65 still has a father alive aged 85, so sub-groups are forming in the older population between older people and the so-called 'very old'. That same man may also feel he has a lot more in common with a 50-year-old than people his father's age, who were young adults during the Second World War, the creation of the welfare state and the years of austerity that followed the war. His world as a young adult, on the other hand, would have been shaped by the dramatic economic and social changes that took place from the 1960s onwards.

---

* Life expectancy continues to increase for both men and women – the average life expectancy for men aged 65 in 2005 increased by 3½ years over the previous 25 years and based on 2005–07 mortality data, they can expect to live for a further 17 years (ONS 2008).

These factors are important because they are likely to affect the way different generations of men will perceive their age, their role and status, and their financial prospects, as well as their mental health and activities or interventions designed to improve it, during what is likely to be, for many, a much longer period of old age than their father's generation would have expected.

Older men will also become an increasingly diverse group for a number of other reasons, including more flexible retirement arrangements, changes in family structures, increased geographical (if not social) mobility, different forms of housing, greater numbers of older men from black and minority ethnic groups (BME) and greater numbers (or greater visibility) of older gay men. All of these factors are important in relation to mental health and well-being and need taking into account if activities or interventions are being planned on a population-wide basis (whether at a local or national level) to promote better mental health and well-being.

Mental health problems – depression, suicide and self-harm

The most common form of mental health problem experienced by older people is depression.[*] Twenty per cent of people aged between 65 and 69 have some symptoms of depression, rising to 40% of people aged over 85 – half of these will meet the clinical criteria for depression (Age Concern 2007). Although statistically, older women are more likely than older men to have depression, above the age of 85 the rates are about the same (McCrone *et al.* 2008). Furthermore, lower rates of depression among older men may mask the extent of the problem as men are less likely to seek help or treatment for mental health problems (women of all ages are almost twice as likely to see their GP for mental health reasons than men), or have mental health problems recognised by themselves, their families or health professionals (Payne 2008).

Certainly, when one looks at male suicide, not least because in many cases it is the most extreme response to depression, a different picture emerges for older men compared to other groups in the population. The suicide rate among men has always been higher than that of women and during the 1970s and 1980s the suicide rate of men aged 75+ was twice that of the national average and increasing, whereas the rate was much lower for older women and falling (Pritchard 1992). Although the suicide rate for older men was overtaken for a time in the 1990s by the suicide rate for young men, it is increasing again for men aged 45–74, and more men between the ages of 50 and 70 take their own life than boys/men between the ages of 10 and 30. Deliberate self-harm among older men also appears to be on the increase (Lamprecht *et al.* 2005).

Key factors causing or contributing to depression among older people are loss of social relationships and being socially isolated (particularly as a result of bereavement), and deterioration in physical health and functioning (especially mobility). These may also be compounded by alcohol misuse (and perhaps greater substance misuse as the 'hippie' generation of the 1960s enter old age). For many men, especially those who for years had put themselves in the role of provider while often

---

[*] For a good overview of depression and older people see Godfrey (forthcoming).

being quite dependent upon others close to them for emotional and domestic support, this isolation can be devastating and compounded by the loss of role, status, good physical health and income associated with retirement and old age.

Yet mental health problems among older people, such as depression, are less likely to be reported or diagnosed, may be incorrectly seen by practitioners as an inevitable part of growing old, or are often not referred to specialist mental health services where appropriate. This is despite the fact that older people are much greater users of health and social care services than younger people, thereby providing more opportunities to identify mental health problems. They visit their GP almost twice as much as younger people, at any one time two-thirds of hospital in-patients will be older people and 72% of people who use social care services are aged 65 and over. Nearly half of all older people who take their own lives visit their GP in the month before the suicide and only a small minority are in contact with specialist mental health services (Age Concern 2007).

BOX 11.2 Older men's mental health problems

> As many as 1 million men over the age of 65 experience depression – half this number will meet the clinical criteria for depression.

> At least two thirds of them have never discussed their depression with their GP – of those that have, only half were diagnosed and receiving treatment.

> 30–40% of older men in general hospitals and care homes are likely to have depression.

> In 2006 1932 men over the age of 44 took their own life in the UK – almost a 7% increase from 1996.

> Older men are more likely to succeed in taking their own life than older women or younger people.

> Deliberate self-harm among older men is increasing faster than among older women.

> Up to half of all older men who take their own life or self-harm will have seen their GP within the previous 4 weeks.

> Men aged over 85 are as likely to have depression as women over 85 and are more likely to be admitted for in-patient treatment for mental illness than women.

Given the stigma attached to mental health problems and a traditional yet widespread view of masculinity that sees seeking help for health problems as a sign of weakness, it is also very likely that many older men will be more reluctant to seek support or help for mental health difficulties than older women, for whom seeking help and talking about health issues may come more naturally. The culture of 'mustn't grumble' or a 'stiff upper lip' would appear still to be very prevalent.

A reluctance to seek help or use services has certainly been observed by organisations providing support to older people, such as Age Concern. In both local and national research undertaken for Age Concern in 2006, traditional notions of gender emphasising the importance for men of independence and self-reliance deterred many from going to a local branch of Age Concern (Age Concern 2006, Ruxton 2006). Groups and activities were often seen by older men as catering primarily for women's needs or for the needs of much more dependent older people. Combined with other reasons, such as problems with health and mobility, limited income and a tendency among many to withdraw in any case, this meant that in many of Age Concern's services and other welfare services older men were invisible or absent. It would seem that the majority of older men, whether or not they experience depression, lead lonely and isolated lives where their options to receive or participate in services that could improve their mental health and well-being appear very limited.

Of course, many older men may have active social lives and being alone may be a choice that some older men make, which should be respected. Nor, despite the commonly held view, is depression an inevitable part of growing old. Yet for the reasons described, being alone and isolated is the *only* choice for many older men, with all that it implies for their emotional health and well-being. To return to our 'grumpy old men' stereotype, grumpiness itself may simply be the frustration and anger born out of real loneliness and increasing depression that many men experience as they grow older, for the reasons described. Lacking both emotional and practical skills to cope, and without either information or the types of support that older men can understand or wish to use, their daily lives are likely to become increasingly bleak.

A note on other mental health problems

While this chapter has focused on depression and both its possible causes and consequences for older men, it is important to remember also that there are other mental health problems that older men may experience. These include the different forms of dementia (Alzheimer's disease being the most common), delirium (acute confusion), and alcohol and substance misuse, as well as more severe and enduring mental health problems, such as schizophrenia and bipolar disorder, which may have begun earlier in their lives but have persisted into old age. Taken altogether, these could affect up to half a million older men. Furthermore, as ageing is the greatest known risk factor for most forms of dementia (1 in 14 people over 65 years of age has some form of dementia, increasing to 1 in 6 people over 80 years of age[*]) it clearly represents a major and growing source of concern for older people and their families, and successive governments, as solutions to this challenge are sought.[†] Unfortunately space does not permit a more detailed discussion of all the issues involved, however, there are two key points to make regarding these other difficulties:

➤ Depression is commonly experienced by people with other mental health problems – for example, up to half of all people with dementia also have depression.

➤ Interventions and activities designed to improve older men's mental health and well-being, including those who experience depression, are likely to be just as

---

[*] Source: Alzheimer's Society England.

[†] In February 2009 the Department of Health published the first ever national dementia strategy for England outlining how this challenge would be met (Department of Health 2009).

beneficial for older men experiencing other mental health problems.*

Part II of this chapter looks at how these challenges can be overcome, with some examples of organisations and projects which are attempting to do this.

PART II – OVERCOMING THE CHALLENGES
Promoting older men's mental health – what works?

Given the problems that many older men experience in relation to their mental health and well-being, there is remarkably little evidence or guidance about what interventions or activities are effective in addressing these problems. The second half of this chapter therefore gives some examples of activities, projects or services that have either been developed in order to specifically meet the mental health needs of older men, or clearly have mental health benefits for older men even if this is not their specific aim.

Reference has already been made to policy and guidance concerning mental health promotion but as already pointed out this is not gender-specific and the women's mental health strategy that was published in 2002 (DH 2002) has not been matched with anything similar for men, let alone older men. Similarly, since the publication of the NSF for Older People in 2001 there have been a number of service improvement guides for mental health services for older people published by the Department of Health, most notably *Everybody's Business* (Care Services Improvement Partnership 2005), though these have not contained specific recommendations or guidance relating to older men's mental health and well-being.

In general, when designing or planning new interventions, activities or services to meet the needs of older men, distinctions may need to be drawn as to the purpose and population it is targeted on. Some of the options, funding permitting, might be:

➤ general health promotion work, including mental health, aimed at all older men in a particular locality

➤ specific mental health promotion work aimed at all older men in a particular locality

➤ specific mental health promotion work aimed at older men who are particularly vulnerable because, for example, they are socially isolated or depressed

➤ activities designed for (and preferably by) older men that are not primarily about mental health promotion but are likely to have mental health benefits, such as men's exercise groups.

The different options are clearly likely to involve different approaches and quite possibly different organisations. The first three options are more likely to be funded and/or led by a statutory organisation such as a primary care trust (PCT) or NHS

---

* It should be noted however that these interventions and activities are likely to need some adaptation, or may not be so appropriate for older men in middle to late stages of dementia.

mental health trust and focus on raising awareness and communicating information about good mental health and well-being and what services are available. The fourth option is perhaps the one most likely to be provided by a voluntary sector organisation, supported (and probably funded) by a PCT and/or local authority. The following are examples of activities, projects and services that broadly come under one of these categories:

➤ *Grouchy Old Men?*: This is a two-year national project that started in 2008, managed by the Mental Health Foundation and funded by the Department of Health. It aims to improve the mental health and well-being of older men, particularly those who are isolated and at risk of depression and suicide, by supporting and promoting a national network as well as local initiatives of organisations seeking to develop services to meet the needs of this group. More information can be found at: www.mentalhealth.org.uk

➤ *Fit as a Fiddle – Age Concern England:* This is a multi-million pound national programme running until 2012, funded by the Big Lottery Fund, which aims to improve the physical and mental health and well-being of older people. Involving a large number of local projects, one key group that it is focusing on is older men. More information can be found at www.ageconcern.org.uk

➤ *The Geezers – East London:* The Geezers are a group of East End men who are 50+ and wanted something akin to traditional working men's club conversations but could also include a holistic approach to health and emotional issues. The group aims to be supportive to men with a range of needs, with the aim that they will need less professional, clinical input. More information can be obtained from www.acth.org.uk

➤ *Men in Sheds – Age Concern Cheshire:* Established in 2009, the aim of this project is to reach older men who may be at risk of becoming isolated and excluded, may have mental and/or physical health issues, or may have recently experienced serious life changes, such as retirement or bereavement. The shed could be used as a haven, a meeting place, a learning experience or a place to share skills with others. It aims to get men 'out of the house, meet over a cup of tea, and put the world to rights'. More information at www.ageconcerncheshire. org.uk

➤ *Men's Activity Group – MHA Live at Home Scheme, Newcastle:* This group for older men in two villages west of Newcastle has 25–30 members meeting every fortnight and was formed because the men did not want to be in groups with women. Supported by a Methodist charity and housing association, visits have been organised to local pubs, the Royal Mail, the Tyne and Wear Metro system and a health information road show. More information at www.mha.org.uk/ Lahs03.aspx

➤ *Hour Bank – Age Concern Bromley (London):* Although not gender-specific, this is a good example of a 'time bank' project with a substantial number of older men that involves a reciprocal skill-swapping scheme where everyone both gives and receives skills. Aimed at tackling social isolation, promoting equality and building self-esteem, skill swaps have included cookery, poetry, DIY and gardening. More information at www.acbromley.org.uk

Drawing upon these examples and others, the second part of this section identifies some key points for anyone working in an organisation that is trying to improve the service it provides to older men with mental health needs.

Making your organisation more 'older-men friendly'

➤ Try to ensure that the physical environment of your organisation isn't off-putting to older men. Think about the décor, any music and facilities, such as a clearly marked male toilet.

➤ Any services need to be physically accessible, as many older people have physical health problems (which can also increase the risk of mental health problems). It is a good idea to make sure that information about local public transport and free bus pass schemes is easily available to make it easier for people to get out and about.

➤ Older men can sometimes feel patronised or disrespected by people they come into contact with, such as shop assistants or call centres. All staff who have direct contact with the public should be made aware of the need to respect and value older people, ideally as part of staff training or induction.

➤ A good way to involve older men in your organisation is to provide opportunities for volunteering – 25% of people over 50 are involved in formal volunteering and it is a good way to use their skills and make them feel valued.

➤ Older men may also wish to maintain some paid employment after traditional retirement age and many companies now have 'age inclusive' recruitment policies. If you employ men nearing retirement age, it's important to have flexible retirement policies and pre-retirement planning because people often find the emotional and practical impact (e.g. loss of status, role and income) difficult to cope with.

Reaching out to isolated older men

➤ Asking for help can be a big step for older men to take, so the first contact they make, or that a service has with them, has to be positive. Putting them off at this stage will make it harder for them to ask again or to approach them again. If services are full or oversubscribed, care must be taken in the management of waiting lists, as these can be very off-putting.

➤ Identifying isolated older men is a challenge and you may need to be quite imaginative in finding ways to find and approach them rather than waiting for them to come to you. It's also important to identify times of transition (e.g. bereavement, retirement, changes to living arrangements) that may be a good time to offer support.

➤ One way to reach isolated older men is to make contact with the people they encounter in day-to-day life, such as publicans, sub-postmasters, owners of corner shops and general practitioners. They may be an older man's main source of interaction and conversation and, if they are given information and properly advised, could be a useful way to direct men to your service or other sources of support. A campaign to raise awareness among older men about prostate cancer, for example, successfully involved providing health promotion information via publicans. You might be able to contact them directly, via your local chamber of commerce, or for example, your local licensed victuallers association.

➤ Another idea that has been suggested to help with this is small contact cards with helpline numbers (or contact details of local groups) left on shop counters/with staff, so services can be signposted in a way that is quick, easy and non-intimidating for an older man who doesn't want to have much interaction.

➤ When giving information about services, a variety of information sources is best. Sometimes it takes a recommendation from a friend or relative of an older man to persuade them that they should take the next step, whilst others prefer being able to read written information in their own time. Increasing numbers of older men are using the internet and the relevant information should always be made available online.

➤ The phrase 'mental health' is often seen by people to be stigmatising and off-putting (perhaps because it is associated with 'mental illness'). For older men who are often reluctant to go and see their GP or seek help elsewhere information needs to be provided in a language and style that they can relate to and doesn't put them off. Rather than talking about mental health in terms of 'problems' or negative feelings, it may be worth trying to use more positive, upbeat language, or encourage them to be active in helping other people.

Developing services for older men

Once an organisation has made contact with the men it wants to provide a service for, the next step is to develop a new service (or adapt an existing one) to meet their needs.

➤ The easiest way to do this is simply to ask the men what they want. If they have been fully involved in the development of the service they are more likely to continue using it and promote it to other older men.

➤ They may prefer a dedicated men's service, or the opportunity to mix with older women. Ask them which they would prefer.

➤ Some older men may find traditional day-centre activities unappealing. It may be better to provide low-intensity 'therapeutic' activities and things for men to do or actively focus on because these may better reflect how many men self-identify in terms of their working lives, hobbies or active interests (e.g. sport), rather than more passive groups where the emphasis is on socialising and chatting. Activities that have been popular with older men have included talks on health advice, benefits or local history; outings to places where they may have worked in the past or connected with particular hobbies or interests; watching DVDs or videos of sports events from when they were younger; IT classes; art and hobbies; gardening; or simply going to the pub.

➤ Physical activities are likely to have positive benefits on men's mental health and well-being as well. Forms of physical exercise such as t'ai chi, walking groups, or swimming have been popular with older men.

➤ Make the most of the skills and knowledge of older men. The evidence suggests that one reason older men don't engage in the services available to them is that it makes them feel like a burden. Giving them opportunities to share their knowledge or volunteer to help others will help to make them feel like an asset instead.

➤ Be careful that your service does not become dominated by more confident, able and younger people. Care must be taken to make sure that the needs of the very old, isolated and frail continue to be met. This may involve finding out about the needs of harder to reach people and communities you have less contact with in your local area and developing your service to meet these needs; for example, by doing more outreach work.

➤ If there is an existing community event that engages older men, this could be used as a vehicle for information to improve quality of life and/or raise mental health awareness. One project, for example, successfully used an annual domino tournament to promote information about prostate cancer to older Caribbean men.

➤ The needs of minority groups should be actively considered. Some black or minority ethnic groups may benefit more from targeted activities and approaches, such as using imams to provide information about local services. The needs of gay older men should also be considered and the importance of long-term partners appreciated.

Other points to consider

The evidence available also raises some points you may wish to consider in the development of your service:

➤ It's good to provide opportunities for mixing between generations wherever possible and younger people can gain as much from this as older people.

➤ Sundays can be a particularly lonely day, as most activities take place during the week and also because Sunday is traditionally a day for family activity.

➤ Poverty among older people continues to be a widespread problem and many people do not take up the welfare benefits that they're entitled to. This information should be promoted and help filling in forms should be offered if needed.

➤ Many older men live in poor-quality housing and may need help with minor repairs to stay in their home. This can be quite simple, such as changing light bulbs, but to the very frail it could help them keep their independence.

CONCLUSION

This chapter has provided an introduction and overview of the key issues involved in older men's mental health and well-being. It has particularly focused on the needs of isolated and excluded older men who are at risk of depression, suicide and self-harm. The chapter has provided some examples of both local and national initiatives that aim to address the needs of this group of older men, as well as practical tips and guidance on how to work more effectively with older men with mental health needs.

Although the chapter has not discussed in any detail older men with other mental health problems or conditions, such as dementia, or wider public health initiatives that could improve the mental health and well-being of older men in general, much of the information contained here is of considerable relevance to these areas of work as well.

What remains more of an unknown is whether older men's perception of their own mental health needs and their use of services may begin to change as men in the so-called 'baby boomer' generation (born in the period between 1946 and 64) move into their 60s and 70s. With very different life experiences from their parents' generation, resulting in many being more comfortable talking about emotions and mental health issues and more assertive and demanding about the type of services they would like to receive, could this result in greater willingness both to seek help and to determine what that help should involve?

Although it seems likely that the pattern and prevalence of mental health problems will change, other factors, such as people adapting positively to living more isolated and independent lives, supported by increasingly sophisticated technology as they grow old, could help us in dealing with these changes. Perhaps successive cohorts of older men with specific mental health needs will demonstrate changing patterns of service use, with corresponding changes in the severity and progression of the mental health problems they experience and in their mental health in general? Yet with an ageing population, the pressures of rapid social and economic change (particularly the potential effects of economic recession) and the persistence of both ageism and major social inequalities, it seems inconceivable that the mental health needs of older people will not remain an enormous challenge for governments and society in general. In this respect alone, understanding and responding positively to the mental health and well-being needs of older men in particular must be a priority.

ACKNOWLEDGEMENTS

I would like to thank Lindsay Jones for her hard work in developing the draft guide for services seeking to work with older men upon which the second half of Part II of the chapter is based. I would also like to thank all the individuals, projects and organisations which contributed to and hopefully benefited from the Mental Health Foundation's 'Grouchy Old Men?' Project.

REFERENCES

Age Concern and Mental Health Foundation (2006) *Promoting Mental Health and Well-being in Later Life*. London: Age Concern England.

Age Concern (2006) *Investigation into the Social and Emotional Well-being of Lone Older Men.*

London: Age Concern Surrey.

Age Concern (2007) *Improving Services and Support for Older People with Mental Health Problems.* London: Age Concern England.

Age Concern (2008) *The Age Agenda 2008.* London: Age Concern England.

Allen J (2008) *Older People and Well-being.* London: Institute for Public Policy Research.

Care Services Improvement Partnership (2005) *Everybody's Business.* London: Department of Health.

Department of Health (DH) (1999) *National Service Framework for Mental Health.* London: DH.

Department of Health (DH) (2001) *National Service Framework for Older People.* London: DH.

Department of Health (DH) (2002) *Women's Mental Health: into the mainstream.* London: DH.

Department of Health (DH) (2004) *Choosing Health.* London: DH.

Department of Health (DH) (2009) *Living Well with Dementia: a National Dementia Strategy.* London: DH.

Foresight (2008) *Mental Capital and Well-being.* London: Government Office for Science.

Godfrey M (forthcoming) Depression and anxiety in later life. In T Williamson (ed), *Older People's Mental Health Today: a handbook.* Brighton: Pavilion Publishing.

Lamprecht HC, Pakrasi S, Gash A and Swann AG (2005) Deliberate self-harm in older people revisited. *Int J Geriatric Psychiatry.* 20: 1090–1096.

Layard R (2005) *Happiness – Lessons from a New Science.* London: Penguin Books.

McCrone P, Dhanasiri S, Patel A, Knapp M and Lawton-Smith S (2008) *Paying the Price: the cost of mental health care in England to 2026.* London: King's Fund.

Mental Health Foundation (2005) *Choosing Mental Health.* London: Mental Health Foundation.

Office for National Statistics (ONS) (2008) *Mortality Statistics: deaths registered in 2007.* London: ONS.

Payne S (2008) Mental health. In D Wilkins, S Payne, G Granville and P Branney (eds), *The Gender and Access to Health Services Study: final report.* London: Department of Health.

Pritchard C (1992) Changes in elderly suicides in the USA and the developed world 1974–87: comparisons with current homicide. *Int J Geriatric Psychiatry.* 7:125–134.

Ruxton S (2006) *Working with Older Men.* London: Age Concern England.

Wilkins D (2006) *Mind Your Head: men, boys and mental well-being.* London: Men's Health Forum.

Wilkins D, Payne S, Granville G and Branney P (2008) *The Gender and Access to Health Services Study: final report.* London: DH.

CHAPTER 12

Combat-related stress

Walter Busuttil

INTRODUCTION

In the UK, veterans include all those who have served for at least one day in Her Majesty's Armed Forces (Regular or Reserve), Merchant Navy Seafarers and fishermen who have served in a vessel at a time when it was operated to facilitate military operations by HM Armed Forces. Psychological symptoms related to military service commonly go unexplored and unnoticed. Ex-servicemen are proud of their military service but are more likely to be ashamed to admit that they have a problem. Moreover, they have come from a 'macho' background where admission of mental health problems is perceived as being a gross sign of weakness. They also tend to feel that 'civvies' may poorly understand their culture and background, making them more reluctant to admit to problems with their psychological health.

Those that have tried to get help through the NHS have often felt let down by a civilian system that they perceive does not understand them. It is estimated that ex-soldiers make up over 75% of those veterans who seek help for mental health problems and that on average each GP in the UK will see an ex-serviceman with a mental health problem in his surgery once every seven years. This makes it more likely that if there is a link between his military service and the mental health problem that this will be missed. There is no automated flagging up system enabling the GP to identify the patient as an ex-serviceman, yet veterans have a unique set of needs and are vulnerable to mental health problems. This chapter will attempt to clarify some of these issues.

HM FORCES

There are approximately 200 000 regular personnel in the armed forces: comprising 100 000 in the Army and 50 000 each in the RAF and the Royal Navy. Additionally, 35 000 serve in the reserve forces (including the Royal Navy Reserve, Royal Marines

Reserve, Territorial Army, Royal Auxiliary Air Force and Regular Reserves). A significant proportion of these reserve forces deploy on operations or active service with the regular forces. Most service personnel are male and have historically been male, reflecting a mainly male veteran population, although recently rates of female personnel have been rising. In April 2004, there were 18390 women serving across the three Armed Forces – 8.9% of all military personnel (10.5% officers, 8.6% other ranks).

Each serviceman or woman is trained to perform a trade or profession within the Services; for example, some are technicians and others are suppliers, cooks, policemen, personnel administrators, medics or infantry front-line soldiers. One-fifth of frontline infantry soldiers are likely to be in close-quarter operational combat or peacekeeping. A much larger number will be involved operationally in a supportive role. Experience of operational situations is therefore very different for front-line and support personnel. It is also very different by virtue of the military service one is part of.

Exposure to significant psychological trauma is more likely in some trades, especially when there is a shortage of personnel. These include medics and logistics personnel, for example. The frequency of operational deployment to a war zone also influences levels of psychological health and is recognised to impact psychologically on the military family and is often a key factor in determining decisions made by members of the armed forces to prematurely terminate their career in the Services.

Recent operational service has been different in that there has been a high intensity of combat operationally as well as an increased tempo and rotational frequency of deployment for some at least. Otherwise it has followed the pattern of the past and has comprised peacekeeping with specific mandates, as well as combat. It should be noted that with the exception of one year, servicemen have died every year since the Second World War while on operational service. Since the Second World War the UK has sent servicemen and women on operations all over the world, including Northern Ireland, Palestine, Aden, Borneo, Rwanda, Kenya, Sierra Leone, Suez, Kenya, Korea, Malaya, Cyprus, the Falklands, the Gulf, the Balkans, Iraq and Afghanistan. The veterans of these operations continue to present with mental health problems related to their service.

MILITARY MENTAL HEALTH SERVICES

The military has its own psychiatric services within the Defence Medical Services (DMS). These comprise Departments of Community Mental Health (DCMHs), which are staffed and run by the uniformed military, as well as hospital-based services, which are contracted out.

Community services

Regular-serving personnel have access to comprehensive uniformed primary care services. Referral for those with mental health problems is usually to a uniformed multidisciplinary community-based occupational mental health service in

Departments of Community Mental Health (DCMH). Access is excellent and the waiting time to see a mental health worker is usually less than 24 hours. Currently there are fifteen of these DCMHs across the UK, in addition there are four in Germany and others in Cyprus and Gibraltar. The DCMHs are similar to NHS Community Mental Health Teams (CMHTs) and are staffed by psychiatrists, psychologists and community psychiatric nurses. Treatments include medical as well as psychological interventions. In combat zones CMHTs, known as Psychiatric Field Teams, deploy with the other support and combat units to the front line. They are primarily staffed by uniformed Community Psychiatric Nurses (CPNs) supported by visiting uniformed military psychiatrists and civilian psychologists employed by the military.

Inpatient services

Until 1994 the Army, Navy and RAF had their own military psychiatric hospitals facilities. (Until the early 1990s the main single-service psychiatric units were situated at the British Military Hospital, Woolwich (Army); Royal Naval Hospital, Haslar and RAF Hospital Wroughton.) The last tri-service psychiatric unit closed at Catterick Hospital in April 2004. At this point inpatient services were contracted out. For five years this contract was held by The Priory Group of private hospitals but in 2009 inpatient services passed from the Priory Group to an NHS Consortium managed by Staffordshire and Shropshire NHS Foundation Trust. Psychiatric services in the UK do not offer treatment to family members of servicemen like they do in places such as Germany.

MENTAL HEALTH PROBLEMS WITHIN THE MILITARY

The rate of reported mental illness seen by the DMS Psychiatric Services is of the order for new referrals of 4.5 per 1000 strength (or 5000 new referrals per year). Serious mental illness (psychosis) is rare in the military. Alcohol consumption is much higher compared to the civilian population, especially in the younger servicemen. A recent study demonstrated that common DCMH presentations included alcohol misuse (33%), depression (19%), anxiety (11%) and adjustment disorders (10%) (Gould *et al.* 2008). Another found that deployment to Iraq and Afghanistan increased the probability of screening positive for post-traumatic stress disorder (PTSD) by 6.3 and 1.6% compared to those who were deployed on ships. This probability is increased by 2.2% for those deployed longer than 180 days (Shen *et al.* 2009). Overall rates of PTSD in personnel who are still serving are reported as being generally low, with figures of between 1% and 8% being reported from recent conflicts. There are anecdotal reports of possible raised suicide rates for young recruits, but overall the suicide rate in service is unremarkable.

Mental health problems within the military can arise from a variety of causes:

➤ *pre-service vulnerabilities:* many join to escape difficult life situations including exposure to all kinds of childhood abuse, inadequate childhood caregivers and role models, poverty, poor housing, poor opportunities and deprivation;

➤ *military life itself:* for example, issues concerning institutionalisation, culturally bound alcohol misuse, effects on marital relations and family life including cyclical peacetime detachments and frequency of operational wartime deployments, alleged institutional and individual bullying, non-operational occupational mental health injury;

➤ *operational service:* exposure to extreme single and increasingly more commonly multiple psychological stressors; including direct involvement in combat, witnessing gruesome events occurring to others, involvement in clearing-up after disasters including body handling, involvement in riot control, and humanitarian aid and peacekeeping;

➤ *earlier onset of physical disorders related to military life:* mainly orthopaedic including knee and lower back joint problems and chronic pain, especially those who undertake repeated long route marches carrying heavy backpacks or other kit; ENT problems, especially for those involved in firing of weapons;

➤ *leaving the service and adjusting to civilian life:* raising the potential of the reactivation of attachment difficulties present prior to joining the military;

➤ *help-seeking issues:* a propensity not to seek help or to drop out of treatment, especially psychotherapy. Issues surrounding being macho, avoidance of seeking help, lack of understanding of and by civilians, shame, stigma, guilt, 'you were not there' etc;

➤ a combination of the above.

Adjusting to leaving the military

Approximately 25 000 personnel leave the regular forces each year. Most leave because they have served their contracted time, others leave because they have resigned – taken preferred voluntary retirement (PVR). These exits are honourable. Others leave administratively because they have got into trouble. Some are therefore discharged 'services no longer required' (SNLR). Some discharges are dishonourable, especially if the exit is the result of the findings of a Court Martial. Some leave on medical grounds. This is a process that involves medical evidence produced at a medical board staffed by medical personnel, including doctors. Each year approximately 1600 leave by means of a medical discharge. Only around 150 leave for mental health reasons. Patients discharged on mental health grounds are helped to access NHS services by means of a liaison service operated by psychiatric social workers employed by the military who ensure referral to NHS CMHTs and other services, including third sector veterans' mental health services, such as Combat Stress. Veterans who are medically discharged for mental health reasons are also given a welfare officer/case worker provided by the Service Personnel and Veterans Agency (SPVA). This worker will remain in contact with them and help them readjust to civilian life.

Currently the average time served for a field soldier is around three and a half years. This brief time is probably a reflection of the current demands placed on the Army and the current wars we are involved in. Leaving the military can be a difficult time for the ex-serviceman. Many will have been in the military for a significant period of their lives. Some would have been born and brought up in a military family before joining up themselves and will have to live in a civilian environment for the first time ever. Resettlement programmes are much better nowadays but have been less so in the past. Recently it was noted that those who leave on mental health grounds have had problems accessing resettlement courses and training and these courses are now deferrable for up to two years after leaving the military.

Many veterans find it difficult to access a career equivalent to their military status or career path. A minority have serious difficulty adjusting to the change. They may feel not only the loss of career when they leave; they will also have lost their rank, self-worth, identity and the familiar system that has enveloped everything they have been used to at work and in their private life. This, for many, might include access to housing and local schooling. They now enter a confusing new system. This is especially the case for those who have joined up in their childhood – as early as 16 years of age (so called 'boy soldiers') and who have served for a maximum time, some leaving the military in their late 40s or 50s. For some, leaving the military may serve to reactivate attachment difficulties that may have existed prior to joining the military.

Some veterans find it difficult to forget their military identity. They find civilian life less intense and less meaningful and find that they have difficulty leading a comparatively disorganised and mundane civilian existence. They miss the excitement, risk taking, camaraderie, team cohesion, friendships and their identity. They find it difficult to relate to civilians who do not have the same sense of organisation, team sprit and urgency about situations. After leaving the armed forces some veterans work in other uniformed 'services' such as the police, fire, ambulance and prison service where there may experience continuing exposure to traumatic events.

The military can feel very much like an institution with its own:

➤ culture
➤ tradition (down to unit level)
➤ reputation (down to unit level)
➤ language and jargon
➤ housing and accommodation requirements and services
➤ timetable and requirements
➤ posting cycle
➤ medical services, rules and regulations, courts and conduct codes.

Institutionalisation into an authoritarian regime can restrict independence by promoting a loss of skills, a loss of individual identity, isolation and social understimulation, the effects of which can all become apparent when a serviceman exits the service.

VETERANS AND MENTAL ILLNESS

While the majority of regular and reserve servicemen and women do not experience mental health problems during or after service, it is recognised that a significant number of ex-servicemen report that they had suffered significant mental health difficulties while still in the Armed Services but felt unable to consult their military GPs and access mental health services while they were in the military. This is linked to feelings of shame and guilt, as well as stigma, and also frequently to a fear that their career might be compromised or even lost.

Veteran population studies – the assessment of need

Population studies enable the assessment of need for mental health services. There have been no British population studies into the mental health needs of veterans, making the planning of services very difficult. It is estimated currently there are about five million veterans in the UK and seven and a half million first-degree dependents.

Military at-risk population studies have been most comprehensively conducted in US Vietnam War veterans, with the gold standard being set by the impressive National Vietnam Veterans Readjustment Study (NVVRS) (Kulka *et al.* 1990). Much can be learnt from this study. The study was set up as part of the Veterans Health Care Amendments (US Public Law 98–160) by the US Congress, which ordered that a systematic and comprehensive study be carried out in order to determine the prevalence and incidence of PTSD and other psychological problems in readjusting into civilian life in Vietnam-era veterans. Before this study was carried out, assessment and treatment facilities for veterans were dispersed, variable and frankly inadequate. Following the study, the Veterans' Agency in the US was able to plan and deliver bespoke mental health services to their veterans. The UK badly needs a similar study to be performed.

The NVVRS study started with a sampling frame of 8 million, which included all persons who served on active (combat) duty (180 days or more) during the Vietnam era (5 August 1964 to 7 May 1975). This represented an estimated 93–94% of the total combat veterans from that war who had returned home. Subjects were randomly selected (n = 1612 males and 736 females) and an age- and sex-matched control group was set up of soldiers who were in the military during the war era but did not serve in Vietnam. Measurements were made using self-report questionnaires and selected structured interviews including the Diagnostic Interview Schedule. NVVRS PTSD prevalence rates are given in Table 12.1.

TABLE 12.1 NVVRS PTSD prevalence rates

	Vietnam veterans		Non-Vietnam veterans	
	Male **(n = 1612)**	**Female** **(n = 736)**	**Male** **(n = 1612)**	**Female** **(n = 736)**
Prevalence at time of study	15.2%	8.5%	2.5%	1.1%
Lifetime prevalence	30.9%	26.9%		

The NVVRS estimated that 1.7 million veterans (or half of all who served in Vietnam) suffered partial or full PTSD at some time since discharge from military service and that 828 000 did at the time of the study. Co-morbidity levels were high – 50% of

Vietnam War theatre veterans with current PTSD had suffered from at least one other diagnosable psychiatric disorder within six months prior to the assessment. The percentage lifetime and current co-morbidity findings in the NVVRS study are shown in Table 12.2. The study also demonstrated high levels of divorce, unemployment and high rates of accidents – including road traffic accident rates 49% higher in combat veterans compared to non-combatants – and suicide rates 65% higher in combat veterans.

TABLE 12.2 Lifetime and current co-morbidity of theatre Vietnam veterans in NVVRS study

	Previous 6 months	Lifetime	Previous 6 months	Lifetime:
	Male (n = 1612) (%)		Female (n = 736) (%)	
Major depression	15.7	26.4	23.0	42.3
Dysthymia	–	21.0	–	33.2
Generalised anxiety disorder	19.8	43.5	19.4	38.2
Panic disorder	4.9	8.2	12.7	20.8
OCD	8.7	10.4	7.5	12.7
Alcohol abuse	22.2	73.8	10.1	28.5
Drug abuse	6.1	11.3	<1	8
Antisocial personality disorder	10.8	–	<1	–
Mania	4.4	5.5	2.5	2.5

In the UK there have been important studies conducted by the King's College Hospital military psychiatry research team into a population of servicemen who participated in Operation Telic (the 2003 war in Iraq) (Hotopf *et al.* 2006; Horn *et al.* 2006). These studies have shown that for serving military personnel the most common disorders are depression, anxiety disorders, substance misuse (mostly alcohol) and psychological trauma-related disorders including PTSD. It is hoped that the Operation Telic studies will evolve into a longitudinal population study in veterans as the servicemen end their military careers. Approximately 25% of this population are now veterans, having left the military since service in Operation Telic. At the time of writing, moves are being made in Scotland to follow the suggestion of the charity Combat Stress for a population study to be conducted there.

While it has been noted above that overall rates of PTSD in personnel who are still serving are reported as being generally low, with figures of between 1% and 8% being reported from recent conflicts, it should be noted that recent UK studies conducted in veteran populations claiming war pensions indicate that these veterans are twice as likely as civilians to develop delayed-onset PTSD after they leave military service. Moreover, it has been shown that 43% of those who present suffering delayed onset PTSD develop it within the first year of leaving the services (Brewin and Andrews 2008). Further research is urgently required into these findings.

Special needs and lack of access to care

While the true mental health needs of the British veteran population are unknown, it is known anecdotally through ex-servicemen's welfare agencies that veterans frequently present to mental health services, especially those in the third sector, with complex mental health problems that have been present for a significant number of years. Veterans usually present to veterans' mental health charities such as Combat Stress (otherwise known as the Ex-servicemen's Mental Welfare Organisation) an average of 14 years after they have left the Services.

The complex psychiatric disorders most commonly comprise co-morbid presentations of PTSD, depression and alcohol disorders including dependence and severe abuse. Moreover, veterans with mental health problems commonly give histories of isolation; social exclusion; social withdrawal; unemployment, including multiple episodes of unemployment; inadequate housing; multiple house moves; multiple employment episodes and employers; and multiple marriages and relationships. They frequently present with behavioural disorders manifested by anger and outbursts. Many have been homeless for long periods of time and significant numbers have been in prison, with ex-servicemen known to be over-represented in these populations.

Veterans are poor at accessing the mental health care that they need and complying with mainstream NHS psychiatric and psychological services – often impulsively removing themselves from waiting lists or failing to attend appointments, especially for psychotherapy and psychiatry. This is because of shame, embarrassment, and a fear that they will not be understood or that they will have to disclose gruesome details of combat to relatively young inexperienced female therapists, mental health workers or psychologists. Many fear they will not be understood. Many have been seen by mental health workers or even their GPs and been told to pull themselves together, with a perceived lack of understanding and sympathy making it more likely that they will be less inclined to ask for help again. Many who have accessed psychotherapy have found it impossible to disclose psychologically traumatic experiences and hide behind statements that the therapist or psychologist cannot be told what has happened because they have not signed the Official Secrets Act. The material is therefore avoided and never disclosed, and trauma-focused psychotherapies for the treatment of PTSD are never engaged in.

Further difficulties can result from a lack of understanding by the mental health worker of the significance of military service, including combat, on mental health presentations, or a lack of understanding of the military culture and a failure by the mental health worker to take an adequate history because of bewilderment of military life and military slang/jargon. Shame felt by veterans at having to disclose terrible psychological trauma to people whom they felt did not want to listen has also prevented engagement in therapy or a therapeutic alliance from being set up for therapy to progress. Sometimes veterans have been included inappropriately in group therapies where they have been told by therapists that their traumatic material was too upsetting to be disclosed in group psychotherapy. Other issues have been difficulties coping with irritable outbursts in the health setting and difficulty controlling frustration generated by a system they could not follow.

Veterans' mental health needs can also be seen as falling between services, with GPs trying to access CMHTs only to be told that the most appropriate service is psychology or psychotherapy, whereas commonly veterans may need expert prescribing of psychotropic medications as well as expert risk assessment in tandem with psychotherapy. It should be noted as well that there is a lack of expertise for the treatment of PTSD generally and a shortage of mental health workers who themselves have served in the military and who therefore have a unique insider understanding of military mental health issues and who, in theory at least, should have less difficulty engaging the veteran patient.*

RECENT GOVERNMENT INITIATIVES

In 1948, the British government decreed that healthcare, including the mental health care needs of veterans, would be provided for by the NHS. However, the mental health needs and the effectiveness of the NHS services delivered to veterans have never been evaluated thoroughly. Recently there has been an increase in popular awareness through the press, because of pressure from ex-service charities and the fact that Britain has been fighting two wars, that veterans with mental health problems have unique needs, making them a unique population. Evidence has also been mounting from overseas, in particular Australia and the US. As a result the Government has taken some steps to try to address this problem:

➤ Efforts have been made to improve access to NHS care by recognising that veterans have difficulty engaging in mental health care, raising awareness of this among NHS staff and providing information on how veterans' health needs differ from those of the population generally.

➤ NHS Trusts and PCTs have been directed that veterans should be fast-tracked and priority given into healthcare, both for physical as well as mental health needs.

➤ From 2007, veterans have had access to a comprehensive assessment of any physical or mental problem they consider is related to their service at the Medical Assessment Programme (MAP) based in London and funded by the Ministry of Defence (MoD). Treatment recommendations are made following assessment and the patient is referred back to his GP for onward specialist NHS referral.

➤ Since 2007, Reservists have had access to a mental health assessment facility at

---

* The UK Trauma Group website gives the addresses of NHS and other clinics in the UK specialising in the treatment of PTSD (www.uktrauma.org.uk).

Chilwell near Nottingham, the Reservists' Mental Health Programme (RMHP) funded by the MoD. Where appropriate, Reservists are offered treatment in Military Departments of Community Mental Health.

➤ The MoD and the charity Combat Stress have set up six veterans NHS pilot sites across the country. These pilots aim to identify the mental health needs of veterans and signpost them into appropriate NHS treatment.

➤ From 1 April 2009 the Scottish Government has commissioned Combat Stress to provide services in Scotland for residential treatment mental health programmes.

➤ As part of the commissioning guidance document of the Improvement into Access into Psychological Treatments (IAPT), veterans have been included as being a vulnerable group that has difficulties accessing care (DH 2008).

EX-SERVICEMEN'S WELFARE ORGANISATIONS

There is a wide range of ex-servicemen's charities designed to help the veteran and their dependents and widows. These include the Royal British Legion (RBL) in England, Wales and Northern Ireland and its equivalent, Poppy Scotland, north of the border; the Soldiers, Sailors, Airmen and Families Association (SSAFA) and the RAF Families Federation. Others specialise depending on target populations; for example, Combat Stress specialises in looking after ex-servicemen and veterans suffering from mental health illnesses (see below); the Officers Association, which helps ex-officers with welfare; St Dunstan's, which specialises in helping blind ex-servicemen; and the British Limbless Ex-Service Men's Association (BLESMA), which specialises in helping the blind and amputees.

Most of these charities emphasise welfare and practical and social needs but are also extremely helpful in identifying those who have mental health needs and also in helping to stabilise crisis situations by having or being able to advise on accessing the resources to find emergency loans, housing and other practical necessities, such as equipping a flat or house with basic furniture or cooking aids. Access to funds can also be made available through the veterans' own regimental funds.

Veterans who develop mental health problems after leaving the services may be eligible for a War Pension or (since 6 April 2005) an award under the Armed Forces Compensation Scheme. The Service Personnel and Veterans Agency (SPVA) is piloting projects to identify vulnerable service leavers before they exit and to provide a mentoring service for six months for Early Service Leavers (those who leave within 4 years of enlistment) to ease their transition from military life. The SPVA is a useful source of information for veterans about welfare issues.

COMBAT STRESS

Combat Stress (also known as the Ex-serviceman's Mental Health Welfare Organisation) is a national charity and the only mental health charity of any size that specialises in treating veterans suffering from mental health disorders. Combat

Stress currently provides mental health welfare multidisciplinary treatments within a combination of community-based services, as well as within residential rehabilitation programmes. The remainder of this chapter describes the work of the charity as an example of how to deliver an ongoing intervention to meet the needs of veterans with mental health problems.

Combat Stress was set up in 1919 after the First World War. It functioned for many years providing residential respite care for mentally ill veterans, but increasingly over the past five years radical changes have been taking place in relation to the services it provides, both within the community and in residential care. Combat Stress is part-funded via the War Pensions system and part-funded by charity (around 60%). The intention is that it will soon be funded through the NHS and indeed this is the case in Scotland from 1 April 2009.

The charity estimates that in the past 89 years over 85 000 veterans and their families have been helped. Currently there are 3680 veterans actively receiving mental health care either in the community or attending residential treatment services, or both, with some further 4800 'dormant cases' – those who are in the process of either accessing care or who have already accessed care and where intervention is completed but who have not as yet been discharged form care. Referral rates have been increasing year on year, from 300–400 annually ten years ago to around 1400 new referrals annually at the time of writing.

While 10 years ago the average age of the veteran was around 60, with a substantial number of Second World War veterans receiving care, now the average age is 43 years and falling (with a range of 20 to 93 years). Ex-Army veterans account for 81.5%, with the remainder equally shared by ex-Royal Navy and ex-RAF veterans and a very small number of ex-merchant navy seamen. Female veterans account for around 3% of the total population.

On average, veterans present 13 years after leaving the military. Most will have served in at least one and usually multiple operational tours of duty, with combat being extremely common; Northern Ireland operations being the most prevalent.

The Combat Stress population

Clinical audit data (*see* Box 12.1 and Table 12.3) supported by analyses of psychometric tests demonstrate that veterans accessing Combat Stress frequently present with multiple co-morbid psychiatric disorders and social, occupational and relationship problems. They also present with co-morbid physical conditions, especially orthopaedic problems and chronic pain, and increased levels of heart disease and diabetes. These findings reflect formal research studies looking at US veterans which have demonstrated higher rates of a large variety of physical illnesses associated with high levels of PTSD compared to the general population.

BOX 12.1 Combat Stress clinical audit data (n = 331) and psychometric data analyses (n = 480) 2005–2008

Psychiatric disorders
➤ Very high levels of chronic psychiatric disorder and co-morbidity, especially PTSD (ranging between 71% for review patients and 81% for new patients) and depression and alcohol-related disorders including psychotic presentations with anxiety, anger, personality difficulties and dissociative disorders.
➤ Very high rates of attachment/abuse problems related to childhood.
➤ Attachment problems regenerated after leaving the military.
➤ Co-morbid presentations of PTSD, depression and alcohol abuse or dependence are the most common presentation.
Behavioural disorders
➤ Aggression, violent behaviour – offending behaviours including Schedule 1 offences.
Physical disorders
➤ Chronic physical disabilities/illness especially orthopaedic and chronic pain problems.
Co-morbidity
➤ Very high levels of psychiatric and physical co-morbidity.
Social exclusion
➤ Dysfunctional relationships, marital and family breakdown.
➤ Unemployment (up to 75% of those of working age).
➤ High percentage live alone and have accommodation problems.
➤ Isolation is a very common problem.

TABLE 12.3 Combat Stress clinical audits 2007

	% New patients (n = 162)	% Review patients (n = 169)
Significant current physical illness: includes diabetes, cardiac disorders	59	86
Physical injury (wounding, or accidental) during military service	45	62
Psychiatric illness as a measure of chronicity – had consulted at least their GP for military-related mental health problems in the past	75	95
Multiple exposure to (military) psychological trauma	95	84

(*continued*)

	% New patients (n = 162)	% Review patients (n = 169)
Past and present history of alcohol and drug dependence and abuse	69	74
Significant attachment difficulties in childhood/adolescence, including child sexual abuse and other forms of abuse	59	39

Clinical pathways into care and referrals

Combat Stress looks after a help-seeking population that has largely tried to become engaged with the NHS in the past but has either not remained engaged or has failed to engage. Around half of the veterans self-refer or are referred by their wives, girl-friends, or partners (*see* Table 12.4). Commonly referral is precipitated by a family, relationship or marital crisis and in many of these cases the veteran is being given an ultimatum to get better by his spouse or girlfriend. Direct referrals from GPs and NHS mental health professionals occur but these are extremely rare.

TABLE 12.4 Referrals into Combat Stress care 2006/7

NHS, social services and military service discharge boards	11% (including approximately 3% NHS)
Service charities, welfare organisations, VA, SPVA	31%
Self referral, referral through family members – wife or partners	46%
Other	13%

Aims of Combat Stress intervention

The main aims of intervention are to assess and treat mental health illness and, with the permission of the veteran, to refer into NHS services. Management may be taken over by the NHS or joint management undertaken depending on the clinical presentation and the veteran's own wishes. Welfare needs are also managed and access to work retraining is encouraged wherever possible.

Once referred, the veteran will receive an initial Regional Welfare Officer (RWO) visit and if a mental health problem exists, with their GP's written consent, veterans are offered a mental health assessment. The RWO is a retired military officer who is not formally trained in mental health, but who has knowledge of mental health problems and who is an integral member of a clinical multidisciplinary team. The RWO is the main portal of entry into care for the veteran. It is hoped that issues of stigma, shame and other civilian barriers can be overcome by the RWOs, who speak the same language as the veterans and are able to gain their trust.

Community services

The Community Welfare arm of Combat Stress employs sixteen (regional) RWOs across the UK and Ireland. A desk officer manages each RWO. After the initial visit the RWO offers welfare support and help. He will also write a referral report for the multidisciplinary team based within a residential treatment centre. The RWO liaises with the SPVA in relation to the veterans' war pension entitlement, as well as with other service charities, and also explores avenues such as retraining for work, if indicated. The RWO follows up and stays in touch as long as the patient's case remains 'active', i.e. help is being delivered for welfare or clinical needs, or both.

Combat Stress is currently in the process of setting up multidisciplinary community services, with the appointment of 16 teams to work alongside the RWOs across the country. Each team will be manned by an RMN, a generic mental health worker who is proficient at delivering therapies including family therapy, and sessional psychiatrists and psychologists. The aims of the community teams are to assess and manage those patients they can within a community setting and to encourage and plug patients into appropriate NHS services via the veteran's GP. They will also refer patients into one of the three treatment centres for bespoke residential treatment programmes. Several community treatments including family groups are being delivered from residential treatment centres. The aim will be to transfer some of these programmes into a community setting in due course.

Residential treatments

Combat Stress owns three residential treatment centres: Tyrwhitt House in Surrey, Audley Court in Newport, Shropshire and Hollybush House in Ayr. Each has around 30 beds as well as some accommodation for spouses.

The treatment centres are run in a manner that is sensitive to military culture. Many but not all the staff are ex-military (mental health workers) themselves. The treatment centres foster a strong therapeutic milieu that an ex-serviceman can easily identify with and encourage a culture of peer support. Most ex-servicemen have no difficulty feeling at ease within this unique setting.

Combat Stress has adopted a recovery model of care in keeping with NICE guidelines for the treatment of veterans (*see* Box 12.2). Most veterans seen within the service have complex presentations and needs. Currently patients are admitted for an initial five-day assessment. This helps the veteran to feel safe and engage with the service. Veterans are then usually offered three two-week admissions or six one-week admissions over a one-year period before their care plans are reviewed. Currently they access a rolling programme comprising group psychoeducation as well as individual trauma-focused therapies, including trauma-focused cognitive behaviour therapy (TF-CBT); eye movement desensitisation and reprocessing (EMDR); rehabilitation activities aimed at socialising them; and access to multidisciplinary interventions with psychologists, OTs, psychiatrists and RMNs.

In the near future, Combat Stress will be able to deliver assessment in the community and will be reorganising its residential bespoke treatment programmes which will be targeted more specifically at the needs of the individual veteran.

As far as treatments for PTSD are concerned, Combat Stress aims to have a bespoke intensive programme lasting four to six weeks in the residential setting, with group and individual psychotherapy that is then followed up and continued in the community. In addition, the aim is to have a bespoke programme for old-age

COMBAT-RELATED STRESS **139**

veterans mainly run in the community and a remedial intensive programme which will be community-based for those who have treatment-resistant chronic PTSD, as well as the current rolling programme and a programme based solely on respite care.

All these programmes will be run with a residential component as well as a community component, will be evidence-based and run on the lines of the US veterans rehabilitation treatment protocols and the Australian veterans' mental health services.*

BOX 12.2 Treatment of PTSD in veterans: basic principles

Multimodal assessment
➤ Clinical history and mental state examination; psychometric tests: subjective and objective.

Stabilise
➤ Prepare for therapy: detox alcohol, drugs.
➤ Address welfare needs – homelessness, isolation, etc.
➤ Prescribe appropriate medications SSRI and related antidepressants, mood stabilisers, anti-impulse, major tranquillisers, medications for pain.

Therapy
➤ *Outpatient* services:
➤ assessment plus TF-CBT
➤ EMDR (single trauma much easier to address!).
➤ Residential specialist services:
➤ initial stabilisation, then disclosure/psychotherapy, then rehabilitation
➤ group programmes: psychoeducation; cognitive restructuring groups; individual TF-CBT; EMDR; psychodynamic including disclosure work; narrative therapy.

Rehabilitation
➤ Needs to commence at the outset – may need to include retraining.

BOX 12.3 Combat Stress Treatment Strategy (Dec 2007); chronic disease management as per 2005 NICE Guidelines for treatment of veterans with PTSD

1	Initial preparation.
2	Stabilisation and safety.
3	Disclosure and working through of the traumatic material and psychotherapy on an individual basis.
4	Rehabilitation and reintegration within society; normalising activities of daily living.

Initial preparation: At Combat Stress this translates to assessment by the RWO and referral meeting

---

* See www.dva.gov.au/HEALTH_AND_WELL-BEING/Pages/index.aspx

with the multidisciplinary team (MDT); gathering of information from GP and NHS team if available; followed by active preparation for initial assessment admission, such as detoxification from alcohol and drugs if needed.

Stabilisation and safety: At Combat Stress this includes psychiatric assessment and the prescription of appropriate medications; engendering trust; engendering safety within a therapeutic milieu; psychoeducation; admission for five-day MDT assessment; subsequent further admissions (current practice); formulation of the Whole Person Care Plan and communication to GP and other agencies working with the veteran. Treatment of co-morbid disorders, such as chronic pain, depression and alcohol dependence is provided before trauma work is undertaken.

Disclosure and working through of the traumatic material and psychotherapy on an individual basis: At Combat Stress this translates to eventually (after engaging in psycho-education of PTSD, alcohol and illicit drugs, coping, anxiety and anger management, etc) when the individual is in the right mental 'space' and able to confront traumatic material, disclosure and working through of the traumatic material and psychotherapy on an individual basis. The best approaches used here include trauma focussed therapies including trauma-focused cognitive behaviour therapy (TF-CBT) and eye movement desensitisation and reprocessing (EMDR).

Some patients just cannot be treated using these techniques. Many patients also have attachment difficulties stemming from childhood, bullying and maltreatment within their service life and loss attachment issues on leaving the services. These patients additionally need psychotherapeutic interventions incorporating long-term psychotherapies. Advice is given to the GP to refer on to the local psychology services for engagement in local TF-CBT/EMDR if available.

Rehabilitation and reintegration within society: This requires occupational therapy assessment and interventions normalising activities of daily living. At Combat Stress rehabilitation starts on admission; welfare support helps reintegration within society, work retraining may be indicated and Combat Stress can refer to agencies that deliver this.

Family and spouse interventions – carers' groups, family and couple therapy

Studies have shown that in US combat veterans the most powerful predictors of ongoing PTSD are first the dose response effect (i.e. dose of exposure to trauma/ combat/time in the front line) and, second, impaired family functioning (which was found to be more powerful than personality and developmental issues). There is also a very strong correlation between PTSD severity and family dysfunction. Studies into treatment outcome for veterans have demonstrated that those who do best in treatment are those who are in a supportive relationship with a female – usually their wife (see Egendorf 1986). Marital support is crucial to adjustment in veterans.

All the Combat Stress treatment centres run regular family and carers groups along the same lines as those run by the Australian Veterans Mental Health Services. Groups are also run in the community in the large cities. Their purpose is to help, educate and support the family members of the veteran accessing the care of Combat Stress.

Combat Stress helpline

Welfare Desk officers offer 9–5 telephone advice and become the named point of contact for each individual veteran that calls. A nursing station also offers out-of-hours advice to veterans – effectively meaning that a 24-hour helpline is available. A bespoke helpline is in process of being set up with the Samaritans.

The Combat Stress website provides information on post-traumatic stress disorder, the services offered by the charity, frequently asked questions and contact details for the support team in each region of the country.

CONCLUSION

While at last the needs of veterans with mental health problems seem to have started to be taken seriously by the government, there is much left to do. A population study is badly needed to identify the size and nature of the problem and aid the planning of services. While referrals to Combat Stress continue to rise, what this charity may be dealing with is only one end of the spectrum. It needs to be acknowledged that some of the problem lies with the veterans themselves, who are very hard to engage. Another difficulty is the failure of the NHS to fully understand and respond to the need, and the traditional reliance on ex-service charities which for years have only offered respite care. The challenge for the future will be to help the NHS to provide adequate services across the country. The model evolving in Scotland, where Combat Stress will be working in partnership with the NHS, may be the model of care that proves to be the ideal long-term clinical service. Joint working between the NHS, CMHTs, the Improving Access to Psychological Therapies (IAPT) programme, Ministry of Defence pilot sites and ex-military charities is probably the best way forward for service delivery and planning.

REFERENCES

Brewin C and Andrews B (2008) Delayed onset PTSD: New research on an Old Controversy. 24th ISTSS Annual Meeting Terror and its Aftermath. Abstract 196022: The Palmer House Hilton. Chicago, USA. November 13–15, 2008. Symposium.

Department of Health (DH) (2008) *Commissioning IAPT for the Whole Community: improving access to psychological therapies*. London: DH.

Egendorf A (1986) *Healing from the War: trauma and transformation after vietnam*. Boston, MA: Shambhala.

Gould M, Sharpley J and Greenberg N (2008) Patient characteristics and clinical activities at a British military department of community mental health. *Psychiatric Bulletin*. **32**: 99–102.

Kulka RA, Schlenger WE,. Fairbank JA, Hough R L, Jordan BK, Marmar CR, *et al*. (1990) *Trauma and the Vietnam War Generation: report of findings from the National Vietnam Veterans Readjustment Study*. New York: Brunner/Mazel.

Horn O, Hull L, Jones M, Murphy D *et al*. (2006) Is there an Iraq war syndrome? Comparison of the health of UK service personnel after the Gulf and Iraq wars. *Lancet*. **367**: 1742–1746.

Hotopf M, Hull L, Fear NT, Browne T *et al*. (2006) The health of UK military personnel who deployed to the 2003 Iraq war: a cohort study. *Lancet*. **367**: 1731–174.

Shen YC, Arkes J, Pilgrim J (2009) The effects of deployment intensity on post-traumatic stress disorder: 2002–2006. *Mil Med*. **174**: 217–23.

CHAPTER 13

Anger management and violence prevention with men

Sue and Pete Dominey

INTRODUCTION

Anger is a natural human emotion that everyone experiences at one time or another. Very mild types of anger can be expressed as distaste, displeasure or irritation. It can be a normal, healthy reaction to feeling frustrated, criticised or threatened. People will either become scared or angry in response to these types of situation – this is known as the 'fight or flight' response. It can also be a secondary emotion that comes straight after feeling scared, sad or lonely. But anger can range from feeling normal annoyance to full-blown rage, which can cloud your thinking and judgement and may lead to actions that are unreasonable and/or irrational.

Examples of common factors that can make people angry are:

➤ losing someone you love (grief)
➤ sexual frustration
➤ being tired, hungry or in pain
➤ physical withdrawal from certain medicines or drugs.

Anger isn't always a bad thing and it can be a helpful emotion when we need it for survival or to protect other people. However, when anger isn't managed properly, it can lead to aggression and the physical, mental and emotional abuse of yourself or other people (Parker Hall 2009). This is shown in many different ways including:

➤ sarcastic comments
➤ swearing
➤ name-calling
➤ bullying
➤ physical violence, e.g. hitting and kicking
➤ self-injury, e.g. cutting yourself or banging your head against a wall.

Help to manage anger may be found through cognitive behaviour therapy, talking treatments or specific anger management or domestic violence programmes. Anger management is a form of counselling to help people cope with any angry feelings they may have that are affecting their health, work, social behaviour or personal relationships.

WHO NEEDS ANGER MANAGEMENT?

Men with anger issues will often believe that their anger is everyone else's fault. It can therefore take others around him to make a man realise that he has an anger problem. Families, workmates or friends may start to let the man know that they are scared of him, perhaps because his behaviour spoils nights out, he's aggressive or abusive towards his partner, he's been a bit tough on the kids, or there have been incidents at work, on the sports field, or road rage.

A man losing his temper is often a clue to other problems – especially stress, and that feeling of being on the edge is common. It could also be that current life events, such as bereavement, relationship problems or trauma through accidents, have impacted in a way to cause a manifestation of powerful feelings. Painful memories and experiences from a man's past or childhood can be 'tapped into' or repressed, and destructive anger 'acted out'.

Admitting that there's a problem is the first step; deciding to get help can be another huge step. It is well known that many men find it difficult to ask for help and it is often a point of crisis that propels a man to seek help.

ASKING FOR HELP

Asking for help about anything can be difficult for many men – it puts them in a position of admitting vulnerability and feeling that it's a sign of weakness. This is tied into the way men 'do' shame, embarrassment, fear of consequences, fear of being judged, denial, minimisation, collusion – 'it's not a problem'.

When men do ask for help, often the first stop is their local health centre – the GP and other health professionals. Occasionally, if their temper/anger has really got them into trouble, they may be signposted by the police, Social Services, Sure Start workers, A&E, mental health services, drug and alcohol services, or Relate (the UK's largest provider of relationship counselling and sex therapy). Men may also search the internet and phone book looking for a source of help, though in the UK, access to help with anger management is better in some areas of the country than in others.

Some of the things that men will commonly say at the first point of asking for help include:
➤ 'I'm losing my temper'
➤ 'I need anger management'
➤ 'I'm losing the plot'
➤ 'She/he/they wind me up'
➤ 'I just saw red/I lost it'

➤ 'I just can't remember but the wife/girlfriend tells me'
➤ 'I just exploded, I can't help it'
➤ 'She/he/they pushed me too far'.

It's important to engage positively with men who present with anger management issues – first impressions count. Building trust and developing a good working relationship are crucial. Aim to be non-judgemental, encouraging, supportive and reassuring (remember they are probably scared).

WHAT NEEDS TO BE MANAGED?

Very often anger is the secondary problem, it's the way men 'do' their emotions that can lead them to being angry a lot. When they feel sad, scared, insecure, emotionally hurt – many vulnerable emotions – they go to anger. Having a blast of anger is a quick release and makes them feel powerful, whereas feeling vulnerable isn't how they're 'supposed' to be feeling as men. The problem is that they don't really feel better after the outburst of anger; it often causes problems that just add to the sense of shame and insecurity that caused the anger in the first place.

Managing anger, for men, can be closely tied to working out how they 'do' their emotions and learning to 'do' them differently. This means having a good look at themselves and working out how they 'work'; this is often tied in with other issues, around childhood and early experiences which can drive how we all behave.

It can also be tied in to how men see the world they live in. If they believe that the world's a hostile place and they are the victim it means they feel entitled to get angry, but it also makes it difficult to do anything about their problems, as nothing is in their power to change. Taking responsibility for themselves is also a big part of managing themselves and their emotions differently. Put simply, managing anger is about much more than learning to keep your temper.

'Anger management' has become a bit of a buzz word. This has meant that increasingly it's seen as acceptable for men to ask for help with anger management, but it's important to be aware that it can be a cover for other emotional and mental health problems.

WHAT WORKS?

The changes needed to manage problems with anger can be helped either through groups or 'one to one' counselling or therapy.

One to one counselling or therapy can get to some of the underlying issues causing emotional problems, providing therapeutic support to recover and heal from early childhood/life experiences. Some types of therapy – especially cognitive behavioural therapy (CBT), which focuses on changing patterns of thinking and behaviour – can be used to help people manage themselves better, but can often miss some underlying emotional issues.

Group work can be very positive, instilling hope and supporting a man by helping him to feel less alone – a problem shared is a problem halved – but many men express anxiety and show a real resistance to joining a group. Admitting they have a problem is tough enough, admitting it to a room full of other men can feel really scary. But the benefits of meeting others with similar problems and sharing solutions and tips are huge. Having men around who've seen improvements in their lives is a real encouragement (Yalom 1995).

As a rule of thumb, adults work better in groups (although they might not choose it) and boys/teenagers work better one to one. This is mainly because the peer pressure among teenagers is so great and can easily over-ride any group ethos set by the facilitators. Adult groups of around ten tend to work, but ground rules should be set together and reviewed occasionally. Groups with teenagers can work, however, the smaller the group the better, and the boundaries have to be firm! What is needed in both groups and one to one is that men are helped to feel safe and build trust with those who are supporting them. No one reacts well, can listen and learn, if they feel scared and uncomfortable or if they feel judged and 'shamed'. So this must be the first job for the facilitator(s) or counsellor(s), after which a curriculum that allows men to examine how they 'work' can be followed (Waring and Wilson 1990).

HOW SHOULD A GROUP SESSION BE STRUCTURED?

At the Brave Project,* a violence prevention and anger management intervention for men in Bradford, UK, we run a two-hour group session, the first half of which is 'the check-in'. The group sits in a circle and facilitators ask each man to 'check in' – describing how their week/fortnight etc has been, the highs and lows, describing any angry incidents that might have happened and analysing what went on. Often it's an opportunity to offload and be respectfully listened to. The group facilitators set the tone for the group and encourage emotional openness, being authentic and honest.

Many men say that they have never heard men speak so openly before and that the group becomes the only place where they can talk like that. We have coined the term 'heart sharing', as the men learn to be honest about how they tell their stories and express their emotions, developing a new language for emotions other that just anger or rage. Most of the men who have attended the Brave Project have shown that underneath the anger they were often feeling a lot of fear and sadness.

The check-in part of the group can often run over an hour as each man has his turn and but we aim to bring this part of the session to a close within 90 minutes to leave time for a short break and then a group exercise or discussion, either from the curriculum or from something that cropped up in the check-in.

When delivering this type of work, it's important to be careful not to challenge the men too early on or you might lose them. Avoid shaming at all costs (check your own attitudes and beliefs) and know your limitations. Facilitators should ask themselves whether they are prepared to go to places they are asking the men in the group to go – looking at their thoughts, feelings and behaviour; sometimes looking deep within.

---

*   www.brave-project.org

WHAT CURRICULUM SHOULD I USE?

As well as having some anger management techniques and strategies, the curriculum/ programme should include exercises to encourage and help the men to understand themselves. There are anger management workbooks available, many of them using visual techniques ('anger-ladder', 'traffic lights', etc) which help the men to remember when those trigger moments come. Staple handouts given to every man should include: 'The Anger Ladder', 'Spotting Anger Signals', 'Emotional Tank', 'Anger Funnel' and 'Time Out'.

It can help if the men can keep an anger diary which will help them to focus on themselves, to see the patterns and drives to their anger and abusive behaviour, and to begin to recognise the consequences of their anger, on themselves and those around them. It's often useful in the groups to do some analysis of angry incidents, to begin to de-mystify what happens and to point out during the episode when different choices could have been made (Waring and Wilson 1990).

It helps to start looking at the way men think about anger. Anger is a natural emotion, and not always damaging. It can be expressed in a positive, assertive, passionate way without harming self or others. It is mostly aggressive rage that does damage. Most men believe they go from 'calm' to 'blind rage' instantly; it's important to help them believe that they do that journey more slowly. They will need to become more aware of the bodily signs – sweaty palms, butterflies in stomach, pumping heart, dry mouth – all of which men find easy to ignore.

Anger is an emotion that makes us focus outwards – 'someone's doing something to me', blaming others and often wanting to punish. We also tend to 'wind ourselves up', have internal voices going on – 'who do they think they are?', etc. It's not difficult to recognise these, and change them to 'wind ourselves down' phrases – 'it's not worth it', 'don't take it personally'.

There are also difficult emotional situations which can trigger our anger; these can be very personal, but common ones are feeling disrespected or disregarded and not being listened to. Some actual situations can also be recognised as danger zones, such as traffic jams, supermarkets, being put on hold on the phone; all these situations can be recognised as our 'triggers' and be prepared for. In fact all of these situations can often be generalised into 'when we feel vulnerable' which takes us back to that 'not measuring up' feeling and the need to help ourselves feel more powerful. Learning new strategies to feel vulnerable or powerless and still be OK is a lot of what's needed to control anger.

Exercises that help to educate men around emotions are always useful, helping to build 'emotional muscle'. It can also help to look at distorted thinking patterns – 'stinking thinking' – and some of the attitudes and beliefs that drive that thinking. We all have self-talk going on in our heads a lot of the time and there are exercises that can turn that self-talk from negative to positive (Heery 2001).

In the beginning it helps with confidence to work from a programme, but eventually, with experience, it can be best to work with what comes up during the check-in.

WHAT ARE SUITABLE APPROACHES FOR WORKING WITH MEN?

A strengths-based approach

A strengths-based approach has a simple premise – identify what is going well, do more of it and build on it. Strengths are positive factors, both in the individual and in the environment, which support healthy development.

A strengths-based approach recognises that each of us has a combination of risk factors and protective factors which shape our development. Some of them are within our control and some beyond. Much attention has been given to the risk factors that have led to young men being over-represented among road crash fatalities, youth suicides, perpetrators of violence and many other negative statistics. What has been given far less attention are the protective factors that mean most young men are not counted among those statistics, and most lead healthy and productive lives posing no risk to themselves or others. Rather than having a problem-based orientation and a risk focus, a strengths-based approach seeks to understand and develop the factors that protect most young people.

A strengths-based approach has three distinct elements:

1 The approach emphasises the resourcefulness and resilience that exists in every-one rather than dwelling on what has gone wrong or placed a person at risk. It affirms that people can grow and change and that everyone has a range of abil-ities and strengths, which, with the right support, can be mobilised to give them a better future.

2 A second element of a strengths-based approach is an acceptance that the solu-tions will not be the same for everyone, that the strengths of individuals and the circumstances are different and that people need to be fully involved in identify-ing their goals and building on their strengths and resources.

3 The third element is the recognition that as individuals we live within famil-ies, communities, a society and a culture and that all these, along with our own attributes, determine our well-being. The strengths of these different environments are just as important to good outcomes as the strengths of individuals.

Strengths are also described as protective factors. Protective factors, as the name suggests, provide a buffer against risk factors. An individual's ability to cope with and manage the balance between risks, stressful life events and protective factors is increasingly described as 'resilience'

Male-focused approaches

Male-focused approaches are built on the understanding that being male is not just the gender into which half of us are born, but is about a set of characteristics, activities, preferences and forms of expression which we associate with it. As well as gender-related traits and preferences, some of which are biologically determined and some culturally, there is a range of explicit and implicit expectations which are placed on boys when they are born and reinforced throughout their lives. Male-focussed approaches accept this and respond to the fact boys and young men face unique challenges and need different responses. A strengths-based, male-focused approach will pay particular attention to the unique strengths which boys and young men have and work to develop them further (Dominey 2005).

WHAT CAN BE ACHIEVED?

Men often feel worse before they start to feel better if they really 'walk the walk' rather than just 'talking the talk'; they need lots of positive reinforcements, positive 'pats and strokes' and encouragement. For men who successfully go through anger management interventions, however, as well as starting to like themselves more, the range of benefits they experience can include:

➤ improved health and well-being
➤ reduced risk of harm to self and others
➤ increased self-esteem and confidence
➤ improved relationships at home and work
➤ reduced stress
➤ better quality of life
➤ improved ability to focus and concentrate (work output)
➤ less road rage
➤ avoidance of conflict
➤ ability to handle stressful situations.

CONCLUSION

Being able to deal with feelings of anger and frustration in a healthy way is essential for achieving a positive state of mental well-being and for not damaging the mental well-being of those around us. Regularly and uncontrollably flying into a rage makes truly healthy and rewarding relationships with others impossible and creates stress and anxiety for all concerned. As well as the negative impact of inappropriately expressed anger, unexpressed anger can also create problems, leading to passive-aggressive behaviour, such as getting at people behind their backs, constantly putting others down or being critical or cynical of everything all the time.

Anger management plays a vital role for men who have difficulties with anger in helping them to learn new strategies to enable them to control both their outward behaviour and their internal responses, dealing with their anger without lashing out, hurting others or themselves, or unhealthily internalising their feelings.

REFERENCES

Dominey S (2005) *Violence Prevention Work with Boys and Young Men.* Winston Churchill Fellowship. Available at: www.brave-project.org/Winston_Fellowship_report_Sue_Dominey_final.pdf

Heery G (2001) *Preventing Violence in Relationships.* London: Jessica Kingsley Publishers.

Parker Hall S (2009) *Anger, Rage and Relationships: an empathic approach to anger management.* London: Routledge.

Waring T and Wilson J (1990) *Be Safe: self-help manual for domestic violence.* Bolton: MOVE.

Yalom ID (1995) *The Theory and Practice of Group Psychotherapy* (4th ed.) New York: Basic Books.

CHAPTER 14

Tackling stress in the workplace

Andrew Kinder and Steve Boorman

INTRODUCTION

It is, perhaps, an often-missed fact that a substantial proportion of our waking lives are spent in the workplace. Whatever the source of stress, its consequences may be felt at work. Employers often worry about sickness absence and the cost associated with people being unable to work due to illness and stress-related illness is often a leading cause for concern. Sick presenteeism is also an important issue – people attending work, but with personal/medical issues which may impair their work performance resulting in accident, lost quality, poor efficiency, etc.

The workplace is a good place to tackle stress as whatever the source – whether an issue is directly work-related or not – its impacts may incur work costs. This chapter describes the reasons why workplace-based approaches can be effective and proposes some practical ways of tackling stress in the workplace.

HUMAN CAPITAL

Many businesses tritely say 'people are our greatest asset' but often fail to measure the value. Costs associated with ill-health may be considerable – the reality of sickness absence of, say, 5% is that one twentieth of the wage bill is going to support people not at work. However, this is not the only cost – sickness may require others to cover or temporary staff may be needed. Individuals less familiar with a job or not there at all may reduce productivity, or impair quality. Lost opportunities may occur and management time is often needed to manage sick employees. These extra costs all add up.

This is, however, only the tip of the iceberg. For every one individual who actually stays home sick, there are others who attend work but underperform due to illness. Particularly with stress-related illness, the consequences may be wide-ranging, including, for example, less creativity, poor memory, impaired problem solving, poor quality, mistakes and accidents. Less obvious consequences may be additional management time, poor workplace relationships, failure to capitalise on opportunities and issues of staff turnover and costs associated with retraining and recruitment.

Stress-related illness is a major contributor to these high costs and is often also an underlying factor in illness recorded due to other causes. An individual with a bad cold or bad back may 'soldier on', but if they are already under stress for other reasons their threshold for remaining at work or succumbing to the role of the patient may be lowered.

A business case can therefore be built up to invest in tackling stress in the workplace, whatever its origin.

EMPLOYERS' DUTIES

Since the passing of the Health and Safety at Work Act in 1974 employers have had clear statutory duties of care. The legislation requires workers' health and safety to be protected 'as far as reasonably practicable' and is reinforced by additional regulations that enforce an approach of identifying and reducing risks. These duties extend beyond simple physical issues of risks and include issues of a psychosocial nature. Enforcing authorities have been relatively slow to act in relation to stress issues, but since the development of Health and Safety Executive (HSE) guidance a number of enforcement notices and prosecutions have arisen and been pursued to conclusion.

Employers may also be subject to civil claims if they cause harm to their workers. Whilst cause and effect may sometimes be difficult to establish without doubt (it is easier to be clear that a broken leg was the result of a fall down a poorly guarded hole, for example), courts have developed experience over recent decades of dealing with stress-related illness in litigation. Compensation claims are possible and in some cases have run to very substantial sums.

Aside from duties under law, most employers would understand a simple moral duty of care for their fellow workers. The HSE also published information emphasising that 'Good Health Equals Good Business' – a tagline promoting the message that happy, healthy people are likely to be more productive and give a better return on investment.[*]

HSE MANAGEMENT STANDARDS

The HSE recommend a five-step risk assessment process, supported by management standards to identify stress hazards:
1 Identify hazards
2 Decide who might be harmed and how
3 Evaluate the risk and take action to avoid or reduce
4 Record the action plan
5 Monitor and review to ensure the plan remains effective.

---

[*] See www.hse.gov.uk for more information.

To assist employers in tackling the issue, the HSE have published a set of management standards defining workplace conditions to help employees avoid stress-related illness. For all these areas the employer is expected to ensure that systems are in place to enable issues to be identified and responded to.

➤ *Demands:* This standard covers issues such as working environment, workload and work patterns and seeks to ensure that employees can cope with the demands of their job.

➤ *Control:* This covers the extent to which individuals can influence their work and are involved.

➤ *Support:* This includes the resources available to encourage and support employees.

➤ *Relationship:* This relates to promoting positive working arrangements and dealing with conflict and unacceptable behaviour.

➤ *Role:* This is about ensuring that individuals understand their roles and are not placed in conflicting situations.

➤ *Change:* This deals with how well change is managed and communicated.

Although the above approach is not a statutory requirement to be followed to the letter, its development and publication by the HSE effectively constitutes the enforcing authority's view of what an employer should reasonably do to avoid stress-related issues arising from work. Support tools based on this model are widely available, either direct from the HSE or from commercial providers of stress control approaches.

WORKPLACE SUPPORT

The HSE approach seeks to reduce the likelihood of workplace stressors causing work-related illness. However, distress is not uncommon and the costs already highlighted make it often worthwhile, particularly for larger employers, to ensure access to employee support services.[*] A wide range of options exist in terms of how these are organised and delivered and it is fair to highlight that their effectiveness can be variable and needs to be measured and monitored.

Where provided, an employer is responsible for ensuring that the services offered are ethical and appropriate. The Association for Counselling at Work (ACW) published guidelines in 2007 which are helpful in understanding what is or isn't ethical and appropriate and in outlining different models of support (Hughes and Kinder 2007).[†]

Mode of delivery is inextricably linked to cost – 'hands on', local support involving highly trained professionals clearly being more costly to sustain than alternative remote approaches, such as telephone support or information delivered via websites. Mode of delivery is also relevant to uptake and usage. Face-to-face delivery is not always better – the anonymity of more remote or technology-based support can

---

[*] See Boorman (2008) for more discussion of this.

[†] This can be downloaded from www.counsellingatwork.org.uk

be preferred in some situations and individuals differ in their personal preferences.

Comprehensive programmes providing a range of support interventions are often termed 'employee assistance programmes' (EAPs). Again, many options exist and these may range from, at their simplest, telephone or e-based advice provision, through to services designed to provide employees with virtually any problem solution (some services extend to the provision of 'concierge' services which can even walk the dog, buy presents or flowers, or diary manage the harassed executive delayed at a late-running meeting!)

Commonly, EAPs provide support for work-related problems, debt or financial issues and for relationship issues. Extended services may also provide legal advice and support. In some circumstances the provision of comprehensive legal support of this nature may become a taxable benefit – particularly if support provided is not directly related to solving issues associated with work and reducing the distress that the individual is experiencing. Guidelines have been released to clarify this (see www.eapa.org.uk).

STRESS ASSESSMENT TOOLS

Structured questionnaire-based tools are often used to score or collate information about stress or other health issues. Many organisations use surveys to gauge employee morale and to gain feedback on issues important to employees and many such surveys collect important data relevant to the areas highlighted within the HSE management standards described above. These approaches are important to monitor stress within the workplace and to evaluate whether the organisation's programme of support is having a significant effect on the causes of stress (see Kinder 2004).

HOW DO YOU SET UP SUPPORT SERVICES FOR MEN?

As described earlier, given the costs to the UK economy of stress in the workplace and the personal impact on individuals, it is imperative for organisations to take action to reduce its effect. The principle is that effective support for employees will increase the psychological health of an organisation. Such support is wide and varied and the remainder of this chapter will outline what is available with a particular focus on the counselling needs of men.

It is often the case that men contact a support service as the 'last resort', such as where their marital relationship has reached the stage where one partner is threatening to walk out or the employee has to attend a dismissal interview in a day's time. Seeking support is counter-culture for many men and therefore it can be associated with a level of shame or a concern of being perceived as 'being weak'. This needs to be taken into account when setting up a service. It is therefore vital that counselling and EAP services provide a variety of ways to access services. Alongside the more traditional face-to-face sessions there are other methods which are popular with men, perhaps because they are anonymous. Some media will be more attractive to younger men (e.g. texting) while others will be used by men who are 'just looking' (e.g. telephone) or seeking advice for a colleague (e.g. self-help guides). Types of media through which support can be accessed include:

➤ online counselling in 'real time'
➤ telephone
➤ texting
➤ interaction with a computer software package, such as computerised Cognitive Behavioural Therapy
➤ bibliotherapy, such as self-help books.

The most commonly used medium is face-to-face but this needs to be carefully considered. If the counselling room is located in the organisation and is situated in a main thoroughfare without a waiting room, it will be no surprise if men will hardly use it due to confidentiality concerns. A private room with a waiting area so that men can slip into the room unnoticed will be much more beneficial. Some men like a reception facility which they report into prior to their appointment, while others will prefer booking their session remotely. Whatever method, it is important to make the experience for the man a discreet one – men are unlikely to want to bump into their boss in the waiting room and certainly don't wish to find that they can overhear what's being said in the next-door counselling room.

HOW DO YOU PROMOTE THE SERVICE?

The general 'feel' of the service is important; for instance, would you prefer to go to a 'well-being clinic' because you wanted to improve your functioning or a 'counselling service' because you were not coping? Branding is more than what marketing people get excited about, it is about what the service needs to convey to potential users in a positive up-beat way. It is worth thinking through what is in a name. 'Mental health', for example, can have a negative association, whereas 'well-being', 'wellness', 'coaching' and action words, such as 'positive step' and 'healthy living', can be used to convey a more up-beat message. Whatever the name, the service needs to develop and actually live the brand. Practitioners, receptionists and everyone associated with the programme needs to be proud of what the service can do and connect to the branding. Sometimes services go for a word which is totally new and doesn't mean anything. A new brand can be created but this takes time and don't be surprised if people keep referring to it as how it was previously known (e.g. one service renamed 'Employee Support' was still being referred to by its old name, 'Welfare', over seven years later). Bear in mind also that change takes time for the people running the service, as well as for the clients of the service.

When setting up a new service there is a great opportunity to use different ways of getting the message across. If there's an existing service, the use of a different, more novel, way of communicating can give it a fresh appeal, such as:

➤ using real case studies of men who are accessing the service (anonymously, of course)
➤ putting posters in places where men are likely to read them (the walls of toilets

can be used to good effect, but it's worth keeping an eye on the posters to ensure that they are not defaced!)

➤ distributing topical newsletters or email cascades (e.g. a headline story such as 'the credit crunch' will capture some interest and can then link in to counselling support for those experiencing relationship breakdown or to services to help men in debt)

➤ developing an internet site with access to telephone numbers or email addresses to ask questions so that men can look at descriptions of the service and access support in the privacy of their home

➤ leaflets which explain the services can be left in leaflet dispensers or given to managers/union officials to give out to employees when needed

➤ giving out cards or fridge magnets with contact details of the service – both are good reminders as they can be put into the wallet 'just in case' or put on the fridge at home and serve as reminders on a daily basis

➤ creating videos – given that many people receive information via the TV, videos can be used to get the message across about what the service provides in an engaging way (but make sure the videos are not too long – each clip should last a maximum of 3 minutes)

➤ creating podcasts – relaxation downloads or 'tips on managing debts', for example, can be a way of communicating with younger men, who almost all have MP3 players and are familiar with downloading TV and radio shows from the internet.

All of these methods for telling men about your service are very good, but perhaps the very best method is by personal recommendation – the 'grapevine' – and this can only be achieved by giving an excellent service that makes a real difference to people's lives!

HOW DO YOU ENSURE CONFIDENTIALITY?

Confidentiality is the cornerstone of any counselling/EAP service. It is what makes the service unique, as men feel that they can say what they are truly feeling without risk of being undermined or made fun of. The importance of this should not be underestimated, since where else can it be found? If a man is having difficulties with their partner, is a secret gambler or facing up to drinking too much, who can they turn to? They could speak with close friends or family but this can create other problems, especially as these people are not neutral and have vested interests.

The process of counselling involves trust and openness. Counsellors develop this by what is known as 'contracting', which is a way of clarifying the limits of the support and the boundaries of confidentiality; for instance, there may be a limit on the number of sessions. Counselling is not about giving advice or directing clients to take a particular course of action, since they will decide this themselves. It should not be seen as conditional; that is, attendance should not adversely affect career progression or status at work and attendance must also be voluntary. Counsellors work to a strict code of ethics and should not judge or exploit their clients in any way.

Confidentiality needs to be explained and 100% confidentiality can never be given. This surprises some people but counsellors need to balance the confidentiality of their client with obligations to society at large. Circumstances where a counsellor may need to break confidentiality include:

➤ where there is risk of harm to self or others
➤ where there is a serious alleged crime
➤ where there is a legal requirement (e.g. protection of children or prevention of terrorism)
➤ where there is a significant threat to the health and safety of those within an organisation.

A counselling service needs to be clear with the paying organisation about what is and what is not confidential, otherwise a different understanding can create unnecessary conflict and confusions. For instance, a counselling service where men self-refer is undermined if the organisation requires the names of people who have used the service. On the other hand, the organisation may set up manager referrals, which are more closely associated with occupational health, where a manager is concerned about an employee's sickness absence. The advantage of manager referrals, where a report is written, is that issues originating in the workplace can be identified, giving the organisation an opportunity to take remedial action. Also, it enables counselling to be provided to employees who may not have considered referring themselves.

WHAT SHOULD THE SERVICE COVER?

We all struggle with a variety of issues at some point in our lives. A counselling support service needs to think through how it can provide support to all these issues or to know how to onward refer men who need more specialist help. There is a credibility issue here; for instance, if a man plucks up courage to contact the service and is greeted with a response which says 'oh, sorry, we can't help you with that here', this is unlikely to build confidence in the service. Don't forget as well that if we experience a poor service we are likely to tell many more people than if we experience a good service.

So a counselling support service needs to consider what issues are likely to be raised, especially by men in employment (e.g. facing redundancy/dismissal etc). The following gives a flavour of the different issues that can be covered:

➤ stress, anxiety and depression
➤ alcoholism
➤ addiction/dependency
➤ bullying/harassment/intimidation/discrimination/conflict at work
➤ financial/legal/tax advice
➤ traumatic incident support
➤ bereavement
➤ relationship issues – divorce/separation/family conflict

➤ care problems related to childcare/eldercare/disability care
➤ neighbour or consumer issues
➤ gay/lesbian/gender issues
➤ domestic violence
➤ ill-health/retirement
➤ government benefits
➤ managerial support in handling staff issues
➤ gambling
➤ debt management
➤ eating disorders
➤ illness of a family member
➤ health, lifestyle and diet
➤ mortgage/repossessions
➤ redeployment/relocation
➤ redundancy.

HOW IS THE SERVICE EFFECTIVENESS MONITORED?

As mentioned previously, confidentiality is a vital component of any support service. This is great on one level, but if you are funding the scheme how do you know it is value for money? How does the service demonstrate its effectiveness? The starting point is to consider using feedback forms for men using the service. These could ask for responses to the following kind of statements along with a rating scale measuring the extent to which the individual agreed or disagreed:
➤ 'My call was answered quickly'
➤ 'The counsellor explained confidentiality clearly to me'
➤ 'I felt the counsellor listened to me effectively'
➤ 'The counsellor helped me to sort out my problems'
➤ 'Overall I am satisfied with the service I received'
➤ 'I would recommend the service to others.'

These questions are fine as far as they go but do not address the 'so what' issue. For instance, a male client may say that they are happy with the service (this is to be expected), but what difference did it make to the life of the client? What happened as a result? Did they get better, i.e. less depressed, more able to contribute at work, move from being off sick to being back at work? A system which looks also at these kinds of outcomes is going to be much more helpful to the managers running the service (i.e. they can see what services make a difference and can plan accordingly) and will allow them to demonstrate to its funders that they are getting value for money. There are a variety of different questionnaires and systems available. One such system is the CORE PC system, which has been used to show the added benefit of counselling services for some time now. Further details are available at www.coreims.co.uk

Other ways of monitoring the service are to put in place Key Performance Indicators around the speed at which calls are answered (you don't want nervous men phoning up for the first time struggling to get through quickly), the speed of getting an initial face-to-face or telephone session and the speed of responding to any query. Measuring the number of complaints or adverse comments made by clients are other important factors. Mystery Shopping should also be considered. This is where an evaluator uses the service as though they had a specific issue or concern and gathers feedback on the quality of their experiences. Lastly, clients can be contacted by telephone to give direct feedback on their experiences. Although this method can be very helpful it is important to bear in mind confidentiality and various ethical considerations. How would you feel, for example, if you were recovering from bereavement, you had used the service and were moving forward when someone phoned you without agreeing this in advance to ask about your past problems/issues? It could be perceived as intrusive. If you're going to use this approach, therefore, it should be contracted with the client beforehand.

Only statistical information on the main themes should be given back to the organisation, rather than names or other personally identifying data, in order to protect confidentiality and encourage men to use the service. The organisation can use such statistics to understand where 'hot spots' occur within the organisation, such as where there are greater perceived issues of work-related stress or perceived bullying/harassment. When overlaid with other data, such as sickness absence, formal grievances, staff turnover and employment relations, the organisation can target further interventions to address these problem issues. Uptake of the service is a good measure of how well it is being used, although organisations need to be confident that the statistics being reported on are not artificially being inflated, e.g. the provider can make the service look well used by counting every contact made whether it is a phone-call or session, rather than counting each individual person.

BOX 14.1 Checklist for setting up a service

> Ensure senior management are clearly supporting the service.
> Identify why the service is being set up – the purpose and outcomes being sought.
> Consider both employee and organisational needs.
> Get stakeholders from around the organisation engaged, including those connected with employee relations, such as unions.
> Plan the best ways to communicate the reasons for having a provision with senior-level endorsement.
> Get a steering group together – those responsible for managing and implementing the service.
> Be clear on the boundaries of confidentiality and define the parameters in relation to stakeholders and the steering group.
> Spend time looking at the best ways of promoting the service.
> Measure service awareness and service usage.

REFERENCES

Boorman S (2008) Employee Support Strategies in Large Organisations. In A Kinder, R Hughes and CL Cooper (eds), *Employee Well-being Support: a workplace resource*. Chichester: Wiley.

Hughes R and Kinder A (2007) *Guidelines for Counselling in the Workplace*. Rugby: British Association for Counselling & Psychotherapy.

Kinder A (2004) Stress Audits: what are they and why bother? *Counselling at Work*. Winter 2004: 14–18.

CHAPTER 15

Gay men's mental health

Justin Varney

INTRODUCTION

When thinking about the mental health of gay men, there is a professional paradox to consider. In all therapeutic encounters the practitioner should consider and explore the individual's relationships and social support structures, and in some this exploration goes further into desire and attraction beliefs and behaviours, however it does not usually define the therapeutic relationship or the context of the interventions provided to the patient. Therefore, an individual who identifies as gay or bisexual should not experience mental health services differently, assuming practitioners do not discriminate or express prejudice. But, and herein lies the paradox, the experience of identifying as gay in most societies leads to significant experiences of discrimination and isolation as well as individual psychic turmoil as the individual seeks to establish an identity other than the pejorative norm, which in turn may lead to poor mental health. Hence, the therapeutic relationship has to consider the impact of a homosexual identity while remaining neutral to the validity of the choice or identity.

THE HISTORICAL CONTEXT

One can't start to discuss gay men's mental health without recognising that in most Western countries homosexuality was classified as a mental disorder for the majority of the last hundred years and that in many countries (*see* Box 15.1) around the world mental ill-health is used as the excuse for the denial of basic human rights, torture, incarceration and murder of gay men; hence, it is an emotive topic.

BOX 15.1 Countries where homosexuality remains criminalised

Illegal
Afghanistan, Bangladesh, Bhutan, Comoros, Fiji, Ghana, India, Kiribati, Lesotho, Malawi, Maldives, Mozambique, Namibia, Nauru, Papua New Guinea, Samoa, São Tomé and Príncipe, Seychelles, Sierra Leone, Solomon Islands, Somalia, Sri Lanka, Togo, Tonga, Tuvalu.

Illegal with prison sentence (many of which can be up to life imprisonment or 10 years of hard labour)
Algeria, Antigua and Barbuda, Barbados, Belize, Botswana, Brunei, Burundi, Cameroon, Djibouti, Dominica, Ethiopia, Eritrea, Gambia, Gaza, Grenada, Guinea, Guyana, Jamaica, Kenya, Kuwait, Lebanon, Libya, Morocco, Myanmar, North Korea, Oman, Pakistan, Qatar, Saint Kitts & Nevis, Singapore, St. Lucia & Saint Vincent and the Grenadines, Syria, Trinidad and Tobago, Tunisia, Liberia, Senegal, Swaziland, Turkmenistan, Uganda, Uzbekistan, Zambia, Zimbabwe.

Illegal with death penalty
Iran, Mauritania, Nigeria, Saudi Arabia, Sudan, UAE, Yemen.

Homosexuality was removed per se from the Diagnostic and Statistical Manual of Mental Disorders (DSM) in 1973. However, it was replaced by the compromise condition of Sexual Orientation Disturbance, which tried to strike a balance between social perceptions of homosexuality as a normal sexual variant and some deep-seated professional views that homosexuality remained a curable, or at least treatable, condition (*see* Box 15.2).

In the third version of the DSM, published in 1980, the category was further revised into Ego Dystonic Homosexuality. However, there continued to be dissatisfaction on both sides of the debate and when DSM III was revised in 1986 all references to homosexuality were removed, with the only remnant being the condition of Sexual Disorders Not Otherwise Specified, which included the state of an individual being in a state of persistent and marked distress about their sexual orientation.

The classification within DSM has been important as it allowed a sect of reparative therapy to develop, i.e. therapeutic interventions designed to change one's sexual orientation (universally from gay to straight). Reparative therapeutic interventions range from psychotherapeutic consultations to extreme aversion therapy with electroshock treatment. To date, all of the evidence from reparative therapy suggests that although repression of same-sex sexual activity is potentially possible it is only a very small minority of highly motivated individuals who achieve sustained suppression (Shidlo *et al.* 2002).

BOX 15.2 DSM definitions of homosexuality

DSM I – Homosexuality categorised as a psychopathic personality with pathological sexuality.

DSM II – Sexual Orientation Disturbance [homosexuality]. This is for individuals whose sexual interests are directed primarily toward people of the same sex and who are either disturbed by, in conflict with, or wish to change their sexual orientation. This diagnostic category is distinguished from homosexuality, which by itself does not constitute a psychiatric disorder. Homosexuality per se is one form of sexual behaviour, and with other forms of sexual behaviour, which are not by themselves psychiatric disorders, are not listed in this nomenclature.

DSM III (pre-revision) – Ego Dystonic Homosexuality is described as: (1) a persistent lack of heterosexual arousal, which the patient experienced as interfering with initiation or maintenance of wanted heterosexual relationships, and (2) persistent distress from a sustained pattern of unwanted homosexual arousal.

BOX 15.3 American Psychological Association Statement on reparative therapies (APA 1997)

The Council of Representatives of the American Psychological Association (APA) has passed a resolution affirming four basic principles with regard to treatments to alter sexual orientation, so-called conversion or reparative therapies.

These principles are:

1   Homosexuality is not a mental disorder and the APA opposes all portrayals of lesbian, gay and bisexual people as mentally ill and in need of treatment due to their sexual orientation.

2   Psychologists do not knowingly participate in or condone discriminatory practices with lesbian, gay and bisexual clients.

3   Psychologists respect the rights of individuals, including lesbian, gay and bisexual clients, to privacy, confidentiality, self-determination and autonomy.

4   Psychologists obtain appropriate informed consent to therapy in their work with lesbian, gay and bisexual clients.

The resolution further states that the APA 'urges all mental health professionals to take the lead in removing the stigma of mental illness that has long been associated with homosexual orientation' (Chicago, 14 August 1997).

BOX 15.4 The American Psychiatric Association position statement on reparative therapy (APA 1998)

The potential risks of 'reparative therapy' are great, including depression, anxiety and self-destructive behaviour, since therapist alignment with societal prejudices against homosexuality may reinforce self-hatred already experienced by the patient.

Many patients who have undergone 'reparative therapy' relate that they were inaccurately told that homosexuals are lonely, unhappy individuals who never achieve acceptance or satisfaction . . . Therefore, APA opposes any psychiatric treatment, such as 'reparative' or 'conversion' therapy, that is based on the assumption that homosexuality per se is a mental disorder or is based on the a priori assumption that the patient should change his or her homosexual orientation.

Since the 1990s there has been growing condemnation of reparative therapies from national psychological and psychiatric professional bodies. In 1997 the American

Psychological Association (*see* Box 15.3) passed a resolution affirming the principles of treatment for gay and lesbian patients and denouncing reparative therapies; this was endorsed by a similar statement from the American Psychiatric Association (*see* Box 15.4) in 1998.

Although there are some countries that still criminalise homosexuality, many countries have gone beyond decriminalisation to enact legislation, which gives legal protection to gay men in the provision of goods and services, including health and psychological services.

RESEARCH AND EVIDENCE BASE

Research into the mental health of gay men, as opposed to research into sexual orientation, has been somewhat limited. The DSM criteria led to a medicalisation of homosexuality which obscured further exploration of mental ill-health. The lack of standardised monitoring of sexual identity in clinical episode statistics or suicide audits and the challenge in sampling a population with a historical distrust of psychological services have also contributed to the lack of a peer review evidence base.

In 2007 the UK Department of Health commissioned a systematic review of the current evidence base relating to the mental health of lesbian, gay and bisexual people. The review (Fish 2007) concluded that:

➤ evidence indicates that the increased risk of mental disorder in LGB people is linked to experiences of discrimination
➤ LGB people are more likely to report both daily and lifetime discrimination than heterosexual people
➤ gay men and bisexual people are significantly more likely to say that they have been fired unfairly from their job because of discrimination
➤ discrimination has been shown to be linked to an increase in deliberate self-harm in LGB people
➤ LGB people demonstrate higher rates of anxiety and depression than heterosexuals.

Throughout much of the research cited there was a common thread that experiences of discrimination on the grounds of an individual's sexual orientation were significant contributory factors to negative self-esteem, depression, self-harm, anxiety and parasuicide, a finding supported by Diaz and colleagues (2001) research in the US and the evidence base of causal relationships between racism and poor mental health (Chakaborty 2002).

Peer review research on the prevalence of discrimination experienced by gay men is limited. However, in a review on homophobic bullying in schools for the Department for Education and Skills (Warwick *et al.* 2004) rates were quoted of between 30–50% of gay men experiencing homophobic bullying in educational settings. The report went on to cite a study finding that 91% of lesbian, gay, bisexual and transgendered (LGBT) students in one American cohort reported verbal abuse based on their sexual orientation or gender identity and another study of school teachers in England and Wales, which found that 82% were aware of verbal homophobic bullying and 26% of physical homophobic incidents.

Despite legislative change, there are still significant challenges in society facing gay young people. A study of young gay people's experiences in the UK (Hunt and Jenson 2007) found that two-thirds of lesbian and gay schoolchildren have experienced homophobic bullying. Ninety-eight per cent of young gay people hear the phrases 'that's so gay' or 'you're so gay' in school and over four fifths hear such comments often or frequently. Half of teachers had failed to respond to homophobic language when they heard it and less than a quarter of schools had told pupils that homophobic bullying was wrong. In a survey of self-identified LGBT students in the US (Kosciw *et al.* 2008) 86% of LGBT students reported experiencing harassment at school in the past year, 61% felt unsafe at school because of their sexual orientation and 33% had skipped a day of school in the past month because of feeling unsafe.

Following publication of the Department of Health briefing paper on LGB Mental Health, a further piece of work funded by the Department of Health was published which was a systematic review and meta-analysis of the prevalence of mental disorder, substance misuse, suicide, suicidal ideation and deliberate self-harm in LGB people (King *et al.* 2008). The review concluded that LGB people are at higher risk of mental disorder, suicidal ideation, substance misuse, and deliberate self-harm than heterosexual people. The meta-analysis drew out some stark findings, in particular:

➤ a twofold excess in suicide attempts in lesbian, gay and bisexual people
➤ an increased risk for depression and anxiety disorders (over a period of 12 months or a lifetime) of at least 1.5 times in lesbian, gay and bisexual people
➤ alcohol and other substance dependence over 12 months was also 1.5 times higher
➤ lifetime prevalence of suicide attempt was especially high in gay and bisexual men.

There is substantial further grey literature which illustrates that the discrimination faced by gay men contributes to higher levels of mental ill-health and substantially higher rates of attempted suicide. However, there is now a growing base of peer review evidence, which should, in time, encourage policy-makers and commissioners to review their approach to services for gay men and ensure that this need is met.

GAY MEN WITH HIV AND MENTAL ILL-HEALTH

Being diagnosed with HIV is a significant life event and the reality is that HIV still disproportionately affects gay men in most Western countries. Although beyond the remit of this chapter, there are of course substantial psychological needs around the time of diagnosis to support individuals to adapt and adjust to their new disease paradigm. Psychological support may also be important to support treatment concordance and transition into an AIDS-defined state.

Declining mental function can occur as a complication of HIV infection, most commonly when an individual's CD4 count falls under 200 cells/ml. Symptoms vary from individual to individual but can include declining cognition, impaired motor function, speech problems and mood and personality changes. The frequency of AIDS-related dementia has substantially reduced since the introduction of highly active antiretroviral therapy (HAART) treatment (Maschkea *et al.* 2000), but it continues to affect around 20% of people living with AIDS.

BOX 15.5 Briefing paper from the UK Royal College of Psychiatrists on Psychiatry and LGB People (2001)

> . . . The evidence would suggest that there is no scientific or rational reason for treating LGB people any differently to their heterosexual counterparts. Socially inclusive, non-judgmental attitudes to LGB people who attend places of worship or who are religious leaders themselves will have positive consequences for LGB people as well as for the wider society in which they live.

GAY MEN'S RELATIONSHIPS WITH MENTAL HEALTH SERVICES

Diagnosis: Homophobic (McFarlane 1998) described a mental health service in the UK which was perceived by many as homophobic, inaccessible and obtuse in its relationships with gay men. On top of that, patients were also discriminated against from within the lesbian, gay and bisexual communities on the basis of their use of mental health services.

Ten years later, in 2008, a survey of 1328 psychotherapists in the UK (Bartlett *et al.* 2009) found that 17% had tried to help their patients reduce or suppress their homosexual feelings at least once in their professional careers and 4% said they would try and help a homosexual or bisexual patient convert to heterosexuality in the future; this is despite several position statements from professional bodies (Box 15.5).

The Department of Health systematic review (Fish 2007) stated that lesbians, gay men and bisexual people use mental health services more frequently than their heterosexual counterparts but report mixed experiences of services, including problems in their encounters with mental health professionals, ranging from lack of empathy about sexual orientation to incidents of homophobia. One-third of gay men and a quarter of bisexual men reported negative or mixed reactions from mental health professionals when they disclosed their sexual orientation. One in five gay men and a third of bisexual men stated that a mental health professional made a causal link between their sexual orientation and their mental health problem.

Although it is difficult to change the fundamental beliefs of any practitioner towards gay men, the vast majority of practitioners are not prejudiced or biased in their approach and therefore the most significant barrier to access is overcoming the perception of discrimination prior to access. The review also highlighted the difficulties for mental health professionals in striking the right balance – whilst some were regarded as insensitive if they placed too much emphasis on sexual orientation in the clinical setting, others were regarded as insensitive if they ignored it.

Diagnosis: Homophobic made over thirty recommendations for good practice with LGB services users. The list echoed previous reports and has been mirrored in reports and guidance since (e.g. Barton 2006). The majority are simple, small changes, which have a significant impact for gay men's perceptions of discrimination and risk related to professional encounters. These include:

1 *Actively tackle homophobia:* clear and visible statements that homophobia is unacceptable and will be dealt with effectively.
2 *Raise the visibility of gay men:* positive images of gay men should be displayed in service settings and literature and advertising, such as websites, should explicitly mention gay men.
3 *Appropriate language:* the language used in assessments should be inclusive, e.g. using partner rather than husband/wife/girlfriend.
4 *Acceptance of non-heterosexual identities/behaviours:* gay men should not be pathologised, ignored or denied and professionals should not make assumptions about 'causes'.
5 *Training and awareness:* mandatory equality training should include sexual orientation and gender identity and should apply to all staff in the organisation.
6 *Monitoring:* include sexual orientation as a demographic identity section in monitoring forms and treat with confidentiality in the same way as other personal information.
7 *Build partnerships:* link with local LGBT community organisations to build referral and support relationships for clients and access local information resources.

It is important that therapists, clinicians and commissioners consider how services are provided to encourage access for gay men and ensure that they receive treatment in a non-judgmental, supportive context.

MODELS OF GOOD PRACTICE

These are a few examples of good practice where services have been developed specifically for gay men or adapted to increase access for gay men.

PACE – LGBT youth project

Regular weekly groups are held offering a range of structured and unstructured time. The groups have an annual 'syllabus', which is broadly:

➤ spring – sexual health
➤ summer – lifestyle, general health, diet, exercise etc
➤ autumn – career, education, aspiration and engagement
➤ winter – mental and emotional health.

Structured group sessions explore issues, discuss ways of getting support and make referrals. Groups are supported by fast-track access to one-to-one emotional support and advocacy with senior youth workers – this can be in person, by phone or text. Groups are also a way to link young people into other PACE services, including counselling and an employment service.

In the first nine months of the project, 82 young people went through the programme. Clients were followed up at one and six months to assess the impact of the intervention. Although only a very small number (n = 17) were successfully tracked for six months, the initial findings showed that 76% had a self-assessed improvement in markers of poor mental health (self-rated scores of isolation, anxiety, self-harm). Despite being a small sample, there is a strong suggestion that this flexible model of group work with young LGBT can have a positive impact on mental health and well-being and build mental resilience.

Further information is available at www.pacehealth.org.uk

Websites to raise awareness of mental health within the LGBT communities

www.healthwithpride.nhs.uk is an NHS website built by NHS Barking and Dagenham to provide a wide range of health information for LGBT people. The site was written by a gay man and includes information on mental health, including substance misuse, eating disorders and signposting to research and other key resources. The website also includes some ground-breaking resources on domestic violence and cancer targeted at LGBT people. In its first month the website recorded over 2000 hits, with positive feedback from a wide range of professionals and community activists.

www.lgbmind-matters.com is a user-created site about mental health for the LGB community. Created by a gay man living with HIV/AIDS who has had experiences of mental ill-health, it was launched in November 2001. The website is a project of community benefit resulting from a Mind, Millennium, Real Lives Real People award.

PACE – evidence-based therapeutic group work for gay and bisexual men

Between 1995 and 2006 the London Gay Men's HIV Prevention Partnership funded over 500 hours of therapeutic group work for gay and bisexual men resident in London. The interventions aimed to reduce HIV sero-discordant unprotected anal intercourse, condom failure and HIV-positive to HIV-negative semen transfer. The group work was solution-focused, combining experiential and therapeutic techniques to support gay men. In 2005 the programme saw 240 participants, providing 530 hours of group work across four broad categories of intervention: self-esteem and identity; relationships and communication; sex and sexuality; and HIV status.

Three-month follow-up questionnaires were used to gather feedback from 163 participants in 2005. Of these, 95 workshop participants responded to a qualitative question on the impact of participation on their lives. The majority of respondents were extremely positive, with key themes being:
➤ increased communication skills
➤ increased confidence and/or reassurance across a range of issues including more at ease with self, own sexuality, own HIV status

➤ increased awareness of self-help, safe sex, meeting men, goals for themselves and new insights into life.

Quantitative evaluation of the programme found that 93% evidenced positive change on a list of 15 variables relating to sexual health behaviour and risk taking. Eighty-two per cent showed positive change on more than 5 of the variables and 62% reported positive change on more than 10 variables. The project illustrates the value of therapeutic evidence-based group work as a constructive intervention for gay men, which can facilitate positive mental health changes.

Further information is available at www.pacehealth.org.uk

Calderdale – ten years of LGB youth work

GAYLIC is an LGBT youth support charity working in Calderdale in West Yorkshire England. GAYLIC was set up following a needs assessment in 1998 of LGBT youth in Calderdale, which found a highly vulnerable group of young people with very little service meeting their needs.

In 2008 a second needs assessment was undertaken which found that little had changed in terms of service provision for LGBT youth but that GAYLIC was having a positive impact on mental health and well-being of the young people accessing it, despite unstable and limited funding. The ten-year review clearly illustrated that there is still significant need but that the youth intervention project is perceived by the users to make a significant positive impact on their mental health and well-being. The study found that homophobic bullying in school had risen from 67% to 76% and the proportion that had dropped out due to homophobia had risen from 13% to 28% between the two surveys. It also showed that 81% of those in contact with GAYLIC felt that it had helped to reduce their feelings of depression and 50% of those with an eating disorder before coming into contact with the service stated that it had reduced or resolved since contact was made.

To find out more about the project and the study go to www.galyic.org.uk

CONCLUSION

Supporting and working with gay men with mental health issues is, in many ways, like working with any other patient group – respect and dignity are key. As practitioners we are trained to assess patients holistically and work with them from their starting point. There is now universal condemnation among professionals of any practice which seeks to change an individual's homosexual identity and increasing evidence that homosexuality, like heterosexuality, is completely compatible with a happy and fulfilling life. Just as with any other group, practitioners should work with gay men to help them achieve a positive state of mental health and well-being.

REFERENCES

Allen K (2008) *International Day Against Homophobia: in Latvia prejudice is ingrained.* Available at: www.bilerico.com/2008/05/international_day_against_homophobia_in.php (Accessed 07/06/09).

American Psychological Association (1997) *Resolution on Appropriate Therapeutic Responses to Sexual Orientation.* Available at: www.apa.org/pi/sexual.html (Accessed 1/10/09).

American Psychiatric Association (1998) *Psychiatric Treatment and Sexual Orientation, Position Statement.* Available at: www.psych.org/Departments/EDU/Library/APAOfficial DocumentsandRelated/PositionStatements/199820.aspx (Accessed 29 September 2009).

Bartlett A, Smith G and King M (2009) The response of mental health professionals to clients seeking help to change or redirect same-sex sexual orientation. *BMC Psychiatry.* 9:11 doi:10.1186/1471–244X-9–11.

Barton P (2006) *Fair for All – The Wider Challenge: good LGBT practice in the NHS.* Edinburgh: NHS Scotland.

Chakaborty A (2002) Does racial discrimination cause mental illness? *Br J Psychiatry.* **180**: 475–477.

Diaz RM, Ayala G, Bein E, Henne J and Marin BV (2001) The impact of homophobia, poverty and racism on the mental health of gay and bisexual Latino men: findings from 3 US cities. *Am J Public Health.* **91**(6): 927–932.

Fish J (2007) *Mental health issues within lesbian, gay and bisexual (LGB) communities.* Briefing 9. London: Department of Health.

Hunt R and Jensen J (2007) *The School Report: the experiences of young gay people in Britain's schools.* London: Stonewall.

King M, Semlyen J, Tai SS, Killaspy H, Osborn D, Popelyuk D and Nazareth I (2008) A systematic review of mental disorder, suicide, and deliberate self harm in lesbian, gay and bisexual people. *BMC Psychiatry.* **8**: 70.

Kosciw JG, Diaz EM and Greytak EA (2008) *2007 National School Climate Survey: the experiences of lesbian, gay, bisexual and transgender youth in our nation's schools.* New York: Gay, Lesbian and Straight Education Network.

Maschkea M, Kastrupa O, Esserb S, Rossc B, Henggeb U and Hufnagel A (2000) Incidence and prevalence of neurological disorders associated with HIV since the introduction of highly active antiretroviral therapy (HAART). *J Neurology, Neurosurgery, and Psychiatry.* **69**: 376–380.

McFarlane L (1998) *Diagnosis: Homophobic: the experiences of lesbians, gay men and bisexuals in mental health services.* London: PACE (Project for Advocacy, Counselling and Advice).

Shidlo A, Schroeder M and Drescher J (2002) *Clinical Sexual Conversion Therapy: ethical, clinical, and research perspectives.* Binghampton NY: The Howarth Press Inc.

Warwick I, Chase E and Aggleton P (2004) *Homophobia, Sexual Orientation and Schools: a review and implications for action.* London: University of London.

CHAPTER 16

Delivering healthy sexuality programmes for young men

Tricia Dressel

INTRODUCTION

The World Health Organization (2004) defines sexuality as a central aspect of being human that encompasses sex, gender identities and roles, sexual orientation, eroticism, pleasure, intimacy and reproduction. More than simply the absence of risk-taking behaviour or its unwanted consequences, healthy sexuality encompasses healthy relationships, sense of intimacy, self-esteem, positive body image, pleasure and feeling happy and confident with the decisions we make around sex.

Teaching young people about healthy sexuality is important not only for its direct link with mental well-being but also as part of effectively promoting safe sex behaviours (Meschke *et al.* 2000). A 1997 review commissioned by the Joint United Nations Program on HIV/AIDS (UNAIDS) concluded that comprehensive sexuality education helps to delay first intercourse and protect sexually active adolescent males from unintended pregnancy and HIV. The review also concluded that responsible and safe behaviour can be learned, and that it's best to start sexuality education before the onset of sexual activity.

Douglas Kirby of the National Campaign to Prevent Teen Pregnancy surveyed the research on teen pregnancy prevention programmes to determine which curricula demonstrated the most success in reducing sexual risk behaviours. In his report, *No Easy Answers: Research Findings on Programs to Reduce Teen Pregnancy*, Kirby (1997) identified six curricula that had demonstrated strong evidence of behaviour change. The successful curricula had a number of characteristics in common, including the following:

➤ successful sexuality education programmes focus on reducing a small number of sexual behaviours

➤ they provide basic information, and give a clear message

> they address social pressures on sexual behaviour
> they employ a variety of interactive teaching methods, including games and small group discussions.

THE MAZZONI CENTER, PHILADELPHIA, US

The Mazzoni Center is one of the oldest public health HIV/AIDS service organisations in the US. Since 1979, we have led sexual health workshops and training in schools, hospitals, mental health institutions and community settings. Our Healthy Sexuality Workshop Series is a comprehensive sexual health programme designed as part of an overall wellness plan, specifically geared to young men. It is important to begin a dialogue with adolescent males around sexual health, as we have found that early discussions around health lead to more active involvement in one's personal and emotional well-being across the lifespan.

An effective sexuality education programme cannot simply discuss the risks of sexual behaviour and explain the ideal behaviour that the teacher would like the students to engage in. It is essential for sexuality educators to directly address the factors that motivate a young person's behaviour – including the role of sexual risk-taking as a part of overall social and emotional development. An interactive approach that incorporates a young person's beliefs and responses as part of the pedagogical strategy is the most effective.

The education services discussed complement existing health programmes for young men and create a true continuum of care for youth and better points of entry to health services. We have been providing risk reduction programmes in schools for a number of years with great success. Over the past decade, through internal tracking and evaluation, we have seen a strong correlation between educational programmes and outreach efforts and the accessing of counselling and medical care services by young men.

Our Healthy Sexuality Workshop Series for middle-school and high-school students is presented in 7 sessions of 45 minutes.

AIMS

The aims of our Healthy Sexuality Workshop Series are to enhance the understanding of young men around sexual health and provide a safe space to discuss feelings and experiences with partners, parents, friends and supporters as part of a comprehensive wellness plan. Often, the burden of responsibility for having a condom, using protection, and initiating conversation is placed on young men – but often little is done to prepare teenage boys for starting this dialogue. Effective healthy sexuality programmes have a positive effect on knowledge, attitudes and behaviours.

> *Knowledge:* Participants will gain more knowledge of anatomy, disease prevention, reproductive health, and gender roles and power dynamics.
> *Attitudes:* Participants will feel that what they learned will help them make informed and empowered decisions about their health and lives.

➤ *Behaviours:* At the end of the series, with increased knowledge of personal healthcare, healthy relationships and human sexuality, participants will reduce their risk of HIV/AIDS transmission and unplanned pregnancy.

WHAT DO THE SESSIONS COVER?

The Healthy Sexuality Workshop Series is geared to adolescents, but the curriculum can be tailored and presented to men regardless of age.

The workshops help young men in a different way. Our sexuality education series goes beyond the typical pregnancy-and-disease education model typically geared toward young women. The comprehensive series includes sessions on relationships, gender roles, sexual orientation and defining consent, looking more deeply at some of the issues that impact sexual decision-making for young men.

The Healthy Sexuality Workshop Series is designed for use in middle and high schools to augment course information on human sexuality. The seven-session curriculum (taught by one or two educators) involves participants in discussions, role-plays and interactive exercises about safer sex.

The workshops work best when using knowledge-based, affective and behavioural goals to break down the barriers that stand in the way of students taking steps to reduce their risk. The factual, knowledge-based elements of the workshops help to challenge the denial and misconceptions that students have about who has HIV, how it works and how it is spread. The affective, emotion-based elements help students to clarify and examine how they feel about HIV and safer sex, and what barriers stand in the way of taking effective steps toward risk-reduction. The behavioural, skills-based elements of the workshops work on developing manageable, incremental strategies that help to make safer sex and risk-reduction easier.

HOW SHOULD I MARKET THE WORK?

Get an active list of every school and community group in your area. Initiate contact with guidance counsellors, health teachers and/or administrators in the schools and community. Often, sexual health workshops are offered in health, physical education or science classes.

Teachers generally welcome the idea of having the sessions because the sexual health curriculum can come over better from a visitor, rather than from a teacher who is in the school full-time. Pupils get close to teachers whether they like them or not and sometimes teachers lose the respect required to talk convincingly on this kind of subject. A lot of discussion around sexual health is between students, rather than students to teachers. Teachers will remain in the room during the workshops, however; this is good because it helps create a safe space for students to discuss sensitive issues with trusted adults.

Be careful to plan ahead and not let the schools all leave sexual health workshops until the end of the year when teachers are wrapping things up and students are busy with exams and final projects. Getting the workshops incorporated into health classes, biology or physical education classes makes it easier to spread them out over the year.

WHO CAN DELIVER THE PROGRAMME?

The series requires one or two health educators, who coordinate the education package within each school, implementing the programme and designing new, expanded lesson plans based on the needs of each group. The educator(s) is also responsible for marketing the programme to schools in the area in order to increase awareness and use of your education services. Once your service becomes known you'll find that schools come to you, as teachers and administrators will tell each other about the service.

WHAT SKILLS AND EXPERIENCE DO I NEED?

The workshops require an interactive teaching style using a variety of methods, including role plays, skits and small groups, so a willingness and ability to effectively deliver these is required. You need to be knowledgeable and comfortable discussing relationships, sexual dynamics, gender roles and sexual health with adults and young people from diverse backgrounds. The main thing is to have an awareness of adolescent health and development, HIV/STIs, gender roles and sexual identities, communication styles and relational dynamics.

It is also important to be able to engage effectively with young people and understand how they interact with each other, so that you know what the issues are at any time and are able to connect with participants. When working with adolescent boys and young men, use inclusive language that allows participants to take both active and passive roles. Aim to create safe spaces that allow young men to feel OK to talk about feelings, ask questions and seek support and guidance. Listen, explore personal biases and initiate conversations around gender and sexual identities.

WHAT EQUIPMENT DO I NEED?

You'll need basic educational workshop supplies, including visual aids, videos, easel paper and materials. When doing role plays you'll need a few props. The idea is to use props and materials with the role plays to try and make the lesson as visual as possible.

WHERE SHOULD I RUN THE SESSIONS?

Most of this kind of work will take place in schools, but you may be asked to run sessions in community centres and community groups. We have presented to groups as small as 5 and as large as 45. If you have more students, two educators would be beneficial for small group facilitation. In school settings, a teacher or monitor should always be present in the workshops. At community settings, the programme manager or site contact should be present.

When working with schools, make sure to review district guidelines for outside presenters inside schools. This may include getting curriculum approval from the City Board of Education, security clearances for staff entering school, permission from an administrator, finding an advisor and/or presenting your workshops to faculty before meeting with students.

HOW LONG SHOULD THE SESSIONS BE?

The workshops each last 45 minutes to one hour, but it's important to stay around for a few minutes afterward in case a student or teacher has additional questions and wants to talk. Students may ask for resources and have questions to ask. Participants may not feel comfortable discussing personal situations (especially ones of a sensitive nature) with the larger group. Schools tend to be quite lenient in that they'll let you have half a lesson or whatever you need to meet a student who wants to see you. Sometimes students will want to talk with their parents and/or the teacher present, but, either way, because of the sensitive subject matter it's important to always have someone with you when the student meets with you, whether it's a teacher, a parent or one of your colleagues. Make sure you have an active referral list of trusted resources and services and make your information available to people for follow-up.

WHAT'S THE STRUCTURE OF THE WORKSHOPS?

Our Healthy Sexuality Workshop Series provides comprehensive sexuality education to adolescents and adults based on the experiential learning style. Seven 45-minute sessions are delivered by one or two trained educators.

The workshops are based on group exercises and classroom activities so that people can learn through experiencing the lesson. Over the course of the series, the educators uses games, role-plays, demonstrations, debates and group discussion to engage participants in thinking about their own sexual and romantic lives.

The seven sessions in the series build on the network of interests and concerns that contribute to a person's sexual decision-making. The programme is used with adolescent males, youth at high risk and adults in community settings. It delivers interactive sexuality and sexual health education, specifically with regard to personal health and information around LGBT and gender-identity issues and is designed to augment the human sexuality curriculum.

Session 1: healthy relationships

The first session focuses on relationships, helping participants to define a picture of what they want out of a healthy relationship. Participants learn how to build healthy relationships and how gender and power roles can influence relationships. They learn what is potentially unhealthy behaviour and how to prevent dating violence and to identify an unhealthy relationship. The theme focuses on self-esteem, respect and safety. We talk about how to set and communicate boundaries with people in order to deal better with peer pressure and potentially coercive situations.

Set up ground rules before each workshop session in order to ensure that group discussions are safe, confidential and respectful. Many groups have a ground rule that no assumptions or labels are used about a group member's sexual orientation. This can help make straight, bisexual, gay, and questioning participants feel comfortable. Always involve participants when establishing ground rules.

Session 2: know your body

The second session focuses on anatomy and physiology, making sure that everybody in the class is up to speed on how their reproductive system works. They learn about the changes that the body goes through during puberty and learn to understand anatomy and function. We discuss the body in specific detail, using visual models, videos and role plays to review changes throughout life.

Session 3: understanding reproduction and birth control

The third session is on reproduction, pregnancy and birth control options, with a specific emphasis on helping young men to understand what behaviours might put them at risk. We review myths and facts about how pregnancy happens, including changes in our bodies during puberty. Activities focus on reducing the risk of teen pregnancy and postponing sexual involvement. There is also a mini-presentation on birth control to explain what the birth control options are and how they work.

Session 4: HIV and sexually transmitted infections (STIs)

The fourth session of the series focuses on HIV and STIs. We provide an overview of sexually transmitted infections and include popular myths about how HIV is transmitted. This session also explains how to stay safe from HIV and other STIs while growing up. Signs and symptoms of STIs are also discussed, along with an interactive discussion around how STIs are treatable and curable in order to destroy stigma around HIV and STIs. We do skits about the impact of disease on the immune system.

Another popular activity used during this session is called 'condom science'. The class performs some simple experiments with condoms to find out how much they can hold, what makes condoms break and how to use them correctly.

Session 5: sexual and gender identity

In the fifth session, we discuss sexual orientation and help students understand how to make sense of their own feelings and thos of people around them. What is homophobia? What is a transsexual? What is a bisexual? What does it mean to be transgender? This session focuses on answering these questions and teaching about sexual and gender identity. This workshop also focuses on helping people to overcome homophobia and heterosexism.

It's important to use gender-inclusive language in the sessions, i.e. do not assume all young people are heterosexual. Young people, particularly young men, often feel pressured to act in 'macho' or overly masculine ways. Intervene when you hear students or teachers using transphobic and homophobic comments.

Session 6: boundaries and consent

The sixth session is about boundaries and consent; many of the students (including young men) that we work with have had experiences with non-consensual sex. We want to help students understand what consent means, so that they're able to protect themselves and avoid harming others. The session focuses on sexual boundaries and consent, and helps participants to develop self-esteem, assertiveness and communication skills in order to decrease the risk of sexual coercion and date rape situations.

Remember that young men are also victims of sexual assault, but rarely report attacks and abuse to authorities. It is especially important to use inclusive language, offer resources and provide safe space for males around this sensitive topic.

Session 7: open

A final session is often set aside for a topic that comes up in the class during the course of the series. Each group has different needs and often we can't predict at the start what the 'hot topic' for that group will be. Having an open final session allows us the flexibility to plan something new, or to move things around, so that we can respond to the students' needs.

CONCLUSION

Healthy sexuality is important for mental well-being and vice versa. Our sexuality is a key aspect of our sense of identity but it exists in a social and cultural context where norms, prejudices, peer pressure, media influences, religion, history, laws and taboos affect how we see ourselves and how our sexuality and the way we express it are judged by those around us. Educating young people about sexuality is about addressing both the physical and mental health aspects of sexual relationships. School-based healthy sexuality workshops have an important role to play in equipping young men to understand and express their sexuality in a way that will enhance their psychological well-being and not be detrimental to the physical or mental health of either themselves or their sexual partners.

REFERENCES

Kirby D (1997) *No Easy Answers: research findings on programs to reduce teen pregnancy.* Washington DC: The National Campaign to Prevent Teen Pregnancy.

Meschke LL, Bartholomae S and Zentall SR (2000) Adolescent Sexuality and Parent-Adolescent Processes: Promoting Healthy Teen Choices. Family Relations. 49(2): 143–154.

UNAIDS (1997) Impact of HIV and Sexual Health Education on the Sexual Behaviour of Young People: A Review Update. Geneva: UNAIDS.

World Health Organization (2004) Sexual Health – a new focus for WHO, No.67. *Progress in Reproductive Health Research.* 67:1–8.

CHAPTER 17

Working with dads and lads

Dennis Jones

INTRODUCTION

During the 1980s and 1990s many articles were written about the 'crisis of fatherhood', with titles like: 'Are fathers getting a fair deal?' (Bothamley 1990) and 'Fatherhood and changing family roles' (Hanson and Bozett 1987). One study ominously began: 'Becoming a father can be considered a risk factor for the onset of psychic disorders and manifestations analogous to those seen in women after childbirth. Such disorders may at times assume psychotic dimensions' (Benvenuti *et al.* 1995: 78).

Putting men under the spotlight in this way was nothing new – feminism had subjected men to its critical gaze since the 1960s as a necessary condition to its aims of understanding gender inequality and focusing on gender politics, power relations and sexuality. The rise of the Women's Liberation Movement and modern feminism entailed a questioning of what it is to be a woman in a patriarchal society. An indirect, but maybe inevitable, consequence of this process has been a growing questioning of what it is to be a man. Often, to put a positive angle on it, women have tried to do this on behalf of men – but there have been diverse attempts at this redefinition by men themselves, from the mythopoetic constructions of Robert Bly (1991) to fathers' rights activists. More broadly, there has been a societal shift that can be seen in a whole range of changes to men's feelings, actions and activities in attempting to redefine their masculinity. In the eighties and nineties this was done in support of gender equity feminism and the anti-sexism men's movement by magazines such as *Achilles Heel*, which exemplified this debate, asking 'What future for men?'* and running articles with titles like 'Should men be accountable to women?' (Blacklock 1993), 'What's it like to be on the receiving end of men's sexism?' (Sweet and Seymour 1993) and 'Why do men abuse and hate women?' (Baker 1993).

---

*   *Achilles Heel*. Autumn 1990. Issue 10. What Future for Men?

By the early years of the 21st century there had been yet another shift in both the public perception of men and, for some, their perception of themselves. No longer were some men prepared to take what they perceived as the unfairness of feminism lying down. An article in a Sunday newspaper announced that 'the militant men's movement has arrived in Britain' under the headline 'Militant fathers will risk jail over rights to see their children' (Hinsloff 2003).

MEN AS FATHERS

This was by no means the case for most men, however. For the majority these social factors and a general lack of confidence in their family roles were coming together to unsettle men's feelings of security and control regarding their relationships with women and their children. One factor in this anxiety surrounded the rise in the use of artificial insemination. Efforts to develop practical methods for artificial insemination began in Russia in 1899 and by the mid-1940s artificial insemination had become an established industry. Improved methods of sperm collection were developed throughout the 1970s and 1980s, with the first commercial sperm bank being opened in the early 1970s. Artificial insemination became an acceptable solution for couples in which the man could not produce sperm adequately enough to fertilise his partner, but its increasing use allowed for a subtle change in male-female sexual relationships. At the same time as male behaviour came under scrutiny in feminist writings, where men were increasingly judged for what they did and didn't do and found wanting, a technology had arrived that effectively dispensed with one of their few biological assets. Writers began using the words 'male' and 'redundant' in the same sentence and because a man's physical presence was no longer required to fertilise a woman, the possibility of doing without men as fathers became very real.

Simultaneously, as the divorce rate began to soar after 1960, another major trend started to emerge that was part of the transformation of the institution of marriage in the 20th century. While rates of marriage decreased, rates of cohabitation increased and so did non-marital births. This non-marital birth rate increase occurred at the same time that women in the West had more contraceptive choice than ever before. After 1960, when the contraceptive pill was introduced, childbearing outside marriage began to climb slowly, but increased dramatically after 1980, reaching 42% in 2004.

Figures from the Office for National Statistics also show that during this time single-mother families in Britain rose from 1% of households with children in 1971 to 11% in 2004 and an analysis of data from 14 European countries found that Britain had by far the highest proportion of single mothers in the European Union (Bartholomew 2004).

On 5 April 1993 the UK Government launched the Child Support Agency (CSA), which was an executive agency, part of the Department for Work and Pensions, responsible for implementing the 1991 Child Support Act and subsequent legislation. From its inception it caused a great deal of controversy, compounding the feelings of anxiety, insecurity and alienation that the media had begun to document concerning the role of men as fathers.

What does all this mean for those men who end up outside of the family where their children are? And what does it mean for their children? In recent years substantial research by organisations dedicated to supporting fathers and the rights of fathers, such as the Fatherhood Institute (Lewis and Warin 2001), has shown that:

➤ where fathers actively engage in supporting and nurturing boys they grow up to enjoy a happy and rewarding life

➤ adolescent boys with a strong paternal bond are less likely to be involved in petty crime and more likely to do well at school; involvement of dads with children aged 7–11 predicts success in exams at 16

➤ where dads are involved before the age of 11, children are less likely to have a criminal record by the age of 21.

There is evidence that men are electing to spend more time with their children. Fathers' involvement in care of under-fives increased from an average of fewer than 15 minutes per day in the 1970s to 2 hours per day (a third of all child care) in the late 1990s (Equal Opportunities Commission 2005).

Becoming a father has changed from being a role that signified abstract authority in the family or the parent who dispensed justice and retribution, or merely the one who went out and brought home the bacon but was content to leave the running of his family to his wife, to being involved in a relationship with one's children.

From what we know of Victorian fatherhood and even up to the 1950s and 1960s, it was enough for a father to be the breadwinner and disciplinarian in a family. Not all fathers were content to live within this stereotype, of course. Current interest in the life of Charles Darwin, both as a scientist and as a man and a father, reveals to us someone who loved to play with his children and was very involved in their lives and this must also have been true of many unsung and forgotten fathers. However, this stereotype has a powerful reality often because men did not have much choice – they worked long hours, were tired when they came home and found the energy and ebullient chaos of their children's lives unfamiliar and difficult to manage.

Being a father is something that you learn to do, not something that you are necessarily born to do. Gaining the necessary skills to be a good enough father involves learning about the self, including the impact of how one was parented, and acquiring capacities to communicate – active listening, expressing feelings and engaging in 'emotion work'.

Many young men struggle with a sense of individual responsibility, deferring instead to the collective responsibility of being with their mates or even of belonging to a gang. When presented with the opportunity to father their own child many are unable to discover the inner resources needed because they haven't experienced it for themselves.

Responsibility is something that is hard to teach outside of a good relationship that includes role modelling as well as instruction, friendship and love. Preferably this comes from your father or possibly a good mentor relationship like the ones in some districts of Australia and New Zealand, such as Boys Alive, which is an eight-week programme for boys 8–12 years old 'who may have a lack of positive male role models, behavioural difficulties, or issues around anger, emotion, relationships, communication, or self-esteem'. The programme involves after school events and three activity days (including an overnight experience). Using the group process, relationship skills are built. The learning from this process links the boys with their own experiences, so they are helped to understand and develop personal responsibility surrounding thoughts, feelings and actions.

When young men lack these skills and insights they will respond to their child with their feelings but often these feelings are overwhelming, possessive and fearful. They focus on rights to the exclusion of responsibilities and they end up with neither. First and foremost the father has to take on responsibility for looking after the mother of his child – giving her a safe place whilst she is nurturing the infant – the male has to rise above his own needs to look after the female when she needs him. Unfortunately, many young men cannot do this because they have no experience of looking after, only of being looked after – by their mum and then in the male pack where irresponsibility is the norm, and then by their girlfriend. When the girlfriend is no longer able to do this because she is looking after her child, often the young man becomes lost and angry. Their success in this task depends upon whether they have been brought up to think and act responsibly.

BOX 17.1

> Sure Start was a British Government programme which aimed to achieve better outcomes for children, parents and communities by:
>
> ➤ increasing the availability of childcare for all children
>
> ➤ improving health and emotional development for young children
>
> ➤ supporting parents as parents and in their aspirations towards employment.
>
> Sure Start Plus was an initiative to support pregnant teenagers and teenage parents under 18. Launched in April 2001, there were 20 Sure Start Plus pilot sites, covering 35 local authority areas, over a 5-year period in England. The aims of Sure Start Plus were to improve health, education, and social outcomes for pregnant teenagers, teenage parents and their children.
>
> Involving fathers was a key feature of Sure Start Plus, support being given to young fathers to encourage their involvement in the upbringing of their children. They were encouraged to take part in one-to-one and group sessions – sometimes with their children, to encourage involvement in the upbringing of their child, and sometimes with other young fathers to support each other and share experiences.

To father a child well you have to make a relationship with him or her – learning from your own responses to your own child. So to be a father you need to have an understanding of yourself as a person who has responsibility and can impose boundaries for the child so that they feel safe. If your child's behaviour makes you feel unsafe then you will not respond well to their insecurities about the world – be serious! Being a dad is a serious business. This doesn't mean that you don't play with your kids – it means that that is not all you do. Get involved with the looking after – when they need feeding, changing, help with school work and help with their problems. You need to be big enough to lean on, not just another kid who runs off when things get tough. So many young mothers leave young men – the father of their child – saying 'it was just like having another kid about the house'.

Many young men I have spoken to often describe themselves as being pushed out – what are they being pushed out from? Mostly they respond with anger and desperation and sometimes learned indifference. They give up because the fight to stay involved seems so unequal – they see their child being pushed in a buggy across the city street and they feel that they have no power to touch them, that the mother has all the power. They are being pushed out of their role because they don't know how to live into it.

Transactional Analysis has a model of relationships that can shed light on the interactions of some young fathers with their children. The model, developed by Eric Berne (1964), divides the human psyche into three parts called ego states following Freud's use of the superego, ego and id: in Berne's version these are the Parent, Adult and Child. These parts of the ego are again sub-divided into ego states with names like Adapted Child, Nurturing Parent, Little Professor and so on to indicate how the personality has developed and adapted to itself, its parents, its peers and the world around it. The healthy adult relationship is of Adult to Adult but so many relationships are Adult to Child where one partner controls aspects of the life of their partner either by the controlling Parent ego-state giving orders, instruction and demands or from the Child ego-state being irrational, demanding or unreasonable. The most desirable ego-state for parenting is of course the Parent because your child needs to feel secure and also needs to learn how to behave in the world. Some young fathers, however, make a relationship with their child by responding to the child's behaviour with their own inner Child. Wanting to play and having a sense of fun is no bad thing in itself but is not the only response required from a parent – your child needs a sense of its own boundaries, not just another playmate.

DADS UNITED

Dads United was set up in order to try to support young fathers in Bradford, UK. We held the first meeting of the group on Monday 5 July 2004 with 11 people present from a variety of agencies but mainly Surestart and Surestart Plus projects (*see* Box 17.1).

For some time there had been good work going on in Bradford around supporting fathers. Up to that time the networks that developed around this were informal. This new group was initiated to promote this important work and to facilitate greater support and the sharing of ideas. At the initial meeting we asked the group to briefly describe the main focus of their work generally and, specifically, the work they do with dads, and to think about the following questions:

➤ Which is the target group that you work with?
➤ What sort of funding can you access?
➤ What examples of good practice do you have in relation to this work?

➤ In 6 months, what would you like to have achieved in relation to working with dads?
➤ If a network such as this could achieve one thing in the next year, what would it be?

This is a sample of some of the examples of good practice that were gathered from this first meeting:

1 *The MASTS project:* The Multi-Agency Supported Tenancies Scheme (MASTS) was formed in 1993 as a project to house and support vulnerable 16–25-year-olds on the Allerton Estate in Bradford, West Yorkshire. It was set up because of the concerns of local people about poverty and homelessness. At the time, young people accommodated by the local authority in single person units on the estate only lasted about 6 weeks in their tenancies. It was felt that the most vulnerable tenants needed support as well as accommodating. MASTS was therefore developed in partnership with the local authority to provide support to young people in council tenancies. MASTS employed two workers to specifically support young fathers through the Dads Matter Group.
   Dads Matter Group:
   ➤ Dads Matter was run as a 12-week programme
   ➤ the project was user-led and began with a consultation phase which was important in getting the dads to trust the workers
   ➤ the sessions were run during the day, which the workers soon realised excluded men who went to work
   ➤ regardless of this, 11 young dads were involved.
   Some important factors for its success:
   ➤ working in partnership – MASTS and Surestart Plus had the benefit of joint funding and joint staffing, so that two people could be present and share expertise and ideas
   ➤ relationships had already been established, through housing support, which was vital in recruiting the young men
   ➤ it was unstructured and user-led; this informal structure, with the absence of stated ground rules, was important because it promoted equality and mutual respect.

2 *Trip to Whitby with dads and sons:*
   ➤ a worker in a fathers' support project in Surestart West Bowling (Bradford) coordinated a trip to Whitby, which was very successful
   ➤ five fathers and sons attended over the weekend, which had a strong focus on activity and working together
   ➤ the difference that the trip made to the relationships between the fathers and sons was extremely significant
   ➤ the worker pointed out the importance of funding from different sources, which spread the considerable cost.

3 *Courses for dads/parents:*
   ➤ the Community Learning and School Support Service was involved in

parenting evenings, with a focus on empowering men for parenthood
➤ a part of this process was to provide parenting skills so that when fathers/ parents had access to children who may be in some form of care, they could demonstrate that they were proactively seeking to improve their ability to be parents.

Dads United Five-a-Side Football Event (9 October 2004)

After this initial exchange of information we held a number of further meetings on a monthly basis which constituted the 'forming' stage of the group development. News went out, the word went round and new recruits began to join, bringing with them many interesting ideas. These provoked the 'storming' stage of the group's development, animating what had been solely a discussion/support group into action.

There was considerable enthusiasm for football as a number of the Surestart workers already played for five-a-side football teams. The idea for a tournament came up in a meeting of the Dads United Network held at the Bradford Health Promotion Service in September 2004 during a discussion about positive ways to involve dads in the lives of their children. We decided to hold an event that would invite all men/ father workers in the Bradford area to participate, giving them an opportunity to network whilst supporting them in an activity that would promote both health and parenting. We agreed that a dads' five-a-side tournament was a positive and practical way to achieve this aim.

Initial planning and structure

At the first meeting we agreed the following points:
➤ the event should be open to any organisation that worked with fathers or fathers to be within the Bradford area.
➤ the event should promote fathers in a positive light as regards to childcare and supervision.
➤ the event should encourage professionals working with men within this area to network and work together.
➤ the event should promote men's health and well-being.
➤ the event should give fathers the opportunity to spend time with their children.
➤ it should be fun.

We decided to contact as many organisations in the district as possible to try to find 16 teams of players and to find a suitable venue and cost for the whole event. An initial date was agreed.

Organisation

We shared the overall organisation of the event between all those involved, with each organisation taking responsibility for small tasks and thus distributing the large amount of work involved in setting up a project of this size.

The initial date was soon found to be unacceptable owing to it clashing with the festival of Ramadan. It was decided to move the event to Saturday 9 October.

A venue was located at a local primary school. This was a new complex with an indoor and an outdoor football pitch, changing rooms, a community room and art studio with ample safe space around the complex. This was particularly important, as we wanted to encourage dads to bring their children and spend time with them rather than just leaving them in a crèche.

The initial contacts had produced a crop of organisations interested in organising teams, including a Healthy Living Project, Sure Starts from the area, the local Gingerbread (a registered charity for the support of lone parents in Britain) and various community associations. Each of these organisations expressed an interest in both putting together a team and funding for the event. They all felt it was a positive way of engaging fathers.

Considerations for the event

We wanted to promote a high degree of father-child interaction, so no childcare was put in place and no food apart from providing fresh fruit and drinks. We hoped that this would motivate fathers to be responsible for their children's needs and make provision for their care and well-being. Children's activities were provided but on a parent-supervised basis only. It was made clear to all parents that they had parental responsibility for their children.

The event

On the day ten organisations brought a team to the event, with approximately 70 men attending. There were also some partners and children. The competition was played in a spirit of goodwill and friendship, with fathers of all ages taking part. The final between Sure Start West Bowling and Sure Start Manningham was won by Sure Start West Bowling by the smallest of margins.

Men's health checks

A worker from the Bradford Health of Men team (see Conrad and White 2007) working for Bradford City Primary Care Trust provided health checks and advice for the men attending the event. These included blood pressure, body mass index and blood sugar levels. These health 'MOTs' for men were well attended and proved popular not only with the men but with their partners, who openly encouraged the men to have a health check.

Children's activities

Children's activities were provided, including two children's art workshops which were well supported by volunteers from the various organisations and by the parents who attended the event.

Refreshments

Refreshments on the day consisted of hot and cold drinks and fresh fruit. The decision not to supply food did not seem to be a problem. Most people visited the many food outlets nearby to buy lunch. This allowed for a flexible lunchtime that did not interfere with the football games. It was mentioned, however, that a shared lunch might have provided more scope for dads and professionals to get together to talk. When we ran the event the year after we took up this suggestion and provided lunch, which did exactly that, and by ordering a buffet this allowed teams to have a flexible lunchtime.

Trophies and medals

Trophies and medals were organised and paid for by one of the Sure Starts. Each player and quite a few supporters received medals at the end of the day and both the finalists received a trophy which was played for at the next and subsequent events.

Volunteers

Volunteers from all the participating organisations worked together to make sure that the event progressed as smoothly as it did, which was illustrated at end of the day by the very little tidying-up which had to be done to ensure we left the venue as we found it.

Referees

Our decision to use experienced referees proved to be an excellent one. They helped organise the fixtures and ensured that the timing of the event and the flow of games went well.

Health and safety

Although St John Ambulance was invited to attend the event, they failed to show on the day. A first aid station was set up in the main reception area and manned by volunteers with first aid certificates. Apart from minor scrapes and bruises no significant injuries were sustained.

Publicity

A press release was written and distributed, extracts from which appeared in the local newspapers. Although because of prior commitments Bradford City Football Club were not able to support the event, they did show interest in supporting future events.

Funding and expenditure

The event was jointly funded by 12 local organisations and although no specific amount was set, it was suggested that each individual organisation give what their budgets would allow. A sum of £100 was suggested, as we agreed that such an amount was not unreasonable for an event of this size. Trophies and medals were paid for in full by a local Sure Start whilst the venue, referees and all fruit was paid for by another of the participating organisations.

Subsequent work

The feel good factor generated by the success of the five-a-side football tournament encouraged the group to organise further events and subsequent tournaments with similar success. It was inspiration from this first tournament that gave the monthly meeting its name: 'Dads United'. Although not all the events that the group ran were about football – we held a ten-pin bowling competition and pizza eating evening – football was a very strong theme.

The sport holds a special place in the male heart and has been given many names accordingly.* Pele's phrase 'The Beautiful Game' comes to mind, as does Alf Garnett's 'working class ballet'. Che Guevara said 'It's not just a simple game. It's a weapon of the revolution.' 'Train the right way. Help each other. It's a form of socialism without the politics,' agreed Bill Shankly, as did the historian Eric Hobsbawm: 'The imagined community of millions seems more real as a team of eleven named people.' 'Life itself is but a game of football,' said Sir Walter Scott. For us in the Bradford Health of Men team, football became a way of engaging young fathers in a manner like no other.

REFERENCES

Baker P (1993) Put up Your Jukes: why do men abuse and hate women? *Achilles Heel*. 16, Winter 93/94.

Bartholomew J (2004) *The Welfare State We're In*. London: Politico's Publishing Ltd.

Benvenuti P, Marchetti G, Niccheri C and Pazzagli A (1995) The psychosis of fatherhood: a clinical study. *Psychopathology*. **28**(2): 78–84.

Berne E (1964) *Games People Play*. New York: Grove Press.

Blacklock N (1993) Called to Account: should men be accountable to women? *Achilles Heel*. 16, Winter 93/94.

Bly R (1991) *Iron John: a book about men*. Shaftesbury: Element Books Ltd.

Bothamley J (1990) Are fathers getting a fair deal? *Nursing Times*. **86**(36): 68–69.

Conrad D and White A (eds) (2007) *Men's Health – How to Do It*. Oxford: Radcliffe Publishing.

Equal Opportunities Commission (2005) *Then and Now: 30 Years of the Sex Discrimination Act*. Manchester: EDC.

Hanson SM and Bozett FW (1987) Fatherhood and changing family roles. *Family & Community Health*. **9**(4): 9–21.

Hinsloff G (2003) Militant fathers will risk jail over rights to see their children. *The Observer*, 20 April.

Lewis C and Warin J (2001) What good are dads? *FatherFacts*. **1**(1). London: Fathers Direct.

Sweet C and Seymour L (1993) Long-lived sexism: What's it like to be on the receiving end of men's sexism? *Achilles Heel*. 16, Winter 93/94.

---

* *See*: www.redpathalbion.co.uk/Philosophy_Page.htm

CHAPTER 18

Tackling racial and cultural bullying in schools

Merv Pemberton

INTRODUCTION

Bullying takes many forms and can be targeted at anything that makes somebody stand out, whether it be height, disability, sexuality, educational attainment, dress or hair colour. Victims can become miserable, fearful and depressed and their progress at school can be severely damaged, whilst perpetrators may develop a false pride in their own strength and superiority (Department for Education and Skills 2004). Although bullying has always been around, we have seen a rise in UK schools in malicious bullying over recent years, with incidents much more commonly escalating to a serious level – even to the point of gang violence. This chapter focuses on one form of bullying that is increasingly becoming a concern and one that schools find particularly challenging (Department for Education and Skills 2006), though of course any form of bullying is damaging to the mental health of the victim (as well as indicating a poor state of mental well-being in the perpetrator).

A survey of pupils' experiences of bullying in Hampshire, UK found that almost a fifth of pupils in Year 9, around a quarter in Years 6 and 7 and over a third in Year 2 had experienced bullying at school in the previous 12 months. The answers to a question in the survey on racial and cultural bullying suggested that in all four year groups virtually every pupil of a minority ethnic heritage had been picked on in school because of their skin colour, religion or because the language that they spoke at home was not English (Department for Education and Skills 2006).

Research conducted in mainly white schools in 2001/02 found that 25% of the pupils from minority ethnic backgrounds in the sample had experienced racist name-calling within the previous seven days. In interviews, a third of the pupils of minority ethnic backgrounds reported experiences of hurtful name-calling and verbal abuse, either at school or during the school journey. Around half of these (one in six overall) reported that the harassment was ongoing or had continued over an extended period of time (Cline *et al.* 2002).

The issue of racial and cultural bullying and the need to overcome the fears or the myths surrounding other cultures should be addressed as a feature of all anti-bullying work with schools. Sometimes, though, there is a need for specific interventions to tackle existing problems.

WHAT FORM DOES RACIAL AND CULTURAL BULLYING TAKE?

It's important to consider not only the nature of the incident or behaviour but also how it makes the recipient feel. Young people can be made to feel unwelcome or left out because of skin colour, ethnicity, culture or religious affiliation. People from travelling communities, refugee families, Muslims and Jews, for example, can all become victims of racist bullying. It's important, though, not to assume that all bullying aimed at people from minority groups is necessarily racist. A useful working definition of racism in schools is: behaviour or language that makes a pupil feel unwelcome or marginalised because of their colour, ethnicity, culture, religion or national origin (Department for Education and Skills 2004).

Bullying can be triggered by something apparently minor and then escalate over time. Pupils may be seen outside of school in different dress which is specific to their religion or culture, for example at a wedding, and then this will be reported back to other pupils along the lines of 'oh we've seen him with funny clothes on this weekend'. Once a perceived difference has been picked out and highlighted, what may start as seemingly low-level teasing can snowball into long running and increasingly serious bullying if the behaviour is left unchecked and the perpetrators appear to be getting away with it.

Bullying can result from gang conflict based on even the most trivial of differences; for example, opposing gangs might be from the same culture but from different villages, where one is seen as higher 'ranked' than another. These perceived 'rankings' are often passed down from parents or grandparents. This happens more within some cultures than others, but with a growing shift towards everyone wanting to be 'top dog' it's something that's becoming increasingly common.

Bullying within friendships

Some young people are bullied because they're in a friendship with someone of a different background, but racial bullying can also occur within friendships. A common trigger is jealousy over material possessions, such as clothes, mobile phones or the latest MP3 player. It's important to get across to young people that just because someone is your friend it doesn't mean that they can't bully you, although often they won't think that this is what they are doing.

Racist language is sometimes used casually in the way that friends communicate with each other. In some cases, the recipient may be uncomfortable with this but unsure how to deal with it and will allow it to continue until the problem escalates. In other cases, both parties are OK with it but other people who are hearing it feel uncomfortable and here there is a judgment call to be made over whether to intervene. We may feel that it shouldn't be happening but it's most important to determine whether the recipient truly is comfortable with it or not. Even where the use of racist language isn't a cause of tension or ill-feeling in a friendship, it's easy for the balance to be tipped. People may be comfortable with certain words and phrases and offended by others and good-natured banter can quickly turn to genuine hostility.

Coming from another area

Almost any perceived difference can form the basis of racial and cultural bullying. People coming to a new school who have moved from a different area can be particularly vulnerable. Even people who've arrived from a different area, let alone a different country, can encounter bullying based on where they're from. A different accent or poorer English can be an easy target for a bully, although sometimes the bully will get a rude awakening when their victim is from a place where people have had to learn to stand up for themselves.

Family influences

The attitudes and behaviours that underlie racial and cultural bullying are often passed down from family members. They get picked up from older brothers or sisters, or adult family members, when children reach a certain age and then they try testing the waters with it. At this early stage, part of the battle is simply about getting young people to understand the offensiveness of half the words and phrases they hear. Often they use certain words without really understand the meaning of them, but they've heard someone else say them and think they sound cool.

Parents may use racist language in the home quite openly without any real underlying malice, although of course some children do grow up in openly racist households where they're encouraged to dislike or avoid people from certain racial or cultural backgrounds. Sometimes pupils won't want to go to certain schools because they have a high proportion of people from a particular background. Where a young person's racist attitudes stem from the influence of someone in the family this can be very difficult to address. You can feel that you're getting somewhere and then they'll go home, talk about what's happening and be told 'Oh that's a load of rubbish. Don't have any part of that. You just stay as you are,' and it knocks it back to square one.

Perpetrators don't always realise that what they're doing is racist and when it is brought to their attention they start to think about what they're doing. With intervention, some bullies do make significant changes, e.g. from not being friends with people from different cultures to then being best friends with them and then they're all going round together. It might not be a big percentage that comes round in that way but every percentage is a bonus.

THE IMPACT OF RACIAL AND CULTURAL BULLYING

As well as the potentially deadly negative psychological effects on the victim that can result from all forms of bullying, racial and cultural bullying can impact on an individual's sense of identity and place and reduce community cohesion. I've had an incident where a boy was being bullied by someone from a different country but a similar cultural background. He told his father, who then came to the school and spoke to the perpetrator of the bullying, saying 'Hang on, we're meant to be supporting each other, looking out for each other,' which was met with the response, 'We're not supporting each other. We're for us and you're for you.'

Racial and cultural bullying is not simply about people being made to feel disconnected from the dominant ethnic and cultural group, it also creates divisions within ethnic and cultural minorities, increasing feelings of isolation and further fracturing communities. Victims of racial and cultural bullying are not only singled out because of perceived differences between themselves and their peers. Differences in home circumstances are a common trigger, with victims bullied on the basis of some attribute of their family; for example, where the parents work, not having a professional job, living in council estates, or not having a car.

AT WHAT POINT DOES THE VICTIM ASK FOR SUPPORT?

Whether people feel able to ask for support depends on the individual rather than there being a pattern of one culture or nationality being more likely to open up. Some people wait until it's got past the stage of no return before they open up about how it's affecting them. Some victims will self-harm before they get to a point where they realise that they need to talk to someone. By the point at which victims decide to ask for help it isn't always easy for them to find a person whom they feel they can get that support from because often they've lost trust in somebody before. It's crucial to tread very carefully at this stage because if the person hasn't been listened to or adequately supported when they last sought help the last thing you want is to blow it as you're making the initial contact.

Nine out of ten times when working in schools I'll get asked if I've been bullied. Sometimes even the parents ask. Sharing your own experiences can help to get victims of bullying to see you as someone that they can open up to and speak about what they've been going through. Some people have been bullied for several years and never dared talk to anyone about it.

WORKING WITH SCHOOLS

In tackling racial and cultural bullying we really need to start at the grass roots – restoring a balanced and effective discipline in schools and a sense of community. Years ago, people in the community looked after each other much more, whereas now it's more common for a sense of 'them against us' to dominate. This attitude crosses over into school life and underpins a lot of this type of bullying.

There's a need to work with primary schools to get to children at a much earlier age. This is the time when we should be making a real effort to get the basic messages across to children, e.g. that it doesn't matter what colour skin we are, or what we wear – we've all got feelings. It's not about getting everyone to be really knowledgeable about everyone else's culture, but just to recognise that we all have different needs within our cultures and to respect those differences. Some primary schools are already doing good work in this area, but there's potential for health professionals to work closer with them to provide schools with the support necessary to have the maximum impact.

Case study

Using theatre is a great way to explore health issues with young people without sending them to sleep. A play developed in Derbyshire, for example, used forum theatre techniques to depict the isolation of minority ethnic people in rural areas and the distress that racist bullying can cause. It also showed how teachers can be unaware of what's going on or fail to respond adequately to the problem.

'Ally Comes to Cumbria' is another example of a piece of forum theatre, specially commissioned for primary and secondary schools in Cumbria. It tells the story of Ally, who arrives from Manchester to start at a new school in Cumbria. Ally is black and faces different reactions from the pupils and teachers at her new school. A workshop following the performance gives pupils the opportunity to practically explore how the characters could have acted differently. Another piece of theatre called 'Just Passing' explores attitudes towards asylum-seekers, Gypsies and Travellers. To find out more about these projects visit: www.globallink.org.uk

---

Sometimes anti-bullying interventions only get to young people just before they're at the point of leaving school and going into workplaces or colleges. By this point we should really be reinforcing an attitude of tolerance and an understanding of other races and cultures, rather than trying to inject it for the first time. If children understand other cultures from an earlier age then they'll carry this through as they get older and it will simply be something that they take for granted.

Schools vary in how well they deal with the issue of racial and cultural bullying. Some are really good at working with parents to address cases at any early stage, whereas some will try sweeping it under the carpet with an attitude that victims should toughen up and accept a certain amount of bullying and racism as a normal part of school life. It's important that there is provision of external anti-bullying support for schools, but also that they are aware of it and have the motivation to make use of it. In some cases, it's not only young people that need educating on the effects of this type of bullying but the teachers as well. Also, don't forget that bullying can be an issue for teachers as well as pupils. A growing problem is pupils using another language to make abusive remarks to teachers, knowing that they can't be effectively challenged because the teacher can't understand what they've said.

Whilst bullying prevention is better than cure, often external anti-bullying support is requested by a school because a specific problem with racist bullying has already developed. Schools will vary in how much time they will give for anti-bullying sessions to be delivered – the majority of schools let you have what you need because they know that they'll benefit from it, whereas others want it compacted and it has to be chopped down to the most important elements. Be prepared for potentially ending up with a lot of follow-up work on your hands when delivering interventions in schools. An intervention may be requested because a couple of pupils have mentioned a problem or a teacher is aware of a specific incident, but once you bring the issue out into the open you suddenly find 20 people saying that it's an issue or that an apparently small incident isn't so small after all.

When dealing with specific cases of bullying, be aware that there can be a danger of other pupils jumping on the bandwagon. Rather than supporting the victim when a case of racial bullying is brought out into the open, some may simply relish it as new source of entertainment for them to get a laugh out of.

WHAT WORKS?

Teambuilding

Taking young people outside of the school environment for teambuilding sessions can help to get them respecting each other, at least on some level. By getting them working together as a team so that they're talking and doing things together rather than being at loggerheads can get them thinking 'Well why do we have to be nasty with this guy? We've worked together on this thing and we came back with a trophy and it was good working with him, so why are we being like that with each other?'

Teambuilding activities can also help people who may have become socially isolated in the school through bullying to build positive links with other pupils. Often we find that when they're back in school a person who is being bullied will be supported by the people they've worked in a team with during the exercises. You can find out more about team-based anti-bullying programmes in the UK by visiting the Beat Bullying website: www.bbclic.com

There are, of course, no guarantees with this type of work. Sometimes the situation will be improved dramatically, other times positive results won't translate to the school environment because once they're no longer working in a team situation they slip back into their old patterns of behaviour. How well a bully responds to intervention work often depends a lot on who's in the background – for example, where they have family members undermining your efforts it can be very hard to produce a sustainable change in attitudes and behaviour.

Using role play

As the case study highlighted, drama can be a really effective tool in anti-bullying work. With age 11 upwards, role play can be used to explore issues around differences in appearance and religious dress. We begin by doing a bit of the role play with the health workers and then get the young people involved so that they take ownership. Also, the other young people watching respect it more coming from kids of their own age rather than the workers. Some have never done any kind of role play before and find that they really enjoy it and are able to use it as a way of exploring their own feelings and behaviour.

When doing role play work, always make sure that young people have permission from home to play certain parts outside of their culture to ensure that it's not going to cause offence.

Class presentations

When asked to do a presentation in school which relates specifically to racial or cultural bullying, or if you're doing a general bullying presentation and want to include this theme, try to use materials which show a very wide range of people – from different ethnicities, religions and cultures, to people with different hairstyles and glasses or braces. Rather than being a preachy lecture on political correctness, the message should be that, however we may look, bullying can affect all of us and we all have feelings.

Class sessions can prompt some pupils to admit quite openly that they feel they are bullying someone or that they have done in the past and now want to try repairing the situation, especially when the bullying has occurred within a friendship. Sometimes, of course, it isn't easy to repair and you need to be honest and say collectively you've got to do quite a lot of work to rebuild the bridges and restore trust and respect. It's a process which requires effort and commitment from both the bully and the victim.

You may get instances where someone will say that their friend is being bullied but also that that friend is in turn bullying them. Often, when you've spent some time with the friend and given them an opportunity to talk about what's been happening and how they're feeling, they will suddenly realise that they are bullying somebody, and that's when they start wanting to change their ways. In all cases of bullying, the sooner the victim can be given support to talk about what's happening and how they're coping with it and to understand it, the better.

A 'WHOLE COMMUNITY' APPROACH

A particular danger with racial and cultural bullying is that it can spill over from schools into the community and vice versa. Increasingly in the UK there are communities with people from several different countries and different religions side by side, where a whole range of tensions and prejudices can build up. Where an incident of bullying involves someone's religion, for example, it can quickly explode into a situation where whole families end up in conflict.

Problems can arise when young people from different cultures become involved in relationships. Families can put a lot of pressure on young people in these situations which they find hard to deal with, e.g. 'you can't live here if you're going to stay with him'. Sometimes it's possible to get the families to sit down and work on the issues and sometimes not. It makes it particularly difficult when one parent wants to engage in discussion and another doesn't want to know. This leaves you working with one parent who wants to support their child and another that is undermining the process. There's no magic solution in these situations – you just have to do what you can and accept that it's not always possible to achieve an ideal outcome, however hard you try.

Some of the work I've done has involved situations where young people have become angry with their own cultures and have caused friction between other people because they don't know how to deal with that anger. There's really a need to get children talking more about different cultures from an early age, not just so that they respect other people's but so that they understand their own cultures properly as well.

Involving fathers in team-building work with young people can be very effective at not only building cohesion in the community but also building bonds between fathers and sons. Sometimes boys will say that the sessions are the first time their father has ever done anything with them. When it works well, the spirit of working together will carry across back into the community, e.g. deciding to let people from other cultures into the football team or other community activities.

Anti-bullying work isn't just about stopping bullying in schools; it's about changing behaviour in adulthood too. The lessons that children learn in schools get carried through into the workplace and the wider community. Tackling racial and cultural bullying in schools is not only important for improving the mental well-being of young people, but also for strengthening communities and improving mental well-being in the whole population.

For more tips on anti-bullying work in schools, see Conrad and White (2007).

REFERENCES

Conrad D and White A (eds) (2007) *Men's Health – How to Do It*. Oxford: Radcliffe Publishing.

Cline T, de Abreu G, Fihosy C, Gray H, Lambert H and Neale J (2002) *Minority Ethnic Pupils in Mainly White Schools: research report RR 365*. London: DfES.

Department for Education and Skills (2006) *Bullying Around Racism, Religion and Culture*. London: DfES.

Department for Education and Skills (2004) Aiming High: understanding the educational needs of minority ethnic pupils in mainly white schools – a guide to good practice. London: DfES.

CHAPTER 19

Working with prisoners and young offenders

James Woodall

INTRODUCTION

Prisons and Young Offenders Institutions (YOIs) are important settings for tackling men's health. Prisons are typically 'male' environments, highlighted by the fact that only 5% of the prison population in England and Wales is female. Men in prison are a vulnerable group in society, with many having been subjected to a lifetime of social exclusion (*see* Box 19.1). Poor education, low income, meagre employment opportunities, lack of engagement with normal societal structures, low self-esteem and impermanence in terms of accommodation and family relationships typify prisoners entering the system (Levy 2005; Senior and Shaw 2007).

BOX 19.1 Men in prison are a socially excluded group

➤ 47% of male sentenced prisoners had run away from home as a child compared to 11% in the general population.

➤ 49% of male sentenced prisoners had been excluded from school (compared to 2% in the general population).

➤ 52% of male prisoners have no qualifications.

➤ 62% of short sentenced male prisoners involved in drug misuse had spent more time unemployed than in work during their life.

➤ 25% of young offenders are fathers.

Source: Social Exclusion Unit (2002)

WHY SHOULD MENTAL HEALTH PROMOTION BE AIMED AT PRISONERS AND YOUNG OFFENDERS?

The mental health of prisoners is a particular concern (Durcan 2008). Mental health problems among the prison population are far more common than those found in the general population (Watson *et al.* 2004). For example, in Western countries around one in seven prisoners have psychotic illnesses or major depression and about one in two men in prison have antisocial personality disorders (Fazel and Danesh 2002). It is true to say that many prisoners 'import' mental health issues into the prison. However, the effect of the prison environment itself may also impact on prisoners' mental health status.

By adopting a philosophy where prisons are seen as important locations or settings for addressing men's health, this allows the opportunity for accessing men who are traditionally difficult to engage in community settings. Typically, men in prison will have had relatively little contact with health promoters and health services prior to their prison sentence. We know that men from working-class backgrounds are less likely than middle-class men to access and respond to health promotion information (Banks 2001). Prison offers the potential to reverse this trend, as the overriding majority of prisoners are male, drawn predominantly from lower socio-economic status groups (Caraher *et al.* 2002).

The importance of promoting positive mental health in prisons and not just promoting the absence of mental illness is crucially important. While it may be difficult to imagine positive mental health among prisoners, prison should provide an opportunity for individuals to be helped towards a sense of personal development without harming themselves or others (World Health Organization 1998). This chapter aims to provide practitioners with practical ideas on how to promote mental health in prisons and YOIs, providing some working principles for practitioners and drawing on lessons learned from research and existing examples of good practice.

UNDERSTANDING THE DIFFICULTY OF MENTAL HEALTH PROMOTION IN PRISON

It seems unusual to start by outlining the difficulties of promoting positive mental health in this setting. However, it is important for practitioners to be fully aware of the barriers in place that act to demote the mental health of men in prison. It is self-evident that health promotion in prison is substantially more complex than for those at liberty – essentially, prisons are not in the business of promoting health (Smith 2000). Their primary function is to protect public safety and maintain the safe running of the establishment. It is apparent that the principles of mental health promotion are in many ways incongruous to prison regimes, which are often disempowering, isolating and focussed on security, surveillance and controlling individuals (Whitehead 2006).

The environment of the prison is also non-conducive to promoting positive mental health. Prisoners are frequently deprived of outside cell contact and individuals are subjected to a lack of privacy and processes of surveillance and control. Men in prison are also taken away from family and friends and only permitted a limited amount of contact time with them. Some of the key issues demoting the mental health of prisoners are highlighted in Box 19.2.

BOX 19.2 Factors which demote positive mental health in prison

> ➤ Long periods of time locked in a cell.
> ➤ Overcrowded conditions.
> ➤ Lack of privacy.
> ➤ Violence and bullying (especially prominent features of YOIs).
> ➤ Conflicts with prison staff.
> ➤ Limited contact with family and friends.
> ➤ Having to adjust to a new environment and coming to terms with strict rules and regimes.
> ➤ Limited autonomy, choice or control.
> ➤ Limited amounts of exercise.

KEY WORKING PRINCIPLES FOR WORKING WITH PRISONERS AND YOUNG OFFENDERS

Before discussing some of the ways in which mental health can be promoted in prisons and YOIs, there are some key principles that practitioners should acknowledge before working in these particular settings:

➤ the security of the prison must never be compromised
➤ always be prepared to attend security training, inductions and tours before working in the prison
➤ always take time to understand the 'procedures' of the prison you are working in and appreciate that these may change from prison to prison
➤ fit in with the regime – don't expect it to fit around you and your work; if in doubt, ask a member of prison staff
➤ always inform a member of staff of what you are doing and how long you intend to be
➤ always be aware of your professional boundaries
➤ never divulge personal information about yourself or your family
➤ never accept gifts from prisoners and never bring anything into the prison for prisoners
➤ be aware of what you can and cannot take into the prison before arriving.
➤ do not bring mobile phones into the prison
➤ dress appropriately – don't wear clothes or footwear that is inappropriate or draws unnecessary attention from prisoners; women should be especially conscious in this regard
➤ the core work of the prison is about protecting the public and maintaining the safety and security of the prison; do be prepared for sessions to be cancelled or re-arranged at the last minute by prison personnel if unforeseen circumstances arise.

GETTING IN

Once you establish yourself as a practitioner within the prison, the organisational make-up of prison regimes means that it is likely that many prisoners will have time available to them and be able to participate in any group activities or sessions you organise. However, establishing how to get in is the first stage in implementing any programme. The local Primary Care Trust may be a first port of call. Since 2006, Primary Care Trusts have been responsible for the healthcare of prisoners in their geographical area.

Working in prison can be a steep learning curve, with lots to take in and lots of jargon related to prison life. Once you get started it's a good idea to take notes and reflect on new things you have learned. This will enable you to track your development as a practitioner and help you to help other practitioners who are starting to work with men in prison.

DOING MENTAL HEALTH PROMOTION IN PRISON

Mental health promotion is a key agenda for prisons, highlighted in the Prison Service Order for health promotion (HM Prison Service 2003) and by the World Health Organization (World Health Organization 1998). However, there are no easy answers in 'doing' mental health promotion, as prisons are complex settings in which to implement change. Ultimately, a 'whole prison approach' and shift in policy will be required, where health promotion is seen as part of the core work of everyone in the institution. External practitioners have a valuable role to play in a whole-prison approach to health promotion; the following sections suggest areas where practitioners may be able to contribute.

PROVIDING SOCIAL SUPPORT MECHANISMS

Prisoners tend to keep problems to themselves. This can result in feelings being bottled up, causing stress and anxiety, especially during periods of solitary cell confinement. There are clear benefits for the mental health of prisoners and young offenders when social support services are in place for sharing problems and concerns. Prisoners can receive social support from a range of agencies in prison such as prison staff, the chaplain, gym officers, healthcare staff and education staff. However, there are a number of barriers which influence prisoners' abilities to seek help from others. These barriers are especially evident with mental health issues, where often a hyper-masculine prison culture exists, in which seeking help exposes weakness to others (Bird *et al.* 1999). In prison, stoic denials of weakness are common, as many prisoners do not want their masculinity questioned by showing more 'feminine' qualities associated with seeking help. Young men in prison can be especially reticent in this regard.

Lessons learnt from research involving young men in prison (Woodall 2007) suggest that support agencies for prisoners are an important outlet for offenders to discuss their problems but must be seen as credible and non-judgemental. Peer support or support services involving ex-prisoners are often effective because these individuals are empathetic and fully understand prison life. For practitioners setting up support services for men in the prison the following key points should be considered:

➤ be non-judgemental – prisoners can magnify issues which may be perceived by practitioners as inconsequential or minor; it is important never to dismiss these problems, however insignificant they may seem to you

➤ always listen carefully – this will help in building trust and rapport

➤ never promise something you can't deliver – often prisoners and young offenders have been let down throughout their lives; always be realistic about what you can achieve

➤ set boundaries – establish with the prisoner the levels of confidentiality you can give to a prisoner as an external practitioner; if prisoners divulge information that may jeopardise the safety of the prison then this must be disclosed to the prison authorities

➤ understand your limits – ask more experienced colleagues or speak to prison staff if you need advice

➤ be a good role model.

Case study: how to tackle bullying in YOIs – a case study in innovative practice

Bullying has now been recognised as endemic in prisons. Victims of bullying experience a range of psychological and psychosomatic symptoms, including anxiety and insecurity, low self-esteem and self worth, as well as being more likely to be unhappy and depressed. Bullying must be eradicated if mental health is to be promoted in prisons.

At HMYOI Castington, an innovative scheme has been delivered to tackle bullying behaviour. The 'tackle it' course is a six week programme designed to develop team working and citizenship skills. Football coaches run the course, using sport as the 'hook' to explore the issue. The 'tackle it' course discusses bullying within football and builds up to discussing the problem in prison. The key is the interactive nature of the course, with lots of interactive games, role plays and worksheets delivered to the young men. Twelve participants attend the course at any one time, a mix of young people that have been bullied, are bullies or have had no involvement in bullying attend each course. This provides a range of perspectives on the issue.

GETTING MEN TO ENGAGE WITH SERVICES IN PRISON

As a practitioner within prison your role may be to support prisoners in taking positive steps to strengthen their resilience and improve their confidence and self-esteem. Depending on the prison you are working in and the individual prisoner, you should consider encouraging the following.

Keeping in touch with family

Contact with family and friends is an important source of support and should be promoted to encourage positive mental health (World Health Organization 1998). Visits are an important part of a prisoners' life, as contact with family and friends can act as a buffer for reducing prison-based stressors, such as solitary confinement (Dixey and Woodall 2009; Woodall *et al.* 2009). The presence of visitors normalises the prison environment and acts as a reminder of the outside world and its associated responsibilities (Hairston 1991; Mills 2005). Regular visits therefore improve the transition back into the community, lowering levels of 'institutionalisation', as prisoners are not completely immersed in the prison sub-culture (Gordon 1999; Codd 2008).

As well as prisoners being isolated from friends and family, some prisoners are isolated from their children, with around one in four young offenders being fathers. Encouraging and supporting men to keep in touch with their children through visits and by telephoning and writing is important for the child and also an important aspect for an offender's mental health, as this contact can reduce the stresses of prison life, especially for younger men (Woodall 2007).

LEARNING NEW SKILLS

There are lots of opportunities in prison for learning new skills and developing self-confidence. Supporting prisoners to access education, vocational courses and prison jobs can provide them with a purposeful sentence which may enable job opportunities and successful resettlement on release.

Case study: the enrichment programme at HMYOI Werrington

Werrington is a juvenile centre for those aged between 15 and 18 years old. The enrichment programme at Werrington started as a small club for 10 young people and has since gone from strength to strength. There is now a full programme of activities for individuals to participate in, including: model club, remote control-car club, computer club and pottery club. These programmes ensure that the young people in custody use their time as constructively as possible, which helps prevent boredom, enables the acquisition of new skills and promotes well-being. Furthermore, initiatives in the local community have been set up to aid the resettlement process. The feedback from the young men is positive and HMYOI Werrington has seen positive effects in the young people's confidence.

From the implementation of the enrichment programme at HMYOI Werrington, some tips for developing similar programmes have been suggested:

➤ delivering sessions in a traditional educational or didactic format are often not received particularly well by young people; try to be innovative and develop, where possible, an interactive, fun approach

➤ recruiting a wide range of staff in delivering activities helps encourage 'whole prison' ownership.

➤ develop and display a clear timetable of activities so that everyone is aware of what is on offer.

Looking after the body

Encouraging prisoners to exercise regularly can help lift an individual's mood and reduce anxiety and stress. Furthermore, food affects mood. Providing basic information on healthy eating can ensure that prisoners have the information to make an informed decision on their dietary choices.

Relaxing

Prisons are stressful environments; encouraging prisoners to unwind is important. Reading, yoga, listening to music and other similar activities are important ways to reduce the anxiety experienced by prisoners.

Providing information to prisoners

Leaflets are useful ways to highlight services, activities and support agencies within the prison that can contribute to promoting positive mental health. Written materials and leaflets are a useful way of communicating with men in prison but should not be used in isolation from face-to-face contact. Low literacy levels and poor educational attainment are common in the prison population and this requires careful consideration when providing information in this way.

Some key lessons have been learnt from using written materials for mental health promotion (e.g. Caraher *et al.* 2000):

➤ don't expect materials to play too many roles – keep the message and aims simple, clear and to the point

➤ the way the information looks is vitally important for prisoners to pick it up – it should be vibrant and appealing

➤ however, the aesthetics should not distract from the message; ensure that the content and the messages are clear and understandable

➤ try to discuss ideas with prison staff and other departments in the prison – their experience and professional expertise may be valuable when coming up with appropriate designs and ideas

➤ acknowledge that men in prison are all different – try, wherever possible, to take into consideration the different needs, ages, cultures and backgrounds of prisoners

➤ always explain to prison staff what the information is for (perhaps using written guidance for staff) – prison staff are likely to have far more daily contact with prisoners than you will have as a practitioner and well-informed staff can provide the materials to prisoners and support this with individual contact

➤ try to involve men in the prison in the design of any resource materials, which could be done through working in collaboration with the education department in the prison; where this is not possible, materials should be piloted or tested with a group of prisoners or young offenders before using them – this will ensure that you are targeting the information correctly and using appropriate language

➤ try to evaluate the impact that the materials have had – this way you can develop the materials to make them more effective in the future

➤ finally, think about using other ways of communicating messages to men in prison; using music maybe one way of drawing interest to an issue and it also overcomes literacy barriers.

REFERENCES

Banks I (2001) No man's land: men, illness and the NHS. *BMJ*. **323**: 1058–1060.

Bird L, Hayton P, Caraher M, McGough H and Tobutt C (1999) Mental health promotion and prison health-care staff in young offenders' institutions in England. *The International Journal of Mental Health Promotion*. **1**(4): 16-24.

Caraher M, Bird L and Hayton P (2000) Evaluation of a campaign to promote mental health in young offender institutions: problems and lessons for future practice. *Health Education J*. **59**: 211–227.

Caraher M, Dixon P, Hayton P, Carr-Hill R, McGough H and Bird L (2002) Are health-promoting prisons an impossibility? Lessons from England and Wales. *Health Education*. **102**: 219–229.

Codd H (2008) *In the Shadow of Prison: families, imprisonment and criminal justice*. Cullompton: Willan Publishing.

Dixey R and Woodall J (2009) *Moving On: an evaluation of the Jigsaw Visitors' Centre*. Leeds: Centre for Health Promotion Research, Leeds Met University.

Durcan G (2008) *From the Inside: experiences of prison mental health care*. London: Sainsbury Centre for Mental Health.

Fazel S and Danesh J (2002) Serious mental disorder in 23 000 prisoners: a systematic review of 62 surveys. *Lancet*. **359**: 545–550.

Gordon J (1999) Are conjugal and familial visitations effective rehabilitative concepts? *The Prison Service Journal*. **79**: 119–135.

Hairston CF (1991) Family ties during imprisonment: important to whom and for what. *J Sociology and Social Welfare*. **18**: 87–104.

HM Prison Service (2003) *Prison Service Order (PSO) 3200 on health promotion*. London: HM Prison Service.

Levy M (2005) Prisoner health care provision: reflections from Australia. *Int J Prisoner Health*. **1**: 65–73.

Mills A (2005) *'Great Expectations?': a review of the role of prisoners' families*. Selected Papers from the British Society of Criminology Conference, Portsmouth, 2004. Available at: www. britsoccrim.org/volume7/001.pdf (Accessed 20 September 2009).

Senior J and Shaw J (2007) Prison healthcare. In Y Jewkes (ed). *Handbook on Prisons*. Cullompton: Willan Publishing.

Smith C (2000) 'Healthy prisons': a contradiction in terms? *The Howard Journal of Criminal Justice*. **39**: 339–353.

Social Exclusion Unit (2002) *Reducing Re-offending by Ex-prisoners*. London: Crown.

Watson R, Stimpson A and Hostick T (2004) Prison health care: a review of the literature. *Int J Nursing Studies*. **41**: 119–128.

Whitehead D (2006) The health promoting prison (HPP) and its imperative for nursing. Int J Nursing Studies. 43: 123–131.

Woodall J (2007) Barriers to positive mental health in a Young Offenders Institution: a qualitative study. *Health Education J.* **66**: 132–140.

Woodall J, Dixey R, Green J and Newell C (2009) Healthier prisons: the role of a prison visitors' centre. *Int J Health Promotion and Education.* **47**: 12–18.

World Health Organization (1998) *Mental Health Promotion in Prisons.* Report on a WHO meeting. Copenhagen: WHO.

CHAPTER 20

Service provision for homeless men

Jo McCullagh

INTRODUCTION

Local Authority data indicate that between April 2007 and March 2007 115 430 people in England were classified as homeless, equating to around 2 per 1000 population (see Diaz 2007). However, estimates regarding the number of homeless people are difficult to validate and under-represent the total population, as not all use formal shelter services (Hwang 2001; Randall and Brown 2002). Many remain hidden away from mainstream services, living in overcrowded conditions, staying with friends (known as 'sofa surfing'), or sleeping rough on the street. Crisis (2004), the national charity for single homeless people, has estimated that in the UK there could be as many as 380 000 concealed people experiencing homelessness, which equates to the entire population of Manchester. The young homeless population is primarily male, by a ratio of around 2:1 (Stephens 2002) and local authority street counts in 2008 found that 87% of rough sleepers in London were male (Homeless Link 2009).

A number of factors contribute to the risk of becoming homeless. Low socio-economic status, family conflict and relationship breakdown, institutional history and poor health can affect an individual's chance of homelessness, with the highest risk among those experiencing multiple difficulties (Ravenhill 2000; Anderson 2001; Social Exclusion Unit 2004). Thirty percent of young single homeless people have been in care and 20% of care leavers experience some form of homelessness within two years of leaving care (Stephens 2002).

Homeless men face an array of issues which reduce their levels of stability, safety and security, negatively impacting their health status and mental well-being. This includes difficulties in securing accommodation (either short-term or long-term), welfare benefits, food and clothing, verbal and physical assault and robbery, and alcohol and drug dependence (Jahiel 1992; Sosin 1992; Kershaw *et al.* 2003; Mental Health Foundation 2006; Canadian Institute for Health Information 2007). A national survey demonstrated that a third of homeless people living in temporary accommodation, and more than half of those sleeping rough, reported having more than one health problem compared with a quarter of the general population (Bines 1997).

This population group face a number of barriers which hinder engagement with traditional NHS services (Wood 1992; Mental Health Foundation 2006), including:

➤ difficulties in registering with a primary care practice resulting from having no fixed abode

➤ experiencing low levels of self-confidence and self-esteem, inhibiting communication and requests for help – particularly when faced with the somewhat judgemental attitude of health service staff and patients

➤ living a chaotic lifestyle resulting from drug and alcohol dependence, which impacts on time-keeping and conflicts with the conventional opening hours and appointment systems of mainstream healthcare services.

A study of 248 homeless people staying in shelters in St Louis, Missouri found that striking gender differences occurred in service utilisation, with women much more likely than men to have received social services (Calsyn and Morse 1990).

HOMELESSNESS AND MENTAL HEALTH

Homeless people face all kinds of difficulties in their day-to-day life that affect their emotional security and stability, including being unable to access accommodation, food, warmth and comfort. Research has clearly demonstrated the relationship between homelessness and compromised mental health (Wong and Piliavin 2001). It creates serious problems in finding or keeping employment, affects access to social capital (especially bridging social capital), undermines sense of identity and exposes men to a wide range of dangers and stressors. Insecure housing impedes emotional growth, degrades self-esteem and increases dependency for young people (Stephens 2002).

Homelessness can be both a cause and a consequence of mental disorder (Canadian Institute for Health Information 2007). A number of predictors for poor mental health are determinants of becoming homeless. Loss of residence can also affect mental well-being and continued homelessness can aggravate mental illness (Mental Health Foundation 2006; Canadian Institute for Health Information 2007). Studies have highlighted that homeless people demonstrate low levels of perceived self-worth and have poorer social support. Moreover, mental illnesses including bipolar disorder and depression, addiction and suicidal behaviour are more common among the homeless than the general population (Meltzer *et al.* 1996; Canadian Institute for Health Information 2007). In addition to the stress associated with struggling to gain access to resources such as clean clothes, comfortable sleeping and a balanced diet, a serious deterioration in physical health resulting from lack of basic resources is likely to lead on to a deterioration in mental well-being (Stephens 2002).

Nationally, it is estimated that between a third and half of people experiencing homelessness have a mental health problem compared with 10–25% of the general population (Warnes *et al.* 2003). This issue is exacerbated among those with no access to shelter compared to their residential counterparts. People living in temporary hostels or bed and breakfast accommodation are eight times more likely to experience a mental health problem, while those sleeping rough on the street are eleven times more likely (Wright 2002). A study of 225 homeless people living in hostels or sleeping rough in Glasgow found that 44% had been diagnosed with a neurotic disorder and 6% with a psychotic disorder (Kershaw *et al.* 2003). Additionally, nearly a third (29%) had attempted suicide at some time in their lifetime.

Studies have also demonstrated a link between substance use and homelessness. Research conducted by Crisis (2002) highlighted that half of the respondents stated drug use as the reason for becoming homeless, while 36% cited alcohol use. During 2004 and 2005, over a third of homeless people contacted by outreach teams in London had a drug or alcohol problem (35% and 32%, respectively; CHAIN 2005). Work undertaken with 389 homeless people in London illustrated that 83% were current drug and alcohol users and levels of dependency increased in parallel to the length of homelessness across all age ranges (Fountain and Hawes 2002). More than half of 225 homeless participants in the Glasgow study (Kershaw *et al.* 2003) were classified as having a hazardous drinking pattern, with hazardous drinking being more prevalent in men than women (60% vs 16% respectively).

DEVELOPMENT OF A HOMELESS MEN SERVICE

In response to these issues, the Salvation Army (Bootle) and NHS Sefton developed a homeless men service in 2002 to offer coordinated support to homeless men who were primarily, although not exclusively, affected by drug and alcohol misuse. This was implemented to facilitate homeless men's engagement and retention in a wider programme of treatment, health and social care support with the aim of integrating them into mainstream society and reducing levels of drug and alcohol use, criminality and homelessness.

The service aimed to improve clients':
- access to primary care
- referral to drug and alcohol treatment programmes
- accommodation status
- levels of physical and mental health
- social inclusion
- social functioning
- rehabilitation of offenders
- employability.

The specific programme objectives were:
- to reduce health inequalities in obtaining information and treatment by improving access rates to health and social care services

➤ to build clients' confidence and self-esteem and encourage the development of personal responsibility
➤ to enable clients to develop the knowledge, skills and motivation for independent living and progress towards educational training and employment.

Service funding

Funding for this programme is short-term and often reliant on in-kind services from collaborative agencies; for example, the men's health clinics and healthy lifestyle programme are funded by NHS Sefton. Although the Salvation Army provided the capital financial support to renovate the community centre building and fund the Core Officer's post, the community coordinator, cook, centre utilities and consuma bles rely on short-term charity grants and private donations. Funding applications are a key component of the community coordinator's role; within the past two years 34 applications have been submitted, with 11 proving successful and raising one-off grants of between £500 and £30,000. This initiative illustrates the importance of multidisciplinary partnership working and the pivotal role of unpaid volunteers in successful service delivery.

What does the service consist of?

The homeless men service is a joint venture between the Salvation Army Bootle and NHS Sefton. The programme is run from the Hope Salvation Army Community Centre three days a week (Monday, Wednesday and Friday) between 10 am and 1 pm. It is coordinated by a multidisciplinary team comprised of a Salvation Army Core Officer, a Community Co-ordinator, a Men's Health Nurse, a part-time cook and fifteen volunteers. Assistance is also provided by partner agencies, including the Citizens Advice Bureau (CAB), Sefton Council, Christian Debt, Sefton Drug and Alcohol Team, SUPPORT, Sefton's local NHS Stop Smoking Service, Sefton Health Improvement Support Service, Sefton Adult and Community Learning Service and Independence Initiative.

A number of collaborative, integrated services are provided.

1 *Healthy meals and food parcels:* Homeless men are routinely provided with a free breakfast, one free cooked meal a month and a subsidised hot breakfast or three-course meal priced at £1.50 and £3.50 respectively. Each client is also issued with a free food parcel containing eight items once a month.

2 *Laundry and shower facilities:* Free shower facilities are available and toiletries including toothpaste, toothbrush, soap and deodorant are issued to each client on a monthly basis. The centre also operates a laundry service at the cost of £1.50 for a wash and dry. New socks and underwear are also issued to assist personal hygiene and prevent foot problems.

3 *Men's health clinic:* A male nurse runs a drop-in health clinic twice a week on a Monday and Wednesday. He offers health advice and support, wound care and referral into other services, including primary care, dietetics, chiropody and alcohol and drug detoxification programmes. An outreach worker from the local drug

service also attends the centre on a weekly basis to facilitate client programme referral and retention.

4 *Healthy lifestyle and peer mentoring programme:* A healthy lifestyle programme, which offers blood pressure, cholesterol and glucose screening, healthy eating, stop smoking and safer drinking advice and stress management techniques is periodically undertaken by a Health Improvement Team. This comprises a Health Promotion Specialist, Health Promotion Officer and Project Officer, Food and Health Workers, Smoking Cessation Support Workers and Stress Counsellor. Clients are also trained as peer mentors to offer healthier lifestyle advice and a supportive network to other homeless men to reduce social isolation.

5 *Welfare rights and housing advice:* Access to housing is an important determinant linked to health and well-being. Assistance is therefore given to clients to complete accommodation and benefit application forms (e.g. Income Support, Incapacity Benefit and Jobseekers Allowance) and arrange appointments. Organisations such as the CAB and Christian Debt also undertake in-house weekly welfare rights and housing advice clinics to raise client awareness and resolve individual issues.

6 *Life and social skills training:* National research has found that only just over a third of people sleeping rough have any educational qualifications compared to two-thirds of the general population (Anderson *et al.* 1993) and around 90% are unemployed (Randall and Brown 1998). In view of this, the Salvation Army and Sefton Drug Action Team have implemented a 'Move On' project, which offers in-house pre-vocational life and social skills training for clients on one afternoon a week. Referral is also offered to the Government-funded Job Centre Plus and Progress To Work programmes.

Who attends the service and why?

The service is offered to all homeless men and is based on flexible definitions of 'homelessness' and 'mental health' in order to reduce barriers to access. Within a year, 79 homeless men utilised the service for a total of 6707 contacts. Their age ranged from 18 to 60 years, with an average of 42 years, and, in line with the population demography of Sefton, all described their ethnicity as White British. Key motivators to accessing the service were the provision of basic life needs – food, personal hygiene and shelter.

Unfortunately, the requirements for temporary housing exceed current provision. Assistance with accommodation is low and reflects the limited availability of temporary shelter and hostels within the borough, which often proves frustrating for the staff. A service questionnaire survey was undertaken with 40 self-selected clients to identify the reasons why they utilised the centre. An overwhelming majority of clients (36/40) rated the friendly, impartial atmosphere as the most important factor, which is in line with the service principle of encouraging men to develop a sense of personal responsibility and respect for themselves and others. The service offers a non-judgemental supportive network for the clients and often a surrogate family for those estranged from their relatives due to their alcohol and drug dependency.

Clients also reported the provision of free or subsidised meals (34/40), access to other health and social care agencies (24/40), free shower facilities (18/40), food parcels (17/40) and the laundry service (15/40) as significant incentives.

Issues affecting client attendance

Homeless men have become mistrustful of services but, by being accessible and approachable in places that they already frequent, it is possible to build up trust and mutual respect. One of the most important factors in engaging homeless men is to strike a comfortable, non-judgemental relationship with them and to talk to them in terms that they can understand. Clients rated the provision of a friendly atmosphere as the most important aspect of this service and this is reflected in the attendance data, with clients on average visiting the service 85 times per year (range 49–142).

Client service utilisation does fluctuate throughout the year with seasonable peaks in the autumn and winter months coinciding with poorer weather conditions and related health problems. Service demand is also higher at the beginning of the week following closure of the centre over the weekend. Mondays are more chaotic as some have been in fights or hospital over the weekend, or not eaten but used drugs or alcohol.

Drug and alcohol dependence also impedes clients' ability to interact with health and social care services. Homeless people can have very chaotic lives and appointments with probation, housing and benefit agencies are often missed. An important role of the programme workers is to act as an intermediary advocate to mediate between clients and mainstream services. Similarly, clients may not always accept or keep a referral for counselling because of the stigma attached to mental health issues, which requires sustained one-to-one support and understanding to de-stigmatise the problem and aid service utilisation.

Case study: the Broadway charity, London

Broadway provide a range of services to meet the mental, physical and social needs of homeless and vulnerably housed adults across London. These include onsite healthcare, showers, laundry and training, alongside structured one-to-one support and group work programmes.

The issue of mental well-being is seen as central to the work that they do. All workers are given a basic introduction to mental health and a Specialist Mental Health Service is available for clients who are feeling stressed, anxious, low or emotionally distressed. A Mental Health Worker works with a caseload of clients, providing solution-based therapy or appropriate referral to other organisations. People with mental health needs can also access Broadway's Healthy Living Centre, where a range of alternative therapies play an important role in reducing stress.

Visit www.broadwaylondon.org for more information.

ACKNOWLEDGEMENTS

Captain Carole Babstock, Commanding Officer, The Salvation Army, Bootle Corps.
Alan Roper, Community Co-ordinator, The Salvation Army, Bootle Corp.

REFERENCES

Anderson I, Kemp P and Guilgars D (1993) *Single Homeless People.* London: HMSO.

Anderson I (2001) *Pathways Through Homelessness: towards a dynamic analysis.* Stirling: Housing Policy and Practice Unit, University of Stirling.

Bines W (1997) *The Health of Single Homeless People: homelessness and social policy.* London: Routledge.

Calsyn RJ and Morse G (1990) Homeless Men and Women: commonalities and a service gender gap. *Am J Community Psychol.* **18**(4): 597–608.

Canadian Institute for Health Information (2007) *Mental Health and Homelessness.* Ottawa, Ontario: Canadian Institute for Health Information.

Combined Homelessness and Information Network (CHAIN) (2005) *Rough Sleeping Report for London 2004/05.* London: CHAIN.

Crisis (2002) *Home and Dry? Homelessness and substance use.* Available at: www.crisis.org.uk/pdf/HomeandDry.pdf (Accessed 20 September 2009).

Crisis (2004) Hidden Homelessness: Britain's invisible city. London: Crisis. Available at: www.crisis.org.uk/pdf/SONreport_HHBIC.pdf (Accessed 20 September 2009).

Diaz R (2007) Homelessness Factsheet: shelter. Available at: http://england.shelter.org.uk/__data/assets/pdf_file/0010/39574/33075.pdf (Accessed 20 September 2009).

Fountain J and Hawes S (2002) *Home and Dry? Homelessness and substance use in London.* London: Crisis.

Homeless Link (2009) Rough Sleeping – Key Facts. Available at: www.homeless.org.uk/policyandinfo/facts/rskeystats1 (Accessed 7 July, 2009).

Hwang SW (2001) Homelessness and Health. *Canadian Medical Association Journal.* **164**(2): 229–233.

Jahiel RI (1992) Services for homeless people: an overview. In RI Jahiel (ed.), *Homelessness: a prevention-orientated approach.* Baltimore, MD: John Hopkins University Press, pp. 167–192.

Kershaw A, Singleton N and Meltzer H (2003) Survey of the health and well-being of homeless people in Glasgow. *International Review of Psychiatry.* **15**: 141–143.

Meltzer H, Gill B and Hinds K (1996) *The Prevalence of Psychiatric Morbidity among Homeless Adults.* OPCS Surveys of Psychiatric Morbidity in Great Britain Bulletin, No 3. London: OPCS.

Mental Health Foundation (2006) *Making the Link between Mental Health and Youth Homelessness: pan-London study.* London: Mental Health Foundation.

Randall G and Brown S (1998) *Homes for Street Homeless People: an evaluation of the rough sleepers initiative.* London: DETR.

Randall G and Brown S (2002) *Helping Rough Sleepers off the Streets: a report to the Homelessness Directorate.* London: ODPM.

Ravenhill M (2000) *Routes into Homelessness: a study by the Centre for the Analysis of Social Exclusion of the paths into homelessness of homeless clients of the London Borough of Camden's Homeless Person's Unit.* London: Centre for the Analysis of Social Exclusion.

Social Exclusion Unit (2004) *Mental Health and Social Exclusion.* London: ODPM.

Sosin M (1992) Homelessness and vulnerable meal program users: A comparison study. *Social Problems.* **39**: 170–188.

Stephens J (2002) *The Mental Health Needs of Homeless Young People*. London: The Mental Health Foundation.

Warnes A, Crane M, Whitehead N and Fu R (2003) *Homelessness Factfile*. London: Crisis.

Wong YLI and Piliavin I (2001) Stressors, resources and distress among homeless persons: a longitudinal analysis. *Social Science & Medicine*. 52: 1029–1042.

Wood D (ed) (1992) *Delivering health care to homeless persons: the diagnosis and management of medical and mental health conditions*. New York: Springer Publishing.

Wright N (2002) *Homelessness: a primary care response*. London: Royal College of General Practitioners.

CHAPTER 21

Working with drug users

Barry Langham and Nick Davy

INTRODUCTION

Drug users often report bad experiences of their interactions with health profession-als, which do little to promote psychological well-being or improve their sense of self-worth. The feelings of being stigmatised by professionals and the public alike have a negative impact on their self-esteem, motivation and willingness to access services, such as needle exchanges (Simmonds and Coomber 2009). This chapter is based on our work with injecting drug users at a needle exchange in Bradford, UK and offers some simple guidance on working with this client group in a supportive and understanding manner.

The Bridge Project needle exchange is a place where injecting users who reside in Bradford can drop in on any weekday for advice, information and to collect clean injecting equipment or to dispose of used equipment. When clients register at the needle exchange, they undertake a risk assessment and health check, so that staff can offer advice on harm reduction and help monitor general health. Clients always have the opportunity to discuss problems they may be experiencing in relation to drug use, in confidence. We provide support to clients who want to address their drug use and direct them to appropriate services, as well as assisting those who continue to inject drugs to minimise the risk.

Clients can expect a friendly non-judgemental welcome and are encouraged to make use of the services available. A physical health nurse is available four days each week and is able to undertake testing for bloodborne viruses, offer advice and treatment for injecting trauma injury and give advice on general and sexual health matters. Hepatitis B vaccinations are also available. Additional services include free fruit, clothing, a resource library containing information about local services and auricular acupuncture.

Now that a lot of other services are clinic- and appointment-based, people may drop in and find that there isn't anyone free to see them. In a needle exchange it's different and people come knowing that someone is always here whom they'll be able to talk to. A needle exchange could be seen simply as somewhere that people come to pick up needles, but it is so much more than that and that's why the skill of the workers in engaging with the clients is so important. There's so much more to meeting the health needs of drug users than 'give me your needles and here's ten in exchange'. Some people do want only to come in, get their needles and go, but if we see an opening to engage with them we'll take it.

WHO ARE THE SERVICE USERS?

Most drug users are no different from anybody else – they just happen to be using drugs. Many people who use drugs lead otherwise perfectly normal lives. One of our clients, for example, was a man with a high-powered job who came to the needle exchange in a suit. Contrary to the popular image, the majority aren't at 'rock bottom' and will be in a good mental state when they come in.

Although there are groups of similar users in terms of their lives, there's no single stereotype and drug users certainly don't see themselves as one group. There's a perceived hierarchy of status among users, with heroin users at the bottom. Cocaine users access services less than heroin users and dislike having to be lumped in with services for heroin users. One client said openly, 'I don't want to go in there. They're all smack-heads; I'm a crack-head'. Steroid users typically don't even see themselves as drug users at all, yet they take a whole range of drugs with little or no understanding of the effects. Tanning injections are becoming increasingly common and another form of drug use which typically isn't seen as such by those who practice it.

THE NEED FOR SUPPORT

Drug users often have little or no family support. Hiding a habit, stealing to fund it and breaking a long stream of promises to change can eventually lead to parents or partners drawing the line and walking away. Although we encourage drug users to try to maintain family support, the reality is that it's often too far down the line.

When a drug user has a substantial social network of other users it would be easy to assume that they have access to social support. Drug users themselves, however, don't see these relationships as friendships – just as a network of co-dependent acquaintances which they have to be a part of in order to survive and feed their habit. When you see a group together it might appear that there's some genuine cohesion there, but the relationships typically offer no real psychological support and drug users are under no illusions about that.

The lack of social support particularly becomes an issue when someone is trying to stop using. Ex-drug users often find themselves in a social vacuum. So many will succeed in giving up drugs only to find that they've lost their focus in life and their former acquaintances. Often all previous relationships with non-users have disintegrated over the course of their drug use, meaning that cutting off contact with drug-using acquaintances means social isolation at a time when support is needed more than ever. Coming off drugs is a lonely business and part of our job is to help to fill the gap and provide that support.

For many users, whether it's medication or street drugs, their habit has become their main reason for living. It's what they think of when they wake up in the morning and what they think of when they go to sleep at night – 'Have I got some for the morning?', 'How am I going to get some?'. Many people struggle with losing that focus and sense of purpose when they quit and it's not uncommon for quitters to reward themselves for not using for a couple of weeks by using.

Case study

One client who had been clean for 6 months reported that on one occasion another user had kept badgering him over and over to have a hit. He became so frustrated that his refusals were ignored that he eventually took the syringe and squirted it out onto the carpet, which was met with predictable outrage.

This example highlights the lack of genuine support that those wishing to quit tend to receive from their fellow drug users and the perceived need that drug users have to maintain their network of fellow users, even if that means pushing quitters back into using.

This is why, when users do want to come off drugs, having an alternative environment away from old haunts and acquaintances is so important. Accommodation is one of the biggest problems for drug users. If they've got nowhere to stay because nothing's been set up, they inevitably end up back staying with drug users. As there's an unwritten rule that if you're staying there you provide for whoever is living in that house; this means being drawn back into acquiring drugs. Most drug users who get out of prison want to change but the odds are against them if they haven't got somewhere safe to go and some support.

GETTING THE CLIENTS TO ENGAGE

Although a common theme in men's health is men's preference for seeking medical help for obvious, serious physical ailments rather than psychological issues (O'Brien *et al.* 2005), with users of the needle exchange it's been the other way around. They're much more likely to see the nurse for psychological support than with a physical problem, although they may not consciously come for psychological support. Whilst as a group drug users have got lots of physical needs, on the whole that's not what concerns them. They can be walking around with quite unbelievable trauma and not see it as a priority. Often, though, spending a bit of time with the client will make them realise that there is something serious which needs attention – because you're taking it seriously.

Sometimes, when it comes to engaging clients, progress is very slow and it's best to think of it as a long-term process rather than expecting a quick win. One guy came in for the first time and said 'just give me some fucking greens and some fucking blues'. We took it as a sign of progress when he stopped saying that he was throwing his used needles in the children's playground.

Although drug users are generally very comfortable using the needle exchange as a place to get psychological support, often on the first visit clients won't have an appreciation of all that the service can offer them. Steroid users are a good example because they don't see themselves as drug users and often don't want to engage at all. In addition, the side effects can make them short-tempered and angry and they will often be in a defensive frame of mind when they come in. A lot of them see themselves as freaks – they're doing something that isn't normal, so they expect a response to that. It's important to remember that stigmatisation occurs among drug users themselves, enforcing a hierarchy of status depending on the drug involved, with steroid users anxious to separate themselves from 'junkies' (Simmonds and Coomber 2009).

It can be very difficult to build a relationship with steroid users because they may only come in once or twice a year, whereas street drug users may come in every day or every week. You learn to judge whether they're listening and whether you're getting anywhere. If not, you just have to back off, give them what they came for and wait for the next time. Sometimes you can see these guys, especially the younger ones, starting to think 'Am I making the right decision?' Maybe they'll come in and something has gone wrong – they might be worried that they're developing a breast or they have itchy nipples. Working with steroid users requires a different approach from working with street drug users. Using humour can be helpful in getting messages across. If somebody young comes in for the first time we'll emphasise the potential side effects, e.g. 'Do you want your balls to shrink to the size of peanuts?' In a way, street drug users find it easier when it comes to sharing their problems and concerns because they're used to telling people about what they're doing; they're not as embarrassed as a steroid user. Steroid users typically won't go to a GP with drug issues, so this kind of service is really the only way to engage them and give them support. Even better would be to have the resources to develop separate services for steroid users, going out to the places where they are.

DEALING WITH DRUG USERS IN A SUPPORTIVE WAY

One of the biggest mistakes that services make is to ask clients a long list of questions as soon as they walk through the door for the first time. Common Assessment Tools for substance-use services in the UK include very personal questions which most of us wouldn't expect to be asked during a doctor's appointment, for example. Collecting a lot of data can be useful, but it doesn't help with engagement. They've come in with a crisis and unless you deal with that crisis they're not going to come back. Asking a long list of questions and then saying, 'Your time's up, come back next week' will get you nowhere.

It's important to approach working with drug users with an appreciation of their circumstances and needs, rather than simply expecting them to conform to a traditional model of how the 'patient' should behave. Street drug users often come in in an anxious or excited state when they've just scored or they're about to go and get that next fix. Those who're coming to get needles because they're just about to score will want to be in and out, but this doesn't mean that they won't want support or be willing to be engaged at another time.

Being non-judgmental is key. Try to get an understanding of the client's psychological state before leaping in with advice. We had one man who was using steroids to bulk himself out before a prison sentence because of the problems he'd had with racist bullying during a previous jail term. When someone says 'Tomorrow I'm going to be on the streets and no one likes me and what's the point in living?' you don't want to be patronising and pat them on the head and say it'll be all right tomorrow when you know that it won't be. You can refer people on who are suicidal but 9 times out of 10 wanting to kill yourself isn't seen as a mental illness. Often there aren't immediate solutions to the clients' problems and you've got to accept that there's only so much that you can do. Sometimes we'll refer someone on knowing that potentially they could end up feeling worse because they'll be denied what they really want, which is safety and security.

Physical health is often of less importance to drug users, so patience is a requirement for those working in this area. We've had people with needles snapped off in their groin and couldn't get them to go to casualty because to them it just wasn't a priority. It takes a lot to get them to keep hospital appointments (although it's important to remember that DNAs are not restricted to drug users). It would be easy to assume when this happens that the client simply doesn't value the advice that you're giving them or the effort you're putting in to try to get them treated. They're usually very apologetic though. If a client says that they'll do something and they don't, they typically feel guilty because they feel that they've let you down. Rather than getting frustrated, you have to make the effort to not let them feel guilty or stupid because usually the last thing that they need is another knock to their self-esteem. That's where the worker's skill comes in. You have to demonstrate that you know what it's like and that you accept that they're not always going to keep appointments. If someone needs something urgently, whether it be a mental or physical health issue, we send them in a taxi. Ideally we'll go with them but that's often not possible. Usually they'll get there but sometimes they just get the driver to take them somewhere else. One guy would never arrive at the other end and eventually we realised that he was only coming in with a problem when he needed to get somewhere else.

When drug users encounter nurses or other health professionals in conventional healthcare settings they often get a very negative response; even if it's just the way that they're looked at. Some of our clients have also used pharmacy-based needle exchange services because it's quicker, but the way they're treated is typically very different. Often the only interaction is 'Where are your returns?' At one point those who regularly didn't return their needles had to fill in a questionnaire, not for any particular purpose or to gather information, but just to inconvenience them. We never take the approach of saying, 'You can only have two because you didn't bring any back last time.' That's not going to achieve anything but make them angry and more likely to throw the used needles away in the street. Generally we find that if workers show respect to service users then the service users have respect for themselves and the community. This is why it's so important to have services which are staffed by people who want to work with drug users and who understand their problems. It is detrimental to their already minimal self-worth to have negative interactions with health professionals. Drug users are used to living in a world where everybody puts them down, and they put themselves down too. We're one of the few services that treat them first and foremost as people. Often someone will come to us a result of a confrontation with a health worker and we'll have to pick up the aftermath, but you have to support your colleagues and avoid taking sides. You can't leap to the conclusion that the client is blameless.

Sometimes clients will get referred on to another service but will still come back because they value the emotional support that we provide. There's a transition period because we treat them well and they don't want to lose that, so we don't turn people away if they want to see us.

IMPROVING MENTAL WELL-BEING

It's typically very hard to build drug users' self-esteem. They often have no self-belief and readily put themselves down quite bluntly, e.g. by casually referring to themselves as 'dirty smack-heads'. By demonstrating a genuine interest in them, it is possible to build relationships over time that promote mental health and which they come to accept as a trusted source of much-needed psychological support. Mental health promotion should be seen as an ongoing part of the job, whether dealing with an immediate crisis or providing long-term routine support.

Frequently we see clients who have come in just to talk. We get a lot of people, for example, who don't even use needles any more but still come in because it's a place where they feel comfortable to come for a chat. In some ways we try to discourage it because being surrounded by the paraphernalia and imagery of injecting, as well as the other service users, can be a real trigger for relapse. On the other hand, we know that this may be the only place which they feel able to come to for informal psychological support.

Although it's an inaccurate stereotype that all drug users are at 'rock bottom', people can be very agitated or very low because of their circumstances when they come in. They might be homeless or have simply had enough of what's going on in their lives and be feeling suicidal. In this situation you can only do your best to try to make them see that there is a point in carrying on, although depending on what's going on in their lives it may be hard to find the positives without sounding patronising or naïve. Life experience helps a lot when it comes to having credibility with the clients. You get asked a lot whether you've used drugs. We have a non-disclosure policy, so we simply say that it's about their drug use rather than ours.

Once, we had a man who was waiting for a couple of hours for his state benefit cheque to be reissued. He was in an agitated state, but rather than being out on the street wandering around and possibly getting into trouble he was in a safe environment being supported by the staff. Although he just walked about shaking his head in disgust, the very informal support that he received was crucial. It's a situation which is quite common and although there's nothing we can do to speed up the process, we can give them access to a telephone and a safe and supportive environment in which to wait. You do have to set boundaries, however, because of the limited staff and space. You can't have someone waiting around all day for a phone call or have everyone in at once when it's busy, but the clients respect the service and are usually happy to wait outside when necessary. Generally the clients appreciate that it's a service for them with dedicated staff, so they respect the place and the workers.

We encourage injecting drug users to have regular blood tests and helping them to deal with the results is another form of psychological support that we provide. Sometimes when a result comes through it's not only the clients themselves to whom we have to give emotional support. One man went to his ex-girlfriend's house and shouted through the letterbox that he was Hepatitis C positive and she came to the needle exchange in a distressed state.

In terms of the workers' own mental well-being, there are easier jobs. It is very rewarding but you have to appreciate the small rewards – 'Are they still alive?' rather than 'Have they stopped using for good?' It can be stressful because you see so much pain. You have to learn not to take it home with you and to support each other as colleagues, to do your job as well as you can and then switch off when you go home.

BOX 20.1 Golden rules

> Your attitude to working with drug users shouldn't be different from working with any other group in any other setting. Whether in a classroom working with boys or giving health MOTs in a workplace, it's all about being respectful, non-judgmental, giving people time and developing a relationship.
>
> ➤ Be non-judgemental.
> ➤ Be respectful. Generally if you treat the clients with respect you get respect back and that's the bottom line with all men's health work.
> ➤ Treat people how you'd want your own relatives or friends to be treated.
> ➤ Be natural. Don't put on an act – drug users are good at sussing people out. They'll know if you're bullshitting, but equally you have to know when they're bullshitting.
> ➤ Don't make promises that you can't keep or you'll very quickly lose credibility.
> ➤ Ask the clients how they feel about the services and get them involved in planning services.
>
> Remember that people don't choose to become drug users; they're there because of circumstances.

REFERENCES

O'Brien R, Hunt K and Hart G (2005) 'It's caveman stuff, but that is to a certain extent how guys still operate': men's accounts of masculinity and help seeking. *Social Science & Medicine.* **61**(3): 503–516.

Simmonds L and Coomber R (2009) Injecting drug users: A stigmatised and stigmatizing population. *International J Drug Policy.* **20**(2): 121–130.

CHAPTER 22

The mental health of men with cancer

Martin Neal and David Conrad

INTRODUCTION

> For several weeks I had put off going to the GP, not out of fear but more the male 'can't be bothered to make an appointment' reason. Finally I'd done it, and now I was being asked to stay behind after the surgery. Little did I know that in less than 10 days I would be being told I had cancer.

> Anonymous reflection by a man living with cancer.

This chapter will look at some of the issues and strategies that can be considered and used by those caring or working with men who have been diagnosed with cancer or who have recovered from cancer. Cancer will affect one in three men, yet it still remains one of the most feared and misunderstood conditions. Even an invitation to be examined for prostate cancer, let alone a diagnosis, has been found to create emotional stress (Gustafsson *et al.* 1995).

The impact of cancer upon men's mental health varies. A study of men with early localised prostate cancer, for example, found that although some men did experience distressing psychological symptoms, there were low levels of psychopathology overall (Bisson *et al.* 2002). About 50% of patients with advanced cancer, however, meet criteria for a psychiatric disorder; the most common being adjustment disorders (11–35%) and major depression (5–26%) (Miovic and Block 2007). Up to 80% of the psychological and psychiatric illness which develops in cancer patients goes unrecognised and untreated. One reason for this is the difficulty in deciding what should be classed as appropriate sadness as patients approach the end of life and what is in fact a depressive illness (Lloyd-Williams 2000).

Under-utilisation of mental health services is known to be a particular issue among advanced cancer patients and mental health concerns of patients with advanced cancer frequently go unaddressed by health professionals (Kadan-Lottick *et al.* 2005). All health professionals working with men with cancer should watch for signs of psychological distress, particularly in patients with poor physical functioning or deficits in social or family support (Balderson and Towell 2003). This chapter aims to provide some basic tips for those working with men with cancer on things to look out for and ways of addressing the emotional aspects of the impact of the disease in a helpful and sensitive way.

HELPING YOUR CLIENT TO UNDERSTAND HIS CONDITION

Many men with cancer initially feel overwhelmed by the amount of information that is given to them upon diagnosis (Gray *et al.* 2000). Helping the person you are working with to understand their condition is critical. It's been demonstrated that assisting men with prostate cancer to obtain information enables them to assume a more active role in treatment decision-making and decreases their levels of anxiety (Davison and Degner 1997). The key to this is being able to direct the person to a source of information that they can understand and is meaningful to them. This might take many forms. However, one central part of this is your ability to moderate, translate and explain any information that the person has found or is searching for. The internet, for example, can be a readily available source of information, support and guidance, but it can also be a source of unfounded and misdirected information. The management of valid and relevant information in order to make it of use to your client is often referred to as 'evidence-based practice'. The language of cancer (oncology) is a highly specialist one and it is worthwhile checking out how much information your clients have about their condition. Men in particular often do not wish to lose face when presented with a barrage of information and this can often leave them with important deficits in the understanding of their condition. Macmillan Cancer Support can provide reliable and easy to understand information in a wide range of formats to help you and your client understand their condition.

BOX 22.1 Our Cancer Year

> The autobiographical graphic novel 'Our Cancer Year' by Harvey Pekar and Joyce Brabner (illustrated by Frank Stack) is an excellent resource for people seeking a man's perspective on the experience of being diagnosed and living with cancer. Harvey Pekar (b 1939) is the author of the comic book series 'American Splendor', in which he which he has written about his daily experiences as a hospital clerk in Cleveland, US, capturing the mundaneness and absurdity of everyday life since 1976. In 1990, he was diagnosed with lymphoma, for which he required chemotherapy. The book tells the story of the practical and emotional realities of living with cancer, from diagnosis to receiving the all-clear, in a frank and accessible way.
>
> *Our Cancer Year* won the 1995 Harvey Award for Best Graphic Album of Original Work.

GRIEVING

Being diagnosed with cancer can be likened to experiencing bereavement. The feelings experienced by people on being diagnosed with cancer are often similar to the stages of grieving. These stages are: anger, denial, bargaining and acceptance (Worden 1991). The feeling of anger is often associated with loss. This loss might be the loss of health, being unable to work (which can be particularly difficult for men) or the perceived or real loss of the ability to have a future, or to see those around them have theirs.

Explain to your client that anger has a place and is a natural reaction, but if it is not acknowledged, validated and mastered it can rapidly become destructive to both them and those around them. The reaction of other people to their anger can be surprising for them; particularly if they are a person for whom anger is not the norm. Being angry can result in people avoiding them or being angry back, which can reflect a frustration at not knowing what to say or a feeling of helplessness. This can result in the person with cancer feeling isolated or feeling more different than ever. Not only have they been unfortunate to have a condition that will impact upon their physical health, but they are likely to find that it also impacts upon their mental health in some surprising ways.

After the anger has begun to subside they may enter denial; in this stage they may begin to deny the presence of their cancer. It is not uncommon for the person to look for alternate explanations to account for why they have cancer or fail to accept that it is cancer. This stage may be accompanied by behaviour and actions that appear strange and illogical to the outside observer. Denial is a mechanism that serves to protect the individual from the harsh reality of their situation. At this time being supportive rather than confrontational is more helpful, although it might be appropriate to discuss with the client about the stages that they are likely to go through.

Following denial, the next stage is that of bargaining; the individual will attempt to change their situation by bargaining, usually through attempting to trade, change or amend behaviour or cognitions. This period can be useful in providing an opportunity to address and reinforce any positive health behaviours that have been adopted. However, false hopes should not be instilled and the role of the support worker is always to be realistic and honest about the changes in behaviour or cognitions.

The final stage of being diagnosed with (or having had) cancer is acceptance. In this stage the person becomes able to acknowledge the reality of their diagnosis and will often be more resigned to and accepting of their condition. Once they have moved to a position of acceptance, individuals are more open to respond appropriately to whatever needs to be done with regard to their cancer.

If you feel that you are unable to provide the psychological support for your client to help them move through these stages, you should help them to find appropriate support from specialist counsellors who are trained to work with individuals who have cancer.

GETTING SUPPORT

Cancer is a subject that many men find hard to talk about. It can be a word that instils fear and worry. Talking to those who are close to them can result in them feeling inadequate or taking on others' fears and concerns on top of their own. For many men the idea of sharing how they feel is alien, but those who choose to ignore these feelings will find that they inevitably become more intense. If true feelings are neglected or denied, the reality of having cancer may come back and manifest itself in other ways, causing psychological problems such as depression, isolation, anger or the adoption of unhelpful coping strategies such as the use of alcohol or drugs.

Male cancer patients and their spouses cited social support as the primary factor facilitating their coping in a study by Keitel and colleagues (1990). There is a lot of mileage in the old adage 'a problem shared is a problem halved' but where do men share the fact that they have cancer? Having cancer can make men feel vulnerable and before they feel that they can disclose the fact to others they need to feel safe enough to do so; this is dependent upon trust. Who they talk to will be dependent upon the support that they have around them. Gray and colleagues' (2000) study of men with prostate cancer found that they tended to restrict both how many people they talk to about their condition and how much. Most of the men only wanted to talk about it where they felt it was necessary, e.g. with family members that they considered had 'a right to know'. Many said that, had it been possible, they would have preferred not to tell anyone other than their spouse.

The point at which clients tell their family, significant others or children about having cancer is often a major source of worry. There is no right or wrong time to do this and, however it's managed, it may well have a major impact upon their future relationships with them. Clients may find it helpful first to discuss their situation with their doctor or specialist cancer nurse. There are several very helpful booklets available from Macmillan Cancer Support on this topic and you can refer your client to their hospital cancer support centre to get these or get them from the Macmillan Cancer Support website (www.macmillan.org.uk).

People can be strange in the way that they react to someone with cancer. Some people are helpful, supportive and show empathy, while others seem to almost go out of their way to do what might be perceived to be the wrong thing. Some might simply keep away for fear of saying the wrong thing. Preparing your client for other people's reactions can help alleviate the sense of bewilderment and isolation that people sometimes feel when they experience this. It can also help them to feel that they have a sense of control, in a situation where control may have been taken away.

Self-help and support groups can be particularly useful in reducing the sense of isolation that is often experienced by people with cancer and there has been a significant increase in the number of groups that are available in recent years. Increasingly these groups focus on a specific type of cancer. Macmillan Cancer Support in the UK or the American Cancer Society in the US will be able to signpost. For people who have been newly diagnosed, sharing their own experiences or listening to the experiences of others can help to alleviate any fears and misunderstanding about their condition and the treatments that they might receive. Many of these groups will have clinical specialists as part of the membership, helping to increase the reliability of the information given. The internet has made finding such groups and identifying the most suitable one a lot easier. Finding a group that they feel comfortable with is essential if men are to feel safe. Get your client to suss out and get a feel for the group before joining and think about whether it offers what they are looking for in terms of support or information.

Some men may prefer a one-to-one approach and choose to see a counsellor to discuss their problems. This might be arranged through their GP or their local cancer centre. Some cancer support organisations will offer telephone support – calling on a regular basis to see how the person is doing, which can help reduce the sense of isolation experienced by some men. What is important is that the person you are working with has a clearly identifiable source of support who they feel that they can access whenever they want to.

EXPLORING FEARS AND WORRIES

Many men with cancer report that fear of the unknown is one of the most destructive aspects of their illness. These fears are very real and might include the fear of dying alone, pain, the future of their significant others or a loss of control induced by their illness or the treatments that they might have. By talking about their fears and worries the client is able to address their personal cancer agenda – not just their illness but the impact that the illness will have upon their life. Clients often have fears that are unfounded and there are many myths about cancer and its treatments. Those finding themselves in an information vacuum will quickly fill it with whatever information is available. One useful strategy to help your client to manage this is to get them to engage with other people who have or have had experience of the same type of cancer. Specific support groups and forums are also particularly helpful for doing this. In the UK, MacMillan Cancer Support has a wide range of materials that aim to address any questions or fears that your client might have. The local and regional cancer centres also serve to provide points at which information is available and you may wish to consider how you will help your client to engage with these.

Cancer impacts and operates on multiple levels and as such does not lend itself to logical and rational thought processes. The use of an appropriate model can help to structure the way that you tackle negative or false perceptions that your client may have about their cancer process and produce a plan that is proactive rather than being reactive to problems only as they arise. Seedhouse's (2002) model of 'Rational Fields' may be useful in helping your client to make sense of their cancer and the complexity of their responses to it.

Helping men to manage the constant worry about the presence of their cancer or thoughts about potential relapse is a central role in supporting the mental health of men with cancer. It is important to help men experiencing this to acknowledge that their worry can be emotionally draining for them. It is not uncommon for men to try to have a stiff upper lip in the face of their cancer, however, repressing such worries can result in them becoming overwhelmed. Helping them to seek support from people who are experiencing similar problems is a particularly useful strategy. It is likely that the worries that they are having have been experienced by someone else in a similar position. Encouraging them to join a support group, or go online and become part of a forum can help reduce the sense of isolation that they might have. The secret of helping men to manage this worry is to help them to prioritise their worries, identifying the most pressing concern. Writing it down can be a way of seeing it in a different way and by rearranging the list they can start to see, as well as think, about what concerns them the most.

MANAGING THE 'EMOTIONAL MINEFIELDS'

An 'emotional mine' is a situation or stimulus that reinforces the man's awareness of their cancer. Having cancer often leaves men feeling isolated, different or inferior. A helpful strategy is to get them to think about how they will respond when asked about their cancer or when they are confronted by situations that drive home the fact they have cancer; examples might be television programmes or adverts, being offered life assurance, or being asked by a charity collector to donate. These situations may make them angry or feel sad; remind them that it's important to remember that they are not directed at them or their cancer. It's helpful if you can get them to rehearse or try to think about when these situations are likely to occur – thinking about what they will do or say without feeling that they have to apologise for the fact that they have cancer.

Some of these emotional mines will occur as a consequence of their illness, e.g. hospital appointments, treatment sessions or side effects of treatments. The key to managing the anxiety associated with these is to spend time preparing for them. Help them look for strategies that they are comfortable with; these might include things to keep them occupied or phrases that they are comfortable with. Explain that they will not know when they will encounter an emotional mine, but when they do they will inevitably be painful. How they manage these emotional mines will help them to avoid becoming anxious, angry or feeling powerless. Simply avoiding situations in which they encounter them can promote the feeling of increased isolation and restrict behaviour through avoidance. As with any minefield, the secret of successfully negotiating it lies with an ability to proceed whilst being mindful of the obvious dangers around you. If they are too cautious they will make no progress, but by not being cautious enough they will step on a mine, leading to unnecessary distress. Being able to recognise the up-and-coming mines allows your client to prepare for them. Explain that the emotional mines of cancer can be exhausting if they choose not to accept that the mines are there.

THAT OLD 'MIND-BODY' THING

Following a diagnosis of cancer it becomes more important than ever to be aware of the links between body and mind. There may be direct impacts upon clients' physical health brought about by their illness, or as a consequence of the treatment they are receiving. How they deal with these will directly impact upon their mental well-being. By accepting the fact that their body has changed, they will be in a better position to manage those changes, allowing them to take back some control of a situation in which they may feel powerless. Finding a language to describe how they are feeling physically to others is an important aspect of managing their condition. Other people may not be able to understand the impact that having cancer has upon someone and sharing how they feel can help those around them realise the importance of both the physical aspects of having cancer and the emotional impacts that occur as a consequence of them.

Several studies have demonstrated the positive acute effects of exercise on anxiety, depression and mood (Guszkowska 2004), and improvements in diet and physical activity have been shown to have a positive effect on our responses to mental stress (Georgiades *et al.* 2000). It's useful, therefore, to review your client's lifestyle and give advice on any changes that might be beneficial, consulting where appropriate with specialists involved with their care, such as dieticians or physiotherapists. Of course, it's important not to lose sight of the impact that the disease is having upon them, but many men with cancer are still able to participate in a surprisingly wide range of activities. By letting the client take control of their lifestyle you are empowering them at a time when their autonomy is being compromised by cancer.

GETTING AWAY FROM THE IDEA THAT THE CANCER DEFINES THE MAN

You may notice that clients become preoccupied with their cancer. Getting them to engage in activities that they've previously enjoyed can help to address this. Keeping busy helps with feeling 'normal' and serves as a distraction from becoming preoccupied with the illness (Gray *et al.* 2000). If they report being embarrassed about symptoms or side effects it might help to direct them to support groups where there are others who have similar problems as a consequence of their cancer.

Many men dealing with cancer will go through periods of being withdrawn and in a depressed mood. Increased irritability during post-surgical recovery is also common. These changes in mood and struggles to control their own emotions can affect how men see themselves (Gray *et al.* 2000). Another factor which can have a detrimental effect on men's sense of their own 'maleness' is sexual dysfunction resulting from prostate cancer treatment. A study of patients' perceptions of quality of life after treatment for early prostate cancer (Clark *et al.* 2003) found that sexual dysfunction was associated with poorer quality of life and a diminished quality of sexual intimacy, sexual confidence and sense of masculinity. Overall, cancer-related outlook – a perception of oneself as having coped well with cancer – was negatively associated with sexual dysfunction while improved outlook was correlated with greater masculine self-esteem.

Helping men stop to consider how they feel about their cancer is an important aspect of helping them come to terms with it. Getting your clients to learn to think and recognise the signs of how they are feeling and behaving at all times can be a helpful strategy. Help them identify the positive as well as the negative behaviours and thoughts that they might have in response to specific situations. We all have a preferred way of thinking – ask them to consider whether they're a 'glass half full or a glass half empty' kind of person. Are they naturally optimistic or are they naturally pessimistic? Being willing and open enough to consider this may help in overcoming the most difficult decisions and choices that they might have to face. It's important to have an understanding and realistic expectations of the condition – being overly optimistic is not sustainable and a self-imposed pressure to remain positive can create more problems than it solves (Yarbro *et al.* 2005).

It may seem a strange thing to say, but it is not uncommon for people to report being diagnosed with cancer as a wake up call, a point at which they reflected upon their current situation. This reflection can result in a readjustment of goals and a reprioritising of what is important. For some men cancer will become an integral part of their life; it will be with them for all of their life. For some men it will represent the point at which they had to review their life and were forced to make the difficult life choices that most men ignore or choose not to reflect on. Being able to find meaning in the experience of having cancer is important to many patients and their spouses and has been associated with improved psychological functioning (see Gray *et al.* 2000).

CANCER MAY NOT BE THE PROBLEM

When diagnosed with cancer it can be very easy for people to lose sight of who they were and how there life was before the diagnosis. They may feel that the cancer is the cause of all of their problems or that it is to blame for every subsequent problem that arises, which is often not the case. This is not to underestimate the impact that cancer has upon people's lives. However, 'bad stuff' continues to happen to people who do not have cancer and if their cancer is successfully treated, things will still happen in the future that have nothing to do with their cancer. Be watchful for clients who attribute all their misfortunes to having been diagnosed with or having had cancer.

LEARNING SOME NEW TRICKS

Being diagnosed with cancer can cause a total disruption of men's lives. The fact that they have cancer means that they have had to stop to reconsider where they are in the world, what their priorities are and what they want their goals to be. By way of the fact that they have or have had cancer their understanding and view of the world will have changed. It might be that their current coping mechanisms may be inadequate or insufficient to address the issues that they face with their cancer. Working with clients to explore alternative ways of thinking and responding can help them to adopt a more flexible approach to new situations. Having cancer may mean that your client are no longer able to do things that they have previously taken for granted. Encouraging them to consider alternative solutions or activities to replace those that have been lost can help to reduce the feeling of helplessness.

The more solutions they can find to the problems they encounter, the more likely they are to overcome them. Encourage your client not to dismiss ideas because they are new or challenging, but rather to try to be open and consider all ideas in a balanced way. De Bono (1999) advocates the use of what he calls the 'Six Thinking Hats' model, which is simple to understand and can provide valuable insights into a client's way of thinking. By becoming a lateral thinker – seeking to find and consider as many alternate solutions as possible, rather than resorting to the same old strategies – they will be more equipped to deal with the unexpected challenges presented to them.

DEPRESSION AND SUICIDE

Being diagnosed with cancer is naturally a frightening experience for anyone. Those who aren't able to talk about how they feel might become depressed and you should take time to assess for this. The presence of depression in association with cancer is well documented and the effective treatment of depression in cancer patients is known to result in better patient adjustment, reduced symptoms and reduced cost of care, and may also influence the course of the disease (Spiegel 1996).

If you believe that your client is becoming depressed, refer them to an appropriate person to assess it more fully if you are not trained to do so. This might be his GP or the consultant who is treating his cancer. Some patients will require treatment and this may take the form of anti-depressant medication, counselling or a combination of both. Regular exercise, if the client is able, can also have a role to play in lifting mood and promoting energy levels. While uncommon, it should always be borne in mind that some people when diagnosed with cancer will contemplate suicide. This may be a consequence of depression or fear of what the cancer might bring in terms of its physical impact. Men who do not have readily identifiable support networks should be watched carefully for signs of depression and suicide.

WORK

Being diagnosed with cancer can cause concern about how employers and workmates may react. Encourage your clients to carefully consider when is the most appropriate time to disclose their cancer to their employers and co-workers. The point at which they disclose their condition is a personal thing, however it might be useful to be conscious of the following:

➤ your client may wish to discuss their diagnosis with the organisation's occupational health nurse
➤ his performance at work may be affected and this may be misunderstood by his workmates

➤ if he have concerns about his job security, ask him to consider seeking guidance from his local cancer centre.

Work has a central role in helping men define who they are; it is natural that if this is threatened that they should feel a sense of concern.

CONCLUSION

Being diagnosed with cancer has a profound effect upon the mental health of men. While the evidence continues to grow of a correlation between cancer patients' mental health and the achievement of positive outcomes, men remain generally less adept than women at expressing their psychological needs, or less inclined to do so, and often have a tendency to neglect them. Meeting the psychological needs of men with cancer is therefore paramount. Taking time to stop and assess the mental well-being of the man with cancer you are working with, or caring for, should be an integral part of any treatment or care that is provided; to fail to do so may be tantamount to neglect.

Cancer is no longer the taboo subject that it used to be, although men may be a little late catching up. Perhaps the next battle to overcoming the fear and stigma associated with cancer will be to bring it out of the shadows and into the open. This will be a real challenge for many men, but as we learn to address and acknowledge the presence of cancer it loses its power to control our lives. The battle against cancer is as much a mental one as it is a physical one.

REFERENCES

Balderson N and Towell T (2003) The prevalence and predictors of psychological distress in men with prostate cancer who are seeking support. *Br J Health Psychology.* **8**(2):125–134.

Bisson JI, Chubb HL, Bennett S, Mason M, Jones D and Kynaston H (2002) The prevalence and predictors of psychological distress in patients with early localized prostate cancer. *BJU International.* **90**(1): 56–61.

Clark JA, Inui TS, Silliman RA, Bokhour BG, Krasnow SH, Robinson RA, Spaulding M and Talcott JA (2003) Patients' Perceptions of Quality of Life After Treatment for Early Prostate Cancer. *J Clinical Oncology.* **21**(20): 3777–3784.

Davison JB and Degner LF (1997) Empowerment of men newly diagnosed with prostate cancer. *Cancer Nursing.* **20**(3): 187–196.

De Bono E (1999) Six Thinking Hats. Ontario: Mica Management Resources Inc.

Georgiades A, Sherwood A, Gullette ECD, Babyak MA, Hinderliter A, Waugh R, Tweedy D, Craighead L, Bloomer R and Blumenthal JA (2000) Effects of exercise and weight loss on mental stress – induced cardiovascular responses in individuals with high blood pressure. Hypertension. 36: 171–176.

Gray RE, Fitch M, Phillips C, Labrecque M and Fergus K (2000) Managing the Impact of Illness: The Experiences of Men with Prostate Cancer and their Spouses. *J Health Psychol.* 5: 531–548.

Gustafsson O, Theorell T, Norming U, Perski A, Öhström M and Nyman CR (1995) Psychological reactions in men screened for prostate cancer. *Br J Urology.* **75**(5): 631–636.

Guszkowska M (2004) Effects of exercise on anxiety, depression and mood [in Polish] *Psychiatr Pol.* **38**: 611–620.

Kadan-Lottick NS, Vanderwerker LC, Block SD, Zhang B and Prigerson HG (2005) Psychiatric disorders and mental health service use in patients with advanced cancer. *Cancer.* **104**(12): 2872–81.

Keitel MA, Zevon MA, Rounds JB, Petrelli NJ and Karakousis C (1990) Spouse adjustment to cancer surgery: Distress and coping responses. *J Surgical Oncology.* **43**: 148–153.

Lloyd-Williams M (2000) Difficulties in diagnosing and treating depression in the terminally ill cancer patient. *Postgrad Med J.* **76**(899): 555–8.

Miovic M and Block S (2007) Psychiatric disorders in advanced cancer. *Cancer.* **110**(8): 1665–1676.

Pekar H and Brabner J (1994) *Our Cancer Year.* Philadelphia: Running Press.

Seedhouse D (2002) *Total Health Promotion: mental health, rational fields and the quest for autonomy.* Chichester: Wiley.

Spiegel D. (1996) Cancer and depression. *Br J Psychiatry Suppl.* **30**: 109-16.

Worden JW (1991) *Grief Counselling and Grief Therapy: a handbook for the mental health practitioner* (2nd ed.). London: Tavistock/Routledge.

Yarbro CH, Frogge MH, Goodeman M, Groedwald SL (2000) *Cancer Nursing: principles and practice* (5th ed.). Boston: Jones and Bartlett Publishers.

CHAPTER 23

Running a counselling service for men

Christian Scambor

INTRODUCTION

This chapter is based on the work of a men's counselling centre in Graz, the capital of the Austrian province of Styria (*see* Box 23.1). At the centre, we understand the term 'health' in the sense of the World Health Organization definition, as physical, mental and social well-being. This perspective is reflected in the aim of our practical work with our clients: to promote men's health by empowerment, identifying and strengthening resources and social integration.

BOX 23.1 A brief history of the centre

In 1996, Men's Counselling Centre Graz was founded in the province of Styria, Austria, as an independent non-profit organisation by initiator J Voitle, B Eilbauer and myself as a charitable association. The three of us had all worked with young people before and realised that there was a deficit, not only in specific psychosocial and health promoting services for male youngsters, but also in a comprehensive service centre for men. A small office was rented at our own expense and we started to work without any funding in the beginning but with much support from many professional workers from psychosocial and health services, among them many women's organisations. Years of struggling for financial resources to build up the centre followed.

The centre was the third of its kind in Austria and many more have emerged since, particularly in the German-speaking countries. In Austria, these centres have either been set up by big social organisations and institutions (such as the Catholic Church), or have developed as independent family counselling centres (like our centre). In both cases, the Family Counselling Centre Funding Act has been an important basis for this development. Originally concerned with family planning and psychosocial services for parents and their children, family counselling centres have diversified and specialised, and men's counselling centres have developed as a result. Most of the centres receive funding not only from the Federal Government for their core activity, namely counselling, but also from other administrative levels, such as city councils, province governments, or the European Union, for various activities and projects concerning health, social projects and youth work.

32 men and women now work for the Men's Counselling Centre Graz, most of them as part-time employees or freelances, sharing approximately 10 full-time-equivalents.

AIMS

The centre's core aim is to provide men and boys with gender-specific services (counselling along with educational work with boys and male youngsters), as well as to engage in networking, adult education and training, fostering the public discussion about gender and men's issues, and conduct research (in the areas of men's studies and gender studies). All in all, the centre combines psychosocial work within a network of regional services, research activities and dissemination (via networking, training, education and participating in public discussion). On the one hand, this approach came from the perspective of focussing on problems (problems that men have or that follow from their behaviour). In this sense, we followed a critical perspective on masculinities and patriarchy in our society. On the other hand, a positive perspective and vision has been developed that can be described as health promotion for men in a broad sense.

Hegemonic constructs of gender are not the only options available to us. One's own socialisation as a man (as well as a woman) can be reflected upon and those restrictions and influences that are detrimental to well-being and lead to behaviour that is self-destructive or harmful to others can be overcome. To broaden the possibilities for the lives of men, beyond narrow and restricting masculine norms, is the overarching aim of our work. All activities of our organisation are part of this approach, e.g. tackling severe problems, such as violence; supporting constructive solutions out of specific problem situations by counselling and group work; or providing positive, pro-social drivers for the development of boys and male youngsters.

WHY DO MEN ACCESS THE SERVICE?

Men seek support to solve the problems that they have. That's why they access a men's counselling service. It's as simple as that – yet there are certain prerequisites that should be considered.

Before most of the men's counselling centres in Austria were founded, family counselling centres found that they were frequented by women and their children, but not by men. This led many political actors to be sceptical about whether male specific services would work. There were general family counselling centres, open for anyone, so why didn't men go there and why should they go to a special service? On the other hand, there were a few pioneer services, like Men's Counselling Centre in Vienna, founded already in the 80s and showing that such centres were frequented by men.

The point is that men have to be addressed in an explicit way. In a society where child-rearing work (including unpaid work in the home, all kinds of caring tasks, being responsible for relationships and emotions) is assigned to the female sphere, with men being responsible for production (paid labour, being the breadwinner and hard, outgoing type), a 'family counselling centre' simply doesn't appeal to men. Of course, social reality is beyond such stereotypes, but in the minds and identities of people, they prevail. Consequently, as far as advertising and promoting services is concerned, a pragmatic approach is needed that takes the inertia of gender stereotypes into account to a certain degree. If it is presented to men in the right way, the service is accepted.

As is the case for many counselling centres, it is easier to reach certain segments of the population than others. For men with a migration background and language difficulties, for example, our centre is not a low threshold service. Here, we try to co-operate with outreach projects that can promote the centre in various communities and refer men to our organisation. At the moment, we are experimenting with a low-threshold contact point in a café (a project called 'Men's Café') to reach men that we haven't reached before. In order to make access to the service as easy as possible, telephone and email counselling should be offered, aside from the more usual personal contacts within a face-to-face-setting.

WHAT ARE THE MEN'S PROBLEMS?

Over the years, the most frequent problem area affecting clients has been relationship break-up, divorce and child custody. Often, questions regarding the legal situation in case of splitting up are the focus of the initial contact, followed later by the more personal, emotional and crisis-prone aspects of a separation situation. In such a case, the centre's lawyers refer the men internally to psychosocial counselling, after having gone through the legal questions. Other relationship and family issues are also a frequent topic, such as insecurities when patchwork families are formed that include one's own and the new partner's children.

The second biggest problem area is mental health problems, including depressive symptoms, crises and over-demanding situations in work and private life, burn-out and social isolation, as well as anxiety disorders or other clinical symptoms. Alcohol and drug addiction fall into this category as well.

In 2007, 681 men and 65 women contacted the Men's Counselling Centre for support. (Each year, between 5% and 10% of our clients are women who contact the centre as relatives or friends of boys, male youngsters or men.) Taking only the men into account, there were 2168 contacts (*see* Box 23.2).

BOX 23.2 Breakdown of male client contacts in 2007

Counselling	
End of relationship, divorce, child custody	26%
Mental health problems and addiction	19%

Questions and problems concerning relationship, family	10%
Health, medical questions, sexuality	5%
Work, economic situation	2%
Victims of sexual abuse and physical violence	1%
Other problems	5%
Work with perpetrators of violence	
Sexual violence	17%
Physical violence	15%

Many of the men with violent behaviour that our organisation works with are not self-referred clients, but agency-referred clients, which means that the contact with our centre is initiated by, for example, the court, the Youth Welfare Authority and similar institutions. They are included in the statistics, but their access to the Centre is in many cases not comparable to the men who seek counselling.

Despite the prevalence of some typical patterns of problems, it is important to remain open to all kinds of problems and be prepared to address less common issues and specific questions, e.g. concerning intersexuality or transsexual men. Not every problem can be dealt with at a counselling centre, not every question answered. But it is important to serve as a contact point for all who ask for support, to listen carefully and to have a good network so that people can be referred to competent relevant services.

HOW TO WORK WITH THE MEN

Thanks to its multidisciplinary team, a wide range of issues and problems can be addressed at the Centre. In many cases, clients are referred to other specialised services (e.g. in the case of alcohol or drug addiction) or professionals (e.g. for physical examinations). The men's problems are often a complex mixture of physical, mental and social aspects that should be addressed in a comprehensive way (*see* example in Box 23.3).

The counselling service at the Centre is free of charge up to the eighth face-to-face counselling session. Experience has shown that many basic counselling processes can be finished within this time (82% of the counselling processes in 2007 could be finished within five sessions and only 8% lasted longer than 10 sessions). Either a satisfying solution is found for the time being that enables the man to take the next steps to tackle his problem, or it has become clear that a referral to a longer-term intervention is necessary. It is not in the interest of our organisation to keep clients as long as possible, but to empower them and to activate their own resources. Restricted funding has enforced this approach, as there are always more men knocking on the door and asking for counselling. However, if someone needs a longer process, this can be provided. Together with the man, the counsellor will look for ways that a long-term intervention can be realised (e.g. there is the possibility to get financial support for psychotherapy by the social insurance). Of course, strict confidentiality is provided and the men don't have to disclose their name or other data.

In addition to face-to-face counselling, group work has been provided for a variety of topics (e.g. becoming a father; social isolation; sexual orientation). At our branch centre in upper Styria, a project has been initiated that deals with prostate cancer. Information and events are organised in cooperation with the local hospital, along with having a self-help group for affected men at the centre.

BOX 23.3 A typical scenario

1	The phone rings, the counsellor picks up. A man introduces himself and says that he has picked up a leaflet about the Men's Counselling Centre at a doctor's suggestion. He has read that he can contact our centre for legal questions regarding divorce and is interested in an appointment with the centre's lawyer.
2	The counsellor asks some questions to get a better impression of what is needed, e.g. why the man had seen the physician. The man says that he has problems with falling asleep and generally feels weak and cannot go to work. The counsellor and the client agree on two appointments at the centre, one with the lawyer and one with a psychologist. The man is informed about the Centre's policies (anonymous and confidential counselling, free of charge up to seven hours).
3	The man and the lawyer discuss the legal questions concerning a possible divorce. It turns out that the man's relationship is in a deep crisis, but it's not clear if there will be a divorce. Rather, the man says that his wife is discontented with the relationship and has mentioned divorce during a quarrel.
4	The counselling sessions with the psychologist during the following weeks reveal depressive symptoms and a burn-out that underlie the man's physical and relationship problems. He is an engineer by profession, working on construction sites abroad under extreme time pressure, with more responsibility than he can handle and little time to spend with his family. After long years of this kind of life, he feels that he is finally 'breaking apart'. When he is at home for the weekends, he can't relax properly, feels nervous and irritable. The couple quarrels a lot.
5	The anamnesis and a psychiatric examination come to the conclusion that psycho-pharmacological treatment is not necessary at the moment, but should be taken into consideration if the man's state deteriorates. In resource-oriented counselling sessions, the psychologist and the man develop alternatives concerning the man's job. A longer process seems indicated and the man is referred to a psychotherapist. The psychologist gives the man information about partner counselling at another organisation to pass on to his wife.

Work with male perpetrators of physical or sexual violence is a special focus of our organisation. Although it's true that the issue of violence can crop up in any work that involves counselling for men, the coordinated psychosocial and forensic work with male perpetrators is a very specialist service. The Men's Counselling Centre provides programmes and psychotherapy for so-called agency-referred men with violent behaviour, in cooperation with various organisations and institutions (e.g. courts, Youth Welfare Office and victim protection organisations). The interest on violence from a public health perspective is quite new in Austria; in 2007, the topic prevention of violence was integrated into the health goals of the province of Styria for the first time.

Men expect male counsellors in a men's counselling centre, on the phone, email and face-to-face – at least for the first contacts. Later on, some men prefer to work with female counsellors; thus, having a good network for referrals is recommended. Also, for work with perpetrators it is important to have women in the team, if this kind of work is provided.

WHAT CAN BE OFFERED TO BOYS AND MALE YOUNGSTERS?

The Men's Counselling Centre offers gender-reflective work with boys and male youngsters from eight to eighteen years. Educators run workshops in schools and youth centres, often in parallel to a women's organisation that works with the girls at the same time. Boys and girls work in homogenous groups for a while (e.g. concerning sexuality) and then come together for discussion in plenary sessions (e.g. on what language or behaviour is regarded as insulting by each group or sub-group).

We have been offering this kind of work with youngsters since 1996. In the beginning, prevention of violence was the focus of the workshops. Today, it's about pro-social relationships among and within the genders and gender sub-groups (like migration background), more flexible gender roles, work-life balance and personal growth. To enable youngsters to find their pathway towards a healthy life, understood as physical, mental and social well-being, is the common purpose of all our work with boys and male youngsters.

The workshops cover the following topics:

➤ love and sexuality
➤ prevention of physical and sexual violence
➤ male identity, gender roles, gender relations
➤ ideas about later work, relationships, work-life-balance
➤ risk behaviour and health.

HOW TO MARKET THE SERVICE

Clear information stating that men are the target group of a service is necessary, as well as promoting specific aspects, such as the provision of male counsellors (a feature that is expected from a male-specific service by many men). Having the terms 'men', 'male' or similar in the name of the service, centre or project helps to make it clear to men that it is for them and likely to be 'male-friendly'.

Disseminating general information through the standard methods (leaflets, press releases, public events) is a necessary part of advertising the service, but the most important strategy is to build up links to other services, organisations and professionals in the region. Most referrals at our centre come from other services, such as family counselling centres, other health and social organisations, lawyers, physicians and so on. Placing the service in a network of other services ensures that men are referred to your service on the one hand and, on the other hand, enables you to refer men on to services and professionals that are specialised in certain fields (e.g. addiction).

PUBLIC RELATIONS

Actively maintaining good public relations is crucial for reaching potential service users. However, PR can be a quite complex task, as it's about communicating a message and an image not only to men as beneficiaries of the service but also to the whole professional field of services and organisations, as well as to political actors. Having a few clear messages, a coherent position and maintaining the focus of marketing the service are key. It's really a job for journalists and professional PR staff.

With 50 to 70 contributions in local and national media per year (newspapers, radio, TV), our organisation tries to play an active role in the public discourse about men, masculinities and gender relations. Violence is a very striking topic in public discourse and the media, so organisations that work with perpetrators of violence tend to be noticed. Although good for profile-raising, this can mean that the whole service becomes associated with 'violence' and 'work with perpetrators'. This makes the counselling and other areas of work less visible and less attractive for potential beneficiaries who don't have a violence problem. Good PR work is needed to ensure that the balance of attention doesn't shift too much to one area of work.

WHAT INFRASTRUCTURE IS NEEDED?

In general, running a counselling centre for men demands the usual infrastructure:
➤ an office and counselling rooms of a certain standard
➤ telephones
➤ computers
➤ filing cabinets that can be locked to store personal data
➤ leaflets, etc.

The costs will be in the range for any comparable service, although there have been some creative attempts to provide services with less infrastructure, thus lowering costs and lessening the dependency on funding agencies.

Case study

In the Austrian province of Vorarlberg, a group of ambitious professionals installed an email-counselling project that worked completely without a base for a long time. The counsellors would provide the counselling service from their home offices, with a schedule of who would be working at any particular time. In this way, they could run the service without an expensive infrastructure of offices and counselling rooms.

QUALITY ASSURANCE AND EVALUATION

A counselling centre is quite a demanding organisation in terms of quality assurance. This is a field where there is not much space to save costs by reducing activity. With any work with people, organisations should strive for high quality and not make compromises. At the Men's Counselling Centre, the quality of the services is assured in various ways that can be regarded as standard, such as defining certain professions and experience for job descriptions, having further education, peer consulting and supervision by external experts. Joining networks of similar services on a regional, national and international level is beneficial in terms of quality assurance. Such networks enable an organisation to learn from others' experiences and new developments can be integrated quickly.

As far as evaluation is concerned, there should be as many activities as possible, to improve the work and to demonstrate that the service's work is meaningful and effective. To a certain extent, public funding agencies demand evaluation and partly base their decisions upon it; however in reality the more important target groups concerning evaluation seem to be the general public, the professional network and the service's staff. First, a service will generally be safer from cut-backs if the general public considers the service to be important. Second, clients will be referred to the service and the service will be supported if the professional network is convinced that it is doing important and effective work. Third, the staff of the service need feedback to improve their work and will be motivated and feel valued by positive evaluation results. As a minimum standard, good documentation systems should be introduced and data should be stored over a long time, so that retrospective analyses can be performed at any time.

DEVELOPING A CONCEPT

A service that deals with men's mental health should consider gender relations as its context, refer to 'gender mainstreaming' and develop a comprehensive concept and mission statement that is based on generally accepted long-term objectives, including:

➤ the WHO definition of health
➤ health equality
➤ gender equality
➤ constructive and tolerant relationships among and within the genders
➤ integration
➤ human rights.

The service's culture, as well as its PR, will benefit from this in the long run. Of course, creating a mission statement based on these core principles doesn't mean that you can't also emphasise more pragmatic arguments to explain the benefits of your service, e.g. reduced expenses for the health system as a result of prevention work and health promotion for men.

Building a service concept should be seen as an ongoing process rather than a one-off exercise. It's important to keep an eye on political papers and strategies for new developments, e.g. is gender health included as a goal on a regional or national level? Within a network of services and organisations, the integration of relevant concepts into political processes can be fostered. Relevant aspects that are on the political agenda should be discussed and integrated into the service's concept, if appropriate.

Over the years, the Men's Counselling Centre has developed a comprehensive approach towards men and masculinities in our society, on the basis of a critical perspective on hegemonic gender roles and patriarchy. To promote alternative – equal – gender relations, we do not only offer services for men, but are also active in terms of 'gender mainstreaming'. In cooperation with the Women's Service, Graz, we run a work group where women and men work together continuously on improving methods, reflecting and evaluating experiences from gender training as well as keeping up with related research and new developments. Training, counselling and projects are delivered in various organisations and offered to the interested public. We also run a research department, where men's studies, gender studies and evaluation projects are undertaken in order to inform our practical work, to further develop the service and to exchange knowledge and good practice on an international level. All of these activities have been realised because having a rather open, comprehensive concept has allowed us to broaden the range of activities over time.

Be aware that it's common for there to be a real lack of comprehensive male specific services in a region and, consequently, when a service does come along it can be swamped with referrals and requests for help from other professionals. Often it turns out to be impossible to meet all of these requests, which leads to disappointment and dissatisfaction with the service. Keeping other professionals well-informed about what you can offer and what is feasible is recommended to help to minimise this problem.

HOW EASY IS IT TO REPLICATE THE PROJECT?

In general, specific services for men should be provided area-wide. In terms of mental health, the demand is there and must be addressed in some way everywhere. When counselling centres are set up that deal with men's mental health, there are some experiences that can probably be transferred from one context to another and others that are more specific where a 'copy and paste' approach across countries and contexts wouldn't be straightforward.

Some issues that should apply in any country include the following.

➤ The team should be multidisciplinary, consisting of various social and health professions (social worker, physician, nurse, psychologist, educational scientist, lawyer, etc). Often, men ask for legal advice first (e.g. concerning a divorce) and the centre's lawyers can refer the man to a psychosocial professional later on.

➤ Men appreciate services which explicitly state that they are 'for men'. A clear information policy is recommended, which includes having 'men' in the name of the centre or project. Many men expect male counsellors, so these should be provided.

➤ Networking with other services and professionals is important. Men are referred from other services to a men's counselling centre and often specialised services are needed to refer men on to. Many problems can be better addressed if organisations co-operate.

➤ Public relations should be taken seriously from the beginning, not only to inform men of the services on offer, but also to keep ongoing contact with the general public, professional networks and political actors to actively maintain a clear, consistent image and message.

Some other aspects of the service will be more country-specific and it might be difficult to transfer them from one country to another. Among these features, the possibilities for funding social and health-related projects are of high importance (*see* Box 23.4). There will also be specific cultural issues, e.g. gender experts from post-communist countries sometimes describe difficulties towards gender-specific services in their countries in general, as a hangover from the communist ideology that gender equality had already been accomplished, on top of male dominance and a male worker ideal. This perspective still functions as a cultural pattern to a certain degree and sometimes leads to a lack of understanding of gender-specific services. On the other hand, similar attitudes can be expected everywhere to some extent, depending, for example, on the respective ideological position of some political actor or on the values and norms in a particular community. Once you start promoting men's mental health or a similar project, resistance of some kind can be expected – it comes with the territory!

BOX 23.4 Finding funding in different countries

According to comparative welfare state analysis done in the late 1980s, Austria and Germany belong to the so-called 'conservative welfare regimes', which are characterised by somewhat more comprehensive social and health policies than 'liberal welfare regimes' (e.g. the UK and US), in which the market is considered to guarantee social security, the state has a rather reactive role, private insurance systems are of high importance and transfer payments are seen as residual. However, in the conservative welfare regimes, social transfer payments are strongly connected to the labour market status of citizens, with a minor impact on re-distribution of resources among people. A third welfare regime has been called the 'social-democratic regime', mostly to be found in Scandinavian countries, with a high quality of health and social systems in general and a philosophy of equality of the highest standards for all citizens.

To what extent these classifications are valid today can be questioned, since they were developed 20 years ago and things have changed in all countries. However, the different welfare regimes can be regarded as historical background patterns which still have a certain influence. As far as Austria is concerned, it can be stated that providing funding for counselling or other services related to health and social issues is still regarded basically as a public duty; services that are mainly funded by donations or private sponsoring are not yet very common. Fostering fundraising for social and health projects from private sources by taxation regulations is a rather new political strategy.

Consequently, when any social or health services in Austria are started, the activities to find resources will still be concentrated on political actors and responsible departments and ministries, rather than on fundraising from private sources. In this respect, there might still be differences between countries. Thus, strategies to find financial resources for the service must take the specific welfare background of a country into account.

CHAPTER 24

Using helplines and the internet

Stephen Anderson

INTRODUCTION

Men's reluctance to access health services in the flesh, particularly with non-physical symptoms, is a familiar theme in the field of men's health. Remote access to health services should ideally be available to everyone, but it's especially important for men with mental health issues. This chapter shows how this can be achieved, using the example of the Breathing Space national telephone and web service in Scotland (www.breathingspacescotland.co.uk).

Undeniably something is 'wrong' for many men. Very simply, Breathing Space tries to help men to address their sorrows by giving them a safe 'space' to talk. It should be noted here that the service does not seek to address the issue of suicide in Scotland; the Choose Life national strategy* gives very strong and positive leadership in that regard. However, Breathing Space aims to address many of the issues that such a depressing suicide statistic indicates in terms of the lived experience of Scottish people's mental health and well-being.

Breathing Space is not alone in this pursuit but compliments the work of other phonelines and agencies which are endeavouring to reduce the suicide rates in Scotland. No telephone service could or should be tackling such deep-rooted health and social issues single-handedly. The service was launched along with other agencies as part of the National Programme for Improving Mental Health and Well-being in Scotland and is funded by the Scottish Government Health Department. As part of this national agenda Breathing Space shares a set of key aims with these other agencies trying to positively influence public mental health in Scotland:

➢ raising awareness and promoting mental health and well-being
➢ eliminating stigma and discrimination in relation to mental ill-health

---

* www.chooselife.net

➤ preventing suicide and supporting people bereaved by suicide
➤ promoting and supporting recovery.

The National Programme works alongside other Scottish Government departments and policies, including those on health improvement, social justice and social inclusion, education and young people, arts and culture, enterprise and life-long learning.

WHAT IS BREATHING SPACE?

Breathing Space is an 'out of hours' service, providing place for people to get help with their problems in the evening and at night time when mainstream services have closed their doors. It provides a free, confidential phone and web-based service available to anyone in Scotland, specifically (but not exclusively) targeting young men who are experiencing difficulties and unhappiness in their lives. Breathing Space was initially launched as a pilot service in Greater Glasgow and western Scotland in 2002 before expanding to become a national service across Scotland in 2004. The service is free, confidential and is backed up by a website which seeks to reinforce the telephone service but also separately deliver for people who cannot currently access support via telephone. We focus on the provision of skilled assistance to help people in difficulty and make a conscious attempt to help people deal with problems at an early stage to prevent problems escalating.

We work with those living with mental health problems and those experiencing emotional distress, including family members, partners and friends who are concerned about their own well-being or that of people they care about. The central belief that underpins the service is that in some way 'talking about it' helps. In this sense, Breathing Space tries to make it easier for people to open up and talk through things, providing a free and anonymous alternative to what people perceive as mainstream services. In essence the service provides a safe space for people to just stop, think and reflect on the distressing 'stuff' in their lives. We seek to do this by providing empathy, understanding and advice, and we always work to try to instil hope even when none exists.

When Breathing Space began, around 400 men a month were calling the service; this has now grown to over 2000.

Breathing Space mission statement

Breathing Space is a free, confidential phone and web-based service for people in Scotland. We are here in times of difficulty to provide a safe and supportive space by listening, offering advice and information. It is our belief and hope that by empowering people they will have the resources to recover.

WHY IS BREATHING SPACE NECESSARY?

Suicide is a leading cause of mortality in those under the age of 35 in Scotland, where the suicide rate is higher than in other parts of the UK. In 2007 there where 838 suicides and undetermined deaths in Scotland and around 75% of those were men. Over the last 20 years, the mortality rate from suicide among Scottish males has risen steadily. This rise in deaths from suicide is particularly significant because figures in England and Wales remained relatively stable over the same period, leading to a widening gap within the UK whereby Scottish males are fairing worse than those in England and Wales. For these reasons, Breathing Space primarily targets young, Scottish men.

HOW DO WE DO IT?

There are two strands to delivering the service. First the delivery of the service as a frontline service available to the public, but second and crucially Breathing Space has a role in raising public awareness of the positive mental health messages carried by Breathing Space and promoting the service and other organisations to all men – not just those who have a need for the service now. There is a core message for men – a call to action – that we promote in all of our communications, to 'open up when you are feeling down'.

The Breathing Space frontline team has 35 phoneline advisors who work on the phone lines Monday to Thursday from 6 pm till 2 am and 24 hours a day at the weekends, from 6 pm on Friday night through to 6 am on Monday morning. The team consists of people who have broad experience of providing frontline mental health services. We have psychiatric nurses and clinical psychologists, but also non-clinically trained staff from person-centred therapy, cognitive therapy, drugs and alcohol work, social work, prison services and support work backgrounds. So the team is not simply a clinical team providing a clinical service; what the team have in common and have demonstrated as part of being recruited is experience of and ability for working with people when they at their very lowest or most distressed. Breathing Space advisors have the experience and ability to offer confident, non-judgemental support to every caller, being able to listen and help people reflect on their issues, even when those issues seem overwhelming and insufferable.

The Breathing Space team has roughly a 50/50 gender balance between women and men. Men are a crucial part of delivering the service, whereas nursing or counselling services tend to be predominantly female and perhaps experienced as 'women's places' by many men. So men's voices are a very big part of our service delivery: comforting, accepting, empathic men's voices encouraging men to engage with their problems through talking about them.

Breathing Space makes a very conscious effort to make the service that we provide welcoming and accepting of men and their differences from women, who are often better versed in talking about problems. The staff work hard to help men find the space to 'open up when they are feeling down'. Often this can be as simple as just being accepting of the men who phone, giving them empathy and being supportive – not rejecting them or judging, perhaps in the way their mates might if they were to disclose that they had been crying or thinking about suicide. Sometimes providing the service can be very difficult as men struggle with anger, distressing events and overwhelming thoughts and feelings. Whatever is happening and whoever phones, we will try to meet them as they are and provide a safe 'space' in which to talk. Perhaps differing from other similar services, and something men seem to like, is that Breathing Space advisors can and will give advice and signposting information to other services. We utilise a database to provide men with details of over 400 agencies across Scotland and this is also available through our website. Many men seem to like this, as they sometimes struggle with conversation as a solution in itself; they engage with conversation in an instrumental way and look to take something definite from it. Ending a call with signposting towards a service can be a way for men to feel that they are progressing with a problem.

Although Breathing Space is a helpline service – free, anonymous and confidential like many others – and although the service we provide may be very similar to other services in some respects, it has been developed specifically with men in mind. The service we provide is shaped to meet people's needs in general, but men's needs in particular, so the voice on the answering machine reading the same message that other services might have is a man's voice. The staff have all gained experience in work with men's mental health.

HOW DOES BREATHING SPACE TARGET MEN?

Since Breathing Space first began as a pilot, the service has engaged with a variety of media in what could broadly be called a social marketing strategy to try to reach a hardly reached audience of young men who are at risk due to their poor mental health and lack of resources. During the early stages of developing the service, marketing campaigns in 'men's places' were used as a way to try to speak to them – male public toilets, football stadia, pubs and clubs all saw Breathing Space materials in the form of posters, leaflets and beer mats. The images and messages used were particularly focused on men – only men were depicted and the images tended to focus on more male subjects, like playing console games with mates, football, etc.

Radio advertising was also a major driver for trying to increase public awareness. The advertising used males voices to discuss feelings, e.g. one of the adverts featured two men in a telephone conversation with one telling the other repeatedly that he felt 'fine' when it was obvious from his voice that he felt far from fine. Slots near male programming were utilised as much as possible and ads tailored to local areas. This regional focus and the intimate nature of radio compared to television worked well in driving calls to the service, which typically got very busy when radio adverts were on. In 2006 Breathing Space began a very limited TV advertising campaign in order to reach a wider audience of men and move from radio adverts intended as an immediate call to action more towards raising general awareness of Breathing Space among the Scottish public. These new TV adverts were voiced by the actor John Hannah – a

Scottish man speaking to Scottish men. We targeted programmes men might tend to watch after 10 pm in the evening, hoping to engage with men when they lacked other sources of support and perhaps when they were isolated and struggling to cope. We also used press advertising on lonely hearts pages or debt sections of newspapers to try to reach men who might be at 'trigger point'.

We sought to generate free publicity by issuing press releases. This seemed like a futile and thankless task at first, with little initial uptake. However, after almost three years of work it is increasingly the case that the media, including national media, come to Breathing Space for comments on mental and emotional issues. Plugging away with stories that were relevant to a national media audience as the profile of men's mental health issues has grown over time has helped us to raise public awareness of the service and promoted positive mental health messages in the long term.

WEBSITE

The Breathing Space website began life as one or two very flat and lifeless web pages which simply acted as a business card on the web and pointed all who found it back to the phone service for support. In 2005, we felt that if we were to offer a proper web service we needed to revisit the website and match its approach to the telephone service. We hoped to provide a sense of 'breathing space' on the web in the same way as we provided a safe space via the telephone.

In developing the Breathing Space website we decided on some central tasks which we wanted it to achieve, with a view to being able to replicate in some way what the phone service offers:

➤ normalise the situation with information that allows the reader to feel 'heard'
➤ offer and advise on self-help
➤ offer signposting to other sources of help
➤ instil hope and a sense of beginning a recovery journey
➤ advertise the telephone service for those ready to speak about their issue.

Achieving these tasks through the web meant that we had to identify key issues for people who were likely to be using the web and being able to talk to them in a way which elicited a 'That's how I feel!' response. We examined the reasons men called the Breathing Space telephone service and used these as a basis for the categories on the website. From there we worked with a web design company to try to capture how the website should look, which was crucial in creating a site where men would feel secure and welcome enough to seek support and advice. We began creating the look and feel of the site with a tortuous discussion over how the home page should look. After much debate we settled on an image of a man in the countryside, which captured the notion of a 'breathing space' – a place to stop and contemplate – while suggesting an onward journey; all in a Scottish context. The rest of the site was then developed to continue this theme and feel, with images of men on each page, in line with our print advertising and literature.

A crucial addition to the site made in late 2008 was the support groups directory which allows anyone to search for local places to find support. These services tend to be the non-statutory services that can compliment people's recovery journey; services such as Depression Alliance; Hearing Voices Network; Citizen's Advice; local counselling; men's health groups and so on. Also in 2008 we began to use Google to advertise Breathing Space as a sponsored link when relevant keywords were searched for by people in Scotland. Thus when someone searches for 'depression' or 'low mood' one of the first results they will see is a link to Breathing Space. Although this can be costly, with web traffic rising to over three times the use of the phone service we have consistently found it to be a productive way to advertise.

THE FUTURE

At the time of writing, Breathing Space is in the process of launching a web service for deaf people which uses webcam technology to allow clients to use British Sign Language. There are 5000 people registered as deaf in Scotland, with 75 000 registered as having hearing difficulties. Working with the Scottish Council on Deafness and Deaf Connections, Breathing Space will provide the same service to a community which can often be isolated and have higher mental health risks than others.

Breathing Space will also play a full part in the new Scottish Government mental and emotional health policy framework – Towards a Mentally Flourishing Scotland. As our growth as a frontline service continues, we hope that Breathing Space can increasingly be part of people's recovery journey and help them to maintain good mental health during times of difficulty.

CONCLUSION

Breathing Space has signed up to some fundamental tasks as part of its remit from the Scottish Government:
➤ raising awareness and promoting mental health and well-being
➤ eliminating stigma and discrimination around mental ill-health
➤ preventing suicide and supporting people bereaved by suicide
➤ promoting and supporting recovery from mental health problems.

In very real terms, Breathing Space tries to take these policy goals and strategic objectives to a place where we do something very simple and fundamentally human: we listen as people talk and we try to support people when they are down and struggling. That we do these things using modern technology in various forms does not change the nature of what we do and does not change the underlying truth that men benefit from being able to find a place and space to talk about the emotions and feelings they have, especially when life gets tough.

CHAPTER 25

Promoting men's mental health services: building from the ground up

Jane Powell

INTRODUCTION

The Campaign Against Living Miserably, CALM, was set up in response to the high suicide rate among men aged 15–35. In England and Wales, suicide has again over-taken road death as the main cause of death in this group.* Getting men into any kind of medical service on their own behalf is tough. Getting them to admit to 'mental health' problems is even harder. Most men who've killed themselves aren't access-ing any service at the time of their death. This is no surprise to most mental health agencies – statutory or otherwise.

Just reaching men is very often seen as an almost impossible target, yet this is something that CALM has regularly achieved with ease since 1997. As both a Department of Health pilot (1997–2006) and as a charity (March 2006 onwards) the helpline that CALM has run has achieved a consistent reach to this audience. As a Department of Health pilot CALM managed to attract a steady 68% of all its calls from men, 60% of whom were aged under 35. As a charity this figure is regularly pushed to 72% and within our 'CALMzones' – areas of the UK where we work in part-nership with NHS Primary Care Trusts – we see figures of up to 100% male callers.

From the start, the ethos behind CALM has been very clear. CALM was set up in response to research undertaken by the Department of Health into why young men weren't accessing helplines for those with depression/mental health problems. The research showed that young men didn't identify with the help that was there; indeed they were turned off by it. The challenge then was to develop a brand that men aged 15–35 would relate to.

---

* Provisional figures for 2008 show suicide for the 15–34 age group at 972 for England and Wales; with road traffic accidents at 876. (Source: ONS.)

WHO'S TALKING?

The brief was to make the helpline look like anything but what it was – a mental health helpline for men. Two young men at the advertising agency Ogilvy came up with the name and the look. The next step was to get music or sports people behind the brand and launch it anywhere but all the usual places (e.g. GP surgeries, drop-in centres, police stations) and get the brand seen where young men would go, such as pubs, clubs and pizza places.

The ads compared the suicide rate in young men with the death rate for all those other things held up as the main threats to society – heroin, AIDS, ecstasy. The visuals were fresh and hard-hitting. With the exception of the drippy 'don't suffer in silence' byline at the bottom, you could see immediately why young men would identify with the ads. They challenged the public to get their priorities (and assumptions about men) straight.

My background is campaigning – not in the world of advertising, but politics with a small 'p'. I've organised meetings, lobbies, leafleted, demonstrated and pretty much tried every avenue there is in order to persuade people to change their minds and actively participate and lobby for change. I'm good at it, but I expect a tough audience. Launching CALM in Manchester I was bowled over by young men's response and I knew just what an incredibly rare and precious thing that was.

The marketing hit the perfect note. With these posters in hand I could traipse around Manchester asking for help to launch the campaign. The response from young guys in the clubs and bars, from the radio stations, the guys sticking out posters on the streets, was instant and inspiring; they wanted to be involved and offered suggestions and ideas and contacts. It helped that music mogul and night-club founder Tony Wilson and his staff backed the campaign and offered to help with the launch. The launch of CALM in Manchester 1997 was a truly combined local effort – people came forward with venues for the party and the press conference, helped out with the promotion, invites for the press conference, DJs for the party and airtime for the ads.

The key was that the audience didn't just put up with the advertising, they identified with it. It was for and about young men, about themselves and their lives, and they were part of delivering the message. From then onwards, we have tried to reach out and involve people in delivering the campaign – mixing the world of health and music. And very often it has been the energy and the support from this 'outside world' that has been critical in keeping CALM going. Guys out there want the line, like the campaign and if you have a minute they'll want to discuss how best they can take the campaign forward. Too often materials are put out there clearly as a message from and on behalf of health professionals. This disempowers the most effective communicators we can have – the audience.

WHERE DO YOU WANT TO BE?

An easy marketing mistake is to fixate on what a problem can look like. 'Bloated? (show a picture of a woman with a ballooning stomach) Then take XXX.' So, put a

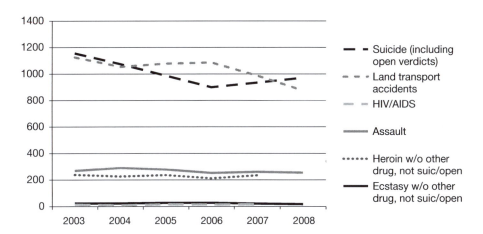

FIGURE 25.1 Number of deaths by cause in men aged 15–34, 2003–2008 (calendar year)

picture of a man holding his head in his hands with a helpline number underneath and, voila, we have a mental health campaign. One of CALM's lowest ebbs came when we had some very beautiful-looking ads with stick figures of men stuck in a box. This may be how it feels to be depressed – but it's sad. Why would someone want to identify with that? Calls to the line reflected the audience's response.

Even if you're down, that isn't how you want to feel. Advertising is about reaching out and finding out where people would like to be, rather than where they are at that moment. Being portrayed as a nameless victim is frankly unappealing. The alternative, however, isn't simply putting a picture up showing a happy-clappy man instead – no one likes to be patronised.

Breast cancer is unapologetically upbeat, it isn't an embarrassed campaign lurking in the corners – it isn't afraid to refer to breasts. There's no reason that a campaign on suicide can't be the same. If you want to attract an audience, then be successful, be upbeat and put it out that this is the campaign to be engaged in.

REMEMBER THE AUDIENCE

Suicide is a strange one. Most people are unaware that their son, brother, husband, father are more likely to kill themselves than be killed. It isn't that 'teenage' suicide is the problem; it's male suicide that is the big issue. This isn't news to any health journalist, though; their response is to ask what's new and ask for a 'case study', someone willing to talk about their depression and suicidal feelings, then slap the story on the health page and put your numbers and website underneath. This is a total turnoff for our audience, even if it does go down a treat with the girlfriends, mums and wives – and, of course, the health industry. If you're lucky, the article may spend a line on the fact that three young men a day kill themselves and perhaps add a vacuous generalisation. Other than that, the journalistic endeavour is concerned with milking the issue dry for every possible emotional nuance and filling in any

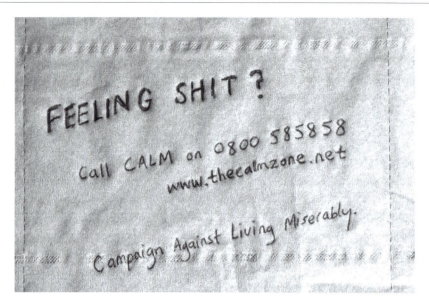

FIGURE 25.2 'Feeling shit?' CALM postcard

gaps with as many pictures and dramatic visuals that can be managed. If the story is on TV or radio, then a weeping relative is *de rigueur*.

If young men are going to identify with us and join the campaign, then exploiting our audience isn't the way to go. We need to show them that we're on their side; we need to pick another angle. We need to be funny, clever, make them think and give them a message in a way which isn't patronising – give them an image of us, of our campaign, which they'll feel comfortable with.

THE ENVIRONMENT

We've tried to make our own news and find our own way of raising the issue by creating ads and events which command respect from our audience – whether by making them laugh, making them think, or using the voices or images of men whom they will listen to. Always keeping sight of our wider agenda of using music, entertainment and comedy as the backdrop to our campaign, we've invited people into CALM by looking for opportunities for them to be involved.

Music has been at the heart of CALM since its inception. Men may not talk about personal issues, but they'll certainly listen to stories of broken hearts, dark depression and splintered lives, provided that they're put to music. So we've looked to music to launch and sustain CALM and to provide the environment in which we operate. We've worked to get our logo on the flyers, beer mats or banners at music events and encouraged musicians and artists to sit with us and promote us.

We have an annual online 'advent calendar' offering a free track each day during the Christmas period, again using our audience's interests and peers to position

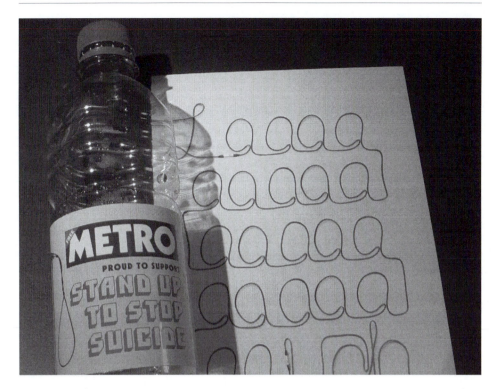

FIGURE 25.3 CALM bottled water, sponsored by the *Metro* free newspaper

ourselves and our message. And again it is a collective exercise, undertaken almost exclusively outside the CALM office, of primarily men who pull this together – asking permission from the record companies, designing the website, picking the tracks and promoting the site.

The comedy night in 2007 is a great example of using men's interests, and men themselves, to create an event and highlight the issue and, again, it brought together individuals and agencies working towards a shared aim.*

One of our latest appeals to raise money for a texting and online service involves looking for companies to support us with £100 each. In return for every £100 we'll put a logo/picture on a t-shirt which we'll use as part of a bid to set a new world record on the number of t-shirts worn by two young men. We're hoping to get 250 t-shirts on each of them. Ogilvy produced a video, with comedians David Baddiel and Stephen Merchant interviewing the guys; Catapult Digital provided the website; Blink created an excellent ad and we got hundreds of logos on the site (www. savethemale.co.uk). Ogilvy also produced some billboards promoting the campaign – Save the Male – and the fashion retailer Top Man helped pay for posting up billboards in London. At the heart of all this work lies the absolute desire *not* to deliver a miserable campaign.

---

* Claire Anstey drove the idea forwards working with Tiernan Douieb and other volunteers, Ogilvy designed the ads, Tullo Marshall Warren provided a fantastic Myspace page and the invites.

START AND STAY WITH THE AUDIENCE

Health professionals are generally useless when it comes to designing ads. They bring with them truckloads of baggage, which they feel needs to be communicated in a leaflet or ideally a booklet. You can virtually see the boxes being ticked as each message, major and minor, is checked off, together with every possible piece of information the public should be told. All this is accompanied by every available logo and corporate slogan with an insistence on using medical terms at every turn – after all the reader really needs to be reminded that these are medical professionals communicating this message. So by the time it hits the streets, whatever spark of an idea started the ad has been well and truly ground into the floor by the full due process of whatever establishment over-generated it.

Men will read leaflets – if it's the insert of a CD they've just bought, or maybe detailing the bike or baseball boots they're going to buy. A leaflet on depression that teenage boys are going to carry around in their jackets, though, lies in the realms of fantasy, even if you do put a car or a road traffic symbol on the front.

Men listen to their peers and their friends (kind of) and young men are invincible (or at least feel the need to behave as if they are). Their image of themselves and what and who they are seen to be in many ways lies at the soul of who they are, which is why branding is so critical. Having a naff image and looking like an inept 'do good' charity staffed by white elderly female volunteers is never going to work, no matter how fantastic the organisation.

To reach our audience we need to be inventive and compete with all those big brands that vie to reach the attention of men. Which means thinking about how they reach the audience and what their materials look like, and, if possible, going to those same agencies and asking for their pro bono help.

To get an agency on board you have to sell the same dream that you're selling the audience. If they're going to work for free, then this has to work for them. They're likely to be male and in their 20s, 30s or 40s. Pretend that they are your audience, as indeed they are; ask them to design the ads that work for them.

In the CALMzones we work on the ground with local funding to find culturally relevant angles for young men to relate to CALM. In Merseyside the local coordinator has been able to purchase a fully branded tent, complete with beanbags and flooring, to take along to local music and lifestyle events. Working with event organisers, the 'CALMzone chill-out tent' has become a standard element of any Merseyside event that attracts young men. It adds value and is wanted and requested by both the organisers and the audience; CALM naturally 'fits' into this arena. It's also not unusual to find CALM materials in record shops, fashion boutiques and chip shops within CALMzones, where our materials sit perfectly alongside posters for club nights and concert listings because of their tone, design and style.

USING NATURAL TALENT

CALM has pretty much managed on fresh air, goodwill and pro bono work. The ads launching the charity in 2006 and shown on MTV featured young men – hip hop artists, DJs and artists – talking direct to camera about how it feels to hit a wall and about the importance of talking. Beat Box artist Killa Kela lays down a soundtrack cutting in between the voices. The stories are chopped so that all you know is that the guys have had their own down days. This was entirely unscripted – we simply asked them to talk to the camera and tell all the guys that listened to them how it could be sometimes.* The cameramen, the director, the studios, editors and sound guys all worked on this pro bono. With the exception of a cab fare and a trip to Tesco, this was directed, compiled and delivered purely from the heart, resulting in an upbeat ad that starts and ends on the side of men.

At the same time that the ads went on MTV, our Iraq War ads went out on billboards and underground trains, comparing the number of British men killed in Iraq with the number that had killed themselves in that same period. This wasn't about dissing the soldiers but about the shocking silence and lack of coverage about another group of men who also deserve our attention.

It really doesn't matter where the idea comes from, as long as you're open to ideas and manage to make them fly – even if it is only with tape and string. We've never been able to pay for advertising space but the quality of the ads, together with the persuasive passion of the agencies and individuals who have come on board, have led to us being offered free outdoor space and airtime.

The ads themselves have brought in more talent, from individuals and from agencies. Students often use CALM for their project – creating media or film proposals for us. The issue facing us isn't how to generate ideas, but how to harness the ever-constant stream of emails from guys wanting to be involved in the campaign.

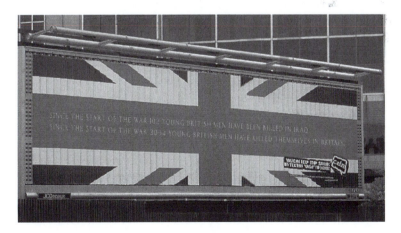

FIGURE 25.4 CALM billboard

---

* Particular thanks here to Dick Carruthers, Tom Woodcraft, Neil Dawson and all the guys in the ad, Killa Kela, Nihal, Rodney P, Skitz, Doc Brown, Benni G and Buggsy Don, Farma G.

OUTCOMES

CALM has always been fuelled by the energy coming from the ground – by creative, talented energetic guys who relate to the campaign and want to be involved and who recommend it to their friends. There can be no better advert than a strong guy telling his mate about the campaign. Then the message isn't 'here's a phone number for the weak and vulnerable', it's 'here's a helpline for all of us to use and get behind'.

At the end of the day we're here to create change, not just to provide a service. It's a change that we have to embed in society that enables people to own the campaign and make it theirs.

As I type this, I'm conscious of being behind in my replies to artists, writers, poets and various 'creatives' in the world of IT, marketing and advertising. There is an astonishing amount of goodwill, energy and creativity out there. To access that you need to be willing to let down some of the barriers that separate you from the audience – the 'us and them'. Your organisation needs to be permeable. One of the biggest obstacles to bringing in the support that is out there is the deep trench that health professionals dig to separate themselves from the audience they serve.

CONCLUSION

Catching up with the 'modern' world isn't simply about being on Facebook and Twitter. It's also about what kind of an organisation you are, your values and ideals, and who you are, who you represent, how you behave and how you respond to your audience. While there is never any simple answer, we are in a society where people increasingly want to see a personal rather than a bureaucratic response; they want to see a campaign about them and need to be able to relate to it. They want a service or an organisation which is worthy of them – critically this includes how the organisation is seen and looks – and they want an organisation which respects them and fits in with their needs, at a time and in a manner that suits.

There is this weird notion held by many statutory and voluntary agencies that 'we don't need all that expensive advertising'. I recently watched a small boy standing

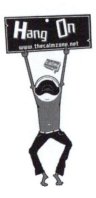

FIGURE 25.5 CALM air freshener, designed by William Wang

in front of the ice cream section at the supermarket who shouted and shouted and shouted at his dad to buy the 'Disney' ice cream. Every parent knows this one. As adults, we may no longer want Disney and we may consider ourselves as way beyond the reach of advertising, but we still want to buy a dream. The question is 'who is selling?'. If we've a message to send to men, then we need to be up there with the best and sell our more vital dreams with conviction and professionalism. There isn't a 'lower rung' which health professionals can stand on and still be relevant. We need to get real and compete with the best of them – and leave all the other baggage behind.

CHAPTER 26

Conclusion

Alan White and David Conrad

When we think of men the image of emotional vulnerability doesn't come immediately to mind and yet the story that seems to be emerging from this book is that there are many men out there suffering (often unrecognised) distress.

There is much that is good about the way men manage their emotions; the relative absence of mood swings and the ability to remain calm in a crisis are often-cited positive attributes of men. The image of masculine bravado, with stories of 'big strong men' who can manage their emotions and keep the 'stiff upper lip' in times of crisis, has perhaps become the epitome of manhood. Many men thrive on the pressure of work and other intellectual, social and physical challenges. Nevertheless it is also evident that there are many men who are struggling and not managing the growing stress that surrounds them – and they need help.

Men's vulnerabilities are most noticeable when we see massive social upheaval, as in the collapse of the Soviet Union, where the rate of suicide approached 120 per 100 000 deaths in Lithuania in 2002 (White and Holmes 2006), or in Busuttil's chapter, where we see the emotional problems in our returning soldiers from armed conflict. Young's chapter highlights that in areas of high social deprivation urban distress has a profound impact on whole communities and the men who live within them. However, it is not just these big societal events that affect men, as Neal and Conrad highlight through their discussion of men's mental health issues when confronted by cancer. But these are still extraordinary events and, as Varney's chapter on gay men's mental health, Robertson and colleagues' discussion on the challenges of living in rural settings, and Williamson's chapter on the impact of ageing demonstrate, many men trying to live normal lives are just as at risk of developing emotional and mental health problems; even becoming a father is potentially fraught with difficulties, as clearly outlined by Madsen and Burgess.

The Mind (2009) survey found that 37% of men are currently feeling worried or low and that the top three issues on our minds are job security, work and money. It is not surprising that stress is now seen as the principle cause of disability from work and the chapter by Kinder and Boorman on men's mental health in the workplace highlights that the benefit of targeted action goes well beyond reductions in absent-eeism. The effect of emotional distress in men is most profoundly seen in the suicide figures – both the chapters by Sayers and Bush on men and suicide and bereavement from suicide highlight the need for urgent action on finding better ways for boys and men to cope.

It would seem from Conrad and Warwick-Booth's chapter that society has created a model of masculinity that makes it difficult for men to manage their emotions effectively and this has left many lacking the personal tools necessary to deal with sudden or sustained life challenges. It has also left a legacy of poor recognition of the signs of men's mental and emotional distress, and, as Branney and White highlight, such a situation has created a situation where men are often left 'on the edge'. The challenges created by men who are not managing their emotions well create the need for a more understanding society and a more understanding health service.

With the challenges being faced in this turbulent world, where stability and structure seem difficult to hold on to, we're going to have to provide men with the tools to survive and provide society, in its many guises, with the ability to recognise and manage men's emotions when they are going askew. This can't just be an issue for the health service.

It is salutary to note the factors that contribute towards the likelihood of a man abusing his partner (*see* Box 26.1). How many of these could be seen to be a consequence of mental distress?

BOX 26.1 Factors associated with a man's risk for abusing his partner

> ➤ Individual factors:
>> ➤ young age
>> ➤ heavy drinking
>> ➤ depression
>> ➤ personality disorders
>> ➤ low academic achievement
>> ➤ low income
>> ➤ witnessing or experiencing violence as a child
> ➤ Relationship factors:
>> ➤ marital conflict
>> ➤ marital instability
>> ➤ male dominance in the family
>> ➤ economic stress
>> ➤ poor family functioning
> ➤ Community factors:
>> ➤ weak community sanctions against domestic violence
>> ➤ poverty
>> ➤ low social capital

> ➤ Societal factors:
>> ➤ traditional gender norms
>> ➤ social norms supportive of violence

Source: Krug *et al.* (2002) p.98

Taking on a whole-population approach to mental health, as advocated within the UK Government's 'New Horizons'* initiative, requires us to look beyond mental illness into those aspects of our lives that affect our emotional stability. As these are many and varied, we need to be looking for a complex solution to what is obviously a complex problem. It requires us to understand how men manage their mental and emotional health if we are wishing to fully comprehend the genesis of the difficulties they face. We then need to adopt a much broader strategy in tackling men's mental health needs.

MEN AND HELP-SEEKING

What is very evident from the work presented in the book is that most of the innovative developments have not come as a consequence of mainstream healthcare providers setting up new services for men. What we see are individual practitioners who have recognised a need and have gone ahead on their own volition to set up services for men. This is not to diminish the work of such bodies as the UK Royal College of Psychiatrists, who produced the leaflet *Men Behaving Sadly* (RCP 1998), for example, but we have not yet seen commissioners of services deliberately going out to purchase work in this area.

Over the past 20 years the care and provision for people with mental health problems has changed dramatically, with the introduction of proven new therapies such as Cognitive Behavioural Therapy (NIHCE 2007) offering effective means of helping prevent emotional difficulties becoming chronic problems. As Kantor (2007) notes, once men are in an environment where they feel that they can trust the therapist not to be disparaging of their experiences, it doesn't take long for them to open up. For some of these men, talking with a mental health professional is the first opportunity they have ever had to fully explore with another person the demons they have been harbouring within.

The positive message that comes across from much of the work on men and their mental health is that once they are engaged in care they do very well, but the challenge remains how to get men aware of their emotional health, especially at times of crisis, and how to get them to the most appropriate care. In part, this is a design issue, with a need for services that are seen to be of the kind that men would be keen to engage with, e.g. web-based or exercise-focused, as suggested by Mind (2009) and outlined here in the chapters by Anderson and Jones on the use of the internet and Dads and Lads. It's also about the way we sell services that already exist, such as CBT

---

*   www.newhorizons-mentalhealth.co.uk

and other talking therapies – and, as Hopkins and Voaden, and Powell highlight, the need to recognise those men at risk and then to be able to market services to them in a way that engages them.

Within the book we have also seen that services can be established that can target men effectively, through imaginative ways of working with familiar masculine pastimes such as Sayers demonstrates with the 'It's a Goal' initiative with young men within a sporting setting . The chapters by Pete and Sue Dominey, Woodall, Langham and Davy, Kinder and Boorman and McCullagh on working with men with anger issues, prisoners, drug users and the homeless illustrate that even the most challenging groups of men will engage with support. It is also possible to set up formal clinics, as shown by the success of the counselling service set up by Christian Scambor in Graz, Austria. Most of the successes outlined in the book are founded on practitioners having an understanding of men and how they live their lives and also on the successful marketing of their services. There is another side to this book and that is the quest for us to get to men and boys before they find themselves in difficulties so that they can be taught how to manage their emotions more effectively. To really make a difference to the mental well-being of the male population, we need to make all our schools truly and comprehensively mental-health promoting. The type of interventions described here by Pemberton, Jones, and Dressel on tackling bullying, getting dads and lads to recognise the benefits of a positive engaged father figure and the work done on getting youngsters to understand how normal relationships and a healthy sexuality can benefit their health and well-being – should be standard features of boys' education experience, rather than isolated beacons of good practice. Delivering this kind of work requires skills in being able to broach potentially embarrassing subjects and this in itself requires attributes that not every practitioner enjoys (Conrad 2007). For us to succeed, we need to nurture those who already have the skills to do this kind of work effectively and educate a new generation of practitioners. Developing basic skills in this area for all those working with men, either from a health or social perspective, will bring lasting benefits (Robbins 2006).

The practical examples in this book illustrate that new ways of thinking about men's mental health require different approaches to the provision of services. These examples will hopefully inspire others to begin planning how to become 'male aware' in their day-to-day work in the field of mental health.

POLICY DEVELOPMENT

Across the globe we have seen a re-focusing of mental health policy onto health and well-being. The WHO's summary report on *Promoting Mental Health* (2005) saw an attempt to sway those whose vision was restricted to psychiatric morbidity towards a broader view of mental health and its promotion as the key goal. This challenge is also being taken up with the new European Pact on Mental Health and Well-being, which hopefully will see more action at the EU and country level on:

➤ prevention of depression and suicide
➤ mental health in youth and education

➤ mental health in workplace settings
➤ mental health of older people
➤ combating stigma and social exclusion.

The forthcoming UK 'New Horizons' policy, guiding action over the next ten years, is also heavily focused on the promotion of health and well-being and hopefully will be a significant part of the drive to see mental health promotion as a goal, as well as the management of mental illness.

These drivers are coupled with the creation of policies aimed at making the needs of men a visible component within policy development and service delivery (Smith *et al.* 2009). The recent Australian and Irish Men's Health Policy and the US 'Men and Families Health Care Act of 2009', which has been introduced with the intention of setting up an Office for Men's Health, are pioneering the development of male-specific policy. Other countries, such as Norway and the UK, have established a more general legal requirement around gender equality.

In the UK, with the passing of the Equality Act in 2006, there has been a legal requirement, known as the Gender Equality Duty, for all public services to meet the needs of men and women. The wording of this is important, removing the obstacle that used to exist of having a 'one size fits all' approach to health service delivery and now requiring men and women's differing requirements to be woven into the fabric of policy and practice development.

The push for change is therefore not just a choice based on a desire to see an improvement in the understanding and care that men receive with regard to their emotional health, it is also one now required through law. All Government policy must now be gender-audited and it is hoped that this will create the impetus for greater change within local health strategy development, both in the commissioning and delivery of services.

Policy development specifically around men's mental health is less evident, but there have been some high-profile campaigns which are striving to get change. In the US, the 'Real men, real depression' campaign (NIMH 2003) launched in 2003 by the National Institute of Mental Health sought to raise awareness of men's mental health through the use of videoed conversations with men from all different walks of life talking about their experiences.

The 2006 Men's Health Week in the UK, organised by the Men's Health Forum, focused on men's mental health under the strap line of 'Mind Your Head'. As part of the activities, a policy paper (Wilkins 2006) was drawn up as a statement about how men's emotional health needs should be addressed. The conclusion to the report offered five recommendations.

1 Public policy should aim to improve men's mental well-being.
2 There must be recognition of male-specific indicators of emotional distress.
3 Services must adapt to meet men's needs more effectively.
4 Mental health promotion aimed at men and boys should take account of 'traditional' masculinity.
5 A national initiative is needed to help men achieve mental well-being.

The UK-based mental health charity Mind had men's mental health as its focus for their campaign week in 2009, called 'Get it off your chest' (Mind 2009). Their action plan listed what they considered the most important recommendations for change, all of which are very laudable and would seem to reflect the emerging findings from the work described in this book:

➤ a national men's mental health strategy is needed
➤ criteria for diagnosing mental health problems need to be expanded
➤ there should be adequate provision of 'male-friendly' treatments, such as computerised therapy or exercise
➤ health services should be advertised in places that men frequent, such as gyms, pubs or the workplace
➤ GP surgeries should be gender-neutral
➤ teacher training must include the issue of boys' emotional development and the signs of distress
➤ employers must do more to support their stressed male employees
➤ the needs of black and minority ethnic men must be recognised
➤ the relationship between sexuality, gender and mental well-being should be a core part of the training given to health and social services professionals.

The Men's Health Forum's *Untold Problems* report on the essential issues in the mental health of men and boys (Wilkins 2010) calls for an approach that takes account of the particular mental health needs of men, in parallel with an approach that takes account of the particular needs of women. Simply being male, it is argued, should be seen as a primary risk factor for several specific mental health problems, including alcohol dependence; drug dependence; aggressive or criminal behaviour associated with underlying emotional distress and behavioural problems in school. The report highlights the need for a cross-cutting approach that goes beyond the simplistic view that improving and maintaining the mental health of men and boys should be the preserve of mental health services.

The challenge that this book poses to practitioners, policy-makers and commissioners of services is to allow their conception of mental health to broaden – to recognise the problems men face with their emotional and mental health and the consequences of lack of action. To truly deliver on these goals requires a serious leap in decision-makers' recognition of the negative impact of poor mental well-being on all aspects of our society and our economy. Crucially, it also requires a willingness to invest heavily in making mental health promotion a fundamental aspect of everyday life, throughout the life course, rather than something we dabble in with one-off projects funded from tiny pots of a woefully inadequate public health budget.

REFERENCES

Conrad D (2007) How to be a men's health worker. In: Conrad D, White A (eds), *Men's Health – How to Do It*. Oxford: Radcliffe Publishing, pp. 151–7.

Kantor M (2007) *Lifting the Weight: understanding depression in men, its causes and solutions*. Westport, Conn: Praeger.

Krug EG, Dahlberg LL, Mercy JA, Zwi AB and Lozano R (2002) *The World Health Organization Report on Violence*. Geneva: WHO.

Mind (2009). *Get it Off your Chest: men and mental health*. London: Mind.

National Institute for Health and Clinical Excellence (NIHCE) (2007) *Anxiety: management of anxiety (panic disorder, with or without agoraphobia, and generalised anxiety disorder) in adults in primary, secondary and community care*. London: NIHCE.

National Institute of Mental Health (NIMH) (2003) Real Men, Real Depression. Available at: www.nimh.nih.gov/health/publications/real-men-real-depression-easy-to-read/real-men-real-depression.pdf (Accessed 1 October 2009).

Robbins A (2006) Biopsychosocial aspects in understanding and treating depression in men: a clinical perspective. *J Men's Health & Gender*. 3(1): 10–18.

Royal College of Psychiatrists (1998) *Men Behaving Sadly*. London: RCP.

Smith JA, White A, Richardson N, Robertson S and Ward M (2009) The men's health policy contexts in Australia, the UK & Ireland: Advancement or abandonment? *Critical Public Health*. 19(3–4): 427–440.

White AK and Holmes M (2006) Patterns of mortality across 44 Countries among men and women aged 15–44. *J Men's Health & Gender*. 3(2): 139–151.

Wilkins D (2006) *Mind Your Head: men, boys and mental well-being*. London: Men's Health Forum.

Wilkins D (2010) *Untold Problems: A review of the essential issues in the mental health of men and boys*. London: Men's Health Forum.

World Health Organization (WHO) (2005) *Promoting Mental Health*. Geneva: WHO.

Index